A Nurse's Survival Guide to Drugs in Practice

Second Edition

T0315331

Titles in this series

A Nurse's Survival Guide to the Ward

A Nurse's Survival Guide to Leadership and Management on the Ward

A Nurse's Survival Guide to Critical Care

A Nurse's Survival Guide to Mentoring

A Nurse's Survival Guide to Acute Medical Emergencies

A Survival Guide to Children's Nursing

At Elsevier, we understand the importance of providing up-to-date and relevant content. For this reason, we are continuously working on updated editions and new titles for the Series. Please visit our website to find out the latest news and the upcoming publications: https://www.uk.elsevierhealth.com/

A Nurse's Survival Guide to Drugs in Practice

Second Edition

Ann Richards BA(Hons), MSc, DipN(Lond), RGN, RNT
Associate Lecturer
Open University

Sharon Edwards EdD, SFHEA, NTF, PGCEA, MSc,
DipN(Lond), RN
Independent Consultant and Advisor for Nurse Education

ELSEVIER

London   New York   Oxford   Philadelphia   St Louis   Sydney   2020

Notices

Practitioners and researchers must always rely on their own experience and knowledge in evaluating and using any information, methods, compounds or experiments described herein. Because of rapid advances in the medical sciences, in particular, independent verification of diagnoses and drug dosages should be made. To the fullest extent of the law, no responsibility is assumed by Elsevier, authors, editors or contributors for any injury and/or damage to persons or property as a matter of products liability, negligence or otherwise, or from any use or operation of any methods, products, instructions, or ideas contained in the material herein.

ISBN: 978-0-7020-7658-9

Printed in Poland
Last digit is the print number: 9   8   7   6   5   4   3   2   1

Content Strategist: Poppy Garraway
Content Development Specialist: Kirsty Guest
Project Manager: Anne Collett
Design: Amy Buxton
Marketing Manager: Samantha Page

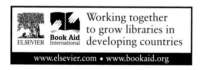

Working together
to grow libraries in
developing countries

www.elsevier.com • www.bookaid.org

Contents

Section 2
Autonomic nervous system

Section 7
Endocrine system

Section 8
Chemotherapy, antimicrobials and the immune system

Section 9
Other areas of pharmacology

Preface

The idea for this small book originated from many years of teaching pharmacology to both pre- and post-registration nurses, paramedics and other healthcare professionals. Detailed handouts describing how the drugs worked, and their side effects and routes of administration, were greatly appreciated. It was suggested that these teaching notes could form the basis for a short text small enough to carry around, which would supplement information given in the British National Formulary and larger pharmacology text books. The Survival Guide was born!

Over the years, not only have many more therapeutic drugs become available but the nurse's responsibility in their administration and prescribing has also increased, making a more detailed knowledge of drug action essential. It is hoped that this book will be especially useful for those involved in nurse prescribing, as well as those administering drugs.

I have always found feedback from students useful and hope that I have continued to incorporate in this short text those areas that my students over the years have found difficult to understand but that are essential in their development as knowledgeable practitioners. The aim has been to provide a user-friendly text where drugs are categorized according to their action on body systems.

For this edition, my fellow author, Sharon Edwards, has joined with me to work together and thoroughly update the content, expanding some areas surrounding nursing practice, such as the possibility of drug errors and how to avoid these. Incorporated within the book, in addition to all the main drug categories, are other important areas such as adverse drug reactions. There are short sections on increasingly popular topics such as herbal remedies.

We realize that in such a small book there will be areas that could be more detailed, but the emphasis has been on making the topic interesting and accessible to nurses at all levels, both pre- and post-registration, as well as all other professions involved in healthcare. It is hoped that the book will become an invaluable companion and essential aid to patient care and to nurse or independent prescribing. Most of all we hope you develop our enthusiasm for this area of study and its application to healthcare.

Ann Richards
Sharon Edwards
2020

Acknowledgements

It would be impossible to mention all those who have had an influence on this short pharmacology text but we would especially like to thank all our students, past and present, for their enthusiasm in the subject that first encouraged me to write the book and Sharon to join me for this edition.

The book would not have been possible without the support of the students and staff at the University of Hertfordshire where I first studied pharmacology at postgraduate level and lectured for over 10 years while writing the first edition of this text.

We would like to thank our husbands and families for their interest in this project and their understanding when it has taken precious hours away from our leisure time together.

Also, I would like to thank all those involved in production, proofreading and publishing at Elsevier for their cooperation when it has not always been possible to keep to the agreed deadlines.

Common abbreviations

bd	Twice daily
tds (tid)	Three times daily
qds (qid)	Four times daily
on	Once daily, in the morning
mane	Morning
midi	Midday
nocte	Night
prn	As required
stat	At once
g	Gram
mcg	Microgram
kg	Kilogram
L	Litre
mL	Millilitre
PO	Oral
SL	Sublingual
IV	Intravenous
IM	Intramuscular
Subcut	Subcutaneous
PR	Per rectum
PV	Per vagina
Gutt	Eye drops
Occ	Eye ointment
ACEI	Angiotensin converting enzyme inhibitor
AIDS	Acquired immunodeficiency syndrome
ARB	Angiotensin II receptor blocker
BP	Blood pressure
COPD	Chronic obstructive pulmonary disease
CPR	Cardiopulmonary resuscitation
CVA	Cerebrovascular accident
DM	Diabetes mellitus
DVT	Deep venous thrombosis
ECG	Electrocardiograph
FBC	Full blood count
GA	General anaesthesia
HIV	Human immunodeficiency virus
HRT	Hormone replacement therapy
LA	Local anaesthesia
LABA	Long acting beta agonist

LTRA	Leukotriene receptor antagonist
LVF	Left ventricular failure
LVH	Left ventricular hypertrophy
MI	Myocardial infarction
MRSA	Methicillin-resistant *Staphylococcus aureus*
NPU	Not passed urine
OA	Osteoarthritis
PD	Parkinson's disease
PEFR	Peak expiratory flow rate
PID	Pelvic inflammatory disease
PMH	Previous medical history
RVF	Right ventricular failure
Rx	Treatment
TIA	Transient ischaemic attack
U&E	Urea and electrolytes
WHO	World Health Organization

Section 1

Principles of pharmacology

Section Outline

1.1 INTRODUCTION TO PHARMACOLOGY

The first recorded systematic register of medicines dates back to the ancient Greek and Egyptian civilizations.

- Man has used drugs since earliest times and there are records of the fermentation of alcohol (ethanol) on pottery from Mesopotamia made around 4200 BCE.
- Today, drugs are used for recreational, religious and medicinal purposes in the most primitive human communities as well as the most developed.

Drugs are usually part of everyday life, from birth, when a child's delivery may often be assisted by the use of drugs, throughout life, due to illness, and during death, when drugs are frequently used to ease suffering at the end of life.

General aspects

Pharmacology is a word that is derived from the Greek *pharmakon* meaning drug and *logos* meaning study. Pharmacology is the study of drugs, their chemical composition, their biological action and their therapeutic application in man. Pharmacology is subdivided into fields according to the types of drugs being studied, e.g. neuropharmacology, psychopharmacology, cardiovascular pharmacology.

Some definitions

A **drug** may be defined as any substance that brings about a change in biological functioning or effects structure or function through its chemical actions on a living organism.

A Nurse's Survival Guide to Drugs in Practice. https://doi.org/10.1016/B978-0-7020-7658-9.00001-9

1

Drugs include:

- substances found within the body, for example hormones, or chemicals not synthesized within the body
- social drugs such as alcohol, nicotine and caffeine as well as illegal drugs such as cocaine
- environmental drugs such as insecticides, metals and food additives.

Toxicology is a branch of pharmacology and studies the adverse effects of chemicals, including drugs, on living systems.

Medicine is a term that tends to be reserved for drugs that are used therapeutically (for treatment of disease and healing).

Drugs may be used to:

- cure disease, for example antibiotics in bacterial infection
- suppress disease, for example methotrexate in juvenile rheumatoid arthritis and steroid inhalers in asthma
- treat symptoms of disease, for example inhalers such as **salbutamol** in asthma
- prevent disease (prophylaxis):
  - **primary prevention** is when the disease is prevented from occurring in a person that is free from the disease, for example the use of antimalarial drugs, vaccination or immunization against infectious diseases
  - **secondary prevention** is the reduction of risk factors when the patient has the disease. An example would be the use of lipid-lowering drugs (statins) in atherosclerosis.

Drug classification

There is more than one way that drugs may be classified. Drugs may be classified according to:

1. *Major clinical or therapeutic use*, for example antidepressant, antimicrobial, antihypertensive, analgesics. Within each of these groups are subgroups; for example the group of antihypertensives includes:
   - calcium channel blockers
   - angiotensin converting enzyme (ACE) inhibitors
   - beta blockers
   - alpha blockers.

   From these subgroups are the individual drugs, for example *amlodipine* is an example of a calcium channel blocker.

2. *Mode of action*, for example ACE inhibitors, which work by inhibiting the enzyme ACE.

3. *Site of action*, for example loop diuretics, which work on the loop of Henle in the kidney.
4. *Molecular action*, for example receptor antagonists such as beta-adrenergic receptor antagonists (beta blockers).
5. *Molecular structure*, for example tricyclic antidepressants, describing their actual chemical structure.

Drug nomenclature (naming of drugs)

During their lifetime, drugs will have four different names.

- The systemic chemical name. This may be very long and describes the chemical structure of the drug.
- The drug company code that is used for secrecy while the drug is being developed.
- An international **nonproprietary name (INN)**. This is the **generic name** given by an official agency, for example the World Health Organization (WHO), when it is decided the drug may be useful, for example *acyclovir.* Countries used to have their own national proprietary name but nowadays it is usual for one drug to have only one official international proprietary name. This is more convenient and also safer. It does mean that some countries have to change the names they had adopted for certain drugs to fall in line with the WHO recommended International Nonproprietary Names (rINN). Examples in the UK are *furosemide* (previously *frusemide*) and *lidocaine* (previously *lignocaine*). The British Approved Name (BAN) for a drug is now the same as the INN with the exception of adrenaline/ epinephrine. The BAN is still *adrenaline.*
- A **proprietary (trade) name**, for example *Ventolin.* This is applied to a particular formulation by a particular drug company when the drug is marketed.

The **generic name stem** gives information as to which class the drug belongs to, for example names ending in −*olol* are adrenoreceptor antagonists and names ending in −*pril* are ACE inhibitors. We can tell *acyclovir* is an antiviral drug because it ends in the −*vir* suffix.

- **In this book generic names are used** but some proprietary names are also given.
- Drugs sold under generic names are usually cheaper than proprietary brands, for example it is cheaper to buy *paracetamol* than *Panadol*, although both are the same drug.
- Using the generic name enables pharmacists to supply whatever version of the drug they have available.

Drug discovery and development

Over the years, many drugs have been discovered by chance. A famous example is the discovery of penicillin by Alexander Fleming. In 1928 Fleming was actually preparing agar plates of staphylococci bacteria in the laboratory and found that contamination of his plates by a mould had occurred. He noticed that there was an inhibition zone around the mould where the staphylococci were not growing. It was very difficult to isolate the active ingredient of the mould and it was not until 1942 that *penicillin* was successfully tested on humans.

Today drug development is a massive industry and computer programmes use molecular modelling in the process of drug development.

Drugs from natural sources

Originally most drugs were derived from plants and throughout history all cultures have used various derivatives from plants including bark, leaves, fruit, roots, flowers and sap. Examples include:

- *atropine* from *Atropa belladonna* (deadly nightshade)
- *ergometrine* from the fungus *Claviceps purpurea*
- *digitalis* from the foxglove
- *opium* from the opium poppy, *Papaver somniferum* (meaning the sleep-bearing poppy)
- *cocaine* from the leaves of *Erythroxylum coca*
- **anticancer drugs** from the periwinkle plant.

There are still many plants whose medicinal value has yet to be discovered and modern day drugs continue to be developed from these sources, for example *paclitaxel*, the anticancer drug used in the treatment of ovarian cancer, was developed from the Pacific Yew tree.

With the availability of screening for biological activity, there has been renewed interest by big drug companies in natural products. Microorganisms in soil and sewage are being examined for potential medicinal use are fungi, plants and animals.

Most of today's drugs are made in the laboratory (synthetic). Once the molecular structure of a natural drug is identified, it often becomes possible to synthesize it instead of extracting it. The drug may also be modified chemically for better absorption, greater effectiveness or fewer side effects.

Rational drug design

This is based on an understanding of drug receptors and biological mechanisms.

- The first drug to be 'purpose built' was the beta-adrenergic receptor antagonist *propranolol* in the early 1960s.

- The rapid development of biotechnology and molecular biology has enabled greater understanding of drug action and allowed new drug targets to be developed.
- The insertion of genes for certain proteins into bacteria and yeast has allowed the development of human insulin.
- Antibodies used as drugs are also increasingly successful.

Preclinical drug testing

Once a drug has survived the initial screening procedure it has to be carefully evaluated for potential risks. Studies may be done on cells, tissues and animals before a drug is tested on fit young adults. Medicines need a marketing authorization before they can be prescribed to patients.

- Major toxicities of a new compound have to be known before it can be used in humans. An assessment of major organ toxicity is performed. Increasingly these tests can be done *in vitro* with isolated cells but animals are still used in some essential studies of drug toxicity.
- Effects on reproductive performance and birth defects are studied.
- The potential of the drug to be a carcinogen (promote cancer) should be investigated if it is to be used for a long period.
- The sequence and mechanism of any toxic action should be investigated.

Once preclinical testing has been completed to the satisfaction of the Medicines and Healthcare Products Regulatory Agency (MHRA) the drug will enter the next stage (clinical trials) and be tested on humans.

Clinical trials

Clinical trials test the new potential medicine on people to see whether it will do more good than harm and to compare the new drug to alternatives already available. The Clinical Trials Unit is part of the Licensing Division of the medicines branch of the MHRA. The unit assesses the applications for clinical trials. Less than one third of drugs tested in clinical trials reach the pharmacy.

- Clinical trials usually begin with a small group (20–50 subjects) of healthy volunteers or volunteer patients. A low dose is used to check it is not harmful.
- Some drug actions, for example anticoagulant effects, may be tested on healthy volunteers but specific actions, for example antiparkinsonian effects, cannot.
- As data are collected the trial is expanded and larger numbers of patients are included in the trial (50–300 subjects).
- In randomized controlled trials the new drug is usually compared with the current treatment. Numbers of subjects range from 250 to over 1000.

- Special groups may need to be studied — if the drug is to be used in the elderly for example.
- If the drug is successful it will be granted a licence.

The whole discovery and development process may take 10—15 years, which explains why new drugs are so expensive and why the drug needs a patent for the first 20 years following registration. Once the patent expires the generic drug can be manufactured by other companies and sold much more cheaply.

Postmarketing surveillance

The work of the MHRA does not finish once the drug is approved. It is also responsible for receiving and assessing pharmacovigilance reports. This ongoing monitoring of safety and usage is not only applicable to newly introduced drugs but all drugs available on the market.

Severe adverse drug reactions (ADRs) to marketed drugs are uncommon and may be unexpected and not recognized until the drug has been on the market for many years. ADRs are discussed in Section 1.7.

The Yellow Card Scheme

This is a spontaneous ADR-reporting scheme in the UK that is run by the MHRA and has been in place for more than 50 years. The scheme acts as an early warning system for the identification of previously unrecognized reactions to prescription medicines, herbal remedies and over-the-counter (OTC) medicines.

- Yellow forms are available in the back of the British National Formulary (BNF) that may be filled in by health professionals. Forms are also available online to submit electronically at the MHRA website (www.mhra. gov.uk).
- Not only nurses, doctors, paramedics and allied health workers are encouraged to use the Yellow Card Scheme but also patients, parents and carers.
- Reports are studied by the Pharmacovigilance Expert Advisory Group of the MHRA to assess possible causal relationships and risk factors.
- This information is studied alongside other available evidence, for example case reports and clinical trials.
- Regulatory action, where necessary, is taken. A drug may be withdrawn from the market.
- Other possible regulatory action includes restrictions in use, reduction in dosage or special warnings and precautions. An example where the dosing schedule of a drug was changed is *Zyban (bupropion)*, a drug licensed as an aid to smoking cessation. Following yellow card reports of an increased incidence of seizures that are a dose-related risk, a lower starting dose was

recommended with a slower increase to the maximum dosage. To further reduce the risk of seizures *Zyban* was contraindicated in certain categories of patient.

The National Institute for Health and Care Excellence

Once a new drug has received a licence from the MHRA, it is usually referred to National Institute for Health and Care Excellence (NICE) who will then decide whether or how this drug should be used within the National Health Service (NHS). While the appraisal is ongoing, NHS organizations locally should decide whether the drug is to be used. Once guidance has been issued by NICE, this replaces local decisions and ensures equality across the country.

- NICE is an independent organization that was set up in 1999 and is responsible for providing national guidance on the promotion of good health and the prevention and treatment of ill health in England and Wales.
- Scotland has its own NHS Quality Improvement Scotland and the Scottish Intercollegiate Guidelines Network (SIGN) but does accept guidance from NICE on drug usage.
- NICE provides clinical guidance on current best practice to healthcare workers and patients. It looks at medicines and the clinical management of medical conditions.
- NICE publishes a simple guide, available on their website (www.nice.org. uk), which explains how decisions about guidance are reached.
- You can suggest a topic for NICE to report on when you visit the website (www.nice.org.uk).
- Guidelines are available on an ever-growing list of conditions (204 in 2019), including hypertension, diabetes, dementia, brain tumours, chronic obstructive pulmonary disease (COPD), Parkinson's disease, prostate cancer. These are all available in full and shortened forms from the website.
- NICE also produces quality standards that aim to improve quality of care. These are available on the website and include those on hearing loss, dementia, sexual health, air pollution and many more (184 in total in 2019, with more in the pipeline).

1.2 THE LAW, DRUGS AND PRESCRIBING

Drugs have the potential to cause adverse reactions, occasionally with fatal consequences. The patient or the healthcare worker may also use drugs inappropriately. These facts have led to legislation to control the manufacture, sale and administration of drugs.

Drugs and the law

There were no legal restrictions on the sale of poisons or drugs before the middle of the 19th century in Britain.

- The Arsenic Act of 1851 was the first statutory control over sales.
- The Pharmacy Act of 1868 introduced a poisons list with 15 entries and this was extended in 1908 to include poisons used for agricultural and horticultural purposes.
- In 1933 the Pharmacy and Poisons Act established a Poisons Board to advise the Secretary of State on what should be included in the poisons list. Poisons were now divided into different schedules but there was no control over the sale or manufacture of other medicines and only those containing poisons were regulated.
- It was not until the Pharmacy and Medicines Act of 1941 that a proprietary medicine had to disclose its composition on the container.
- Legislation only developed as it was needed, and when antibiotics were discovered in 1947, the Penicillin Act was passed to control their sale and supply.
- In 1959 as more and more medications became available, a working party was set up by the Government to examine the need for new controls.
- The Medicines Act of 1968 was based on this, and was designed to replace all earlier legislation relating to medicines.
- In Britain today, the Medicines Act 1968 and the Poisons Act 1972, together with the Misuse of Drugs Act 1971, regulate the use of all medicines and poisons.
  - The Medicines Act 1968 controls the manufacture and distribution of medicines.
  - The Poisons Act 1972 regulates the sale of non-medicinal poisons.
  - The Misuse of Drugs Act 1971 deals with controlled drugs and the abuse of drugs.
- All hospital and community trusts have their own procedures and policies in addition to these acts.

The Medicines Act 1968

This Act regulates the manufacture, distribution and importation of all medicines for human and animal use.

Although most herbal remedies are still exempt from licensing requirements, the Medicines Act 1968 does have a section on homeopathic medicines and there are lists of substances of plant origin that can only be sold by registered pharmacies.

There are three classes of product under the Medicines Act 1968.

1. General sales list (GSL) medicines

Sold to the public without the supervision of a pharmacist.

- They may be available in a wide range of shops such as supermarkets, newsagents and petrol stations.

- There are certain conditions that apply to their sale; for example, the largest pack of paracetamol that may be sold in a supermarket is 16 tablets. Packs of 32 tablets may be sold in a pharmacy.
- If a product contains paracetamol it must be labelled with the words 'if symptoms persist, consult your doctor' and 'do not exceed the stated dose'.
- Often, only low strengths of the medicine are available. Ibuprofen may be sold in a supermarket in 200 mg tablets whereas it may also be sold in 400 mg tablets in a pharmacy.

2. Pharmacy (P) medicines

   May only be sold under the supervision of a pharmacist.

- The pharmacist usually checks that it is safe for the person to take the medication by asking if the client takes any other medicines or has any medical conditions. An example would be the sale of some nasal decongestants that contain ephedrine (a sympathomimetic) and the purchaser will be asked if they have hypertension before the drug is sold.
- The pharmacist may also offer advice; for example when chlorphenamine, an antihistamine, is purchased the client will be warned that the medication may make them drowsy and that they should not drive while taking the drug.

3. Prescription-only medicines (POMs)

   Sold or supplied in accordance with a prescription given by an appropriate practitioner.

- There are some exemptions from POM status and these include all preparations of insulin and some controlled drugs below a stated strength.
- There is a list of medicines for use by parenteral administration that is exempt from this restriction when administered to save life in an emergency. This list includes adrenaline (epinephrine), atropine, glucagon and promethazine.
- There are other exemptions and the restrictions on sale and control of some POMs do not apply to a registered midwife in the course of her professional practice.

Patient information

There are regulations that promote the safety of medicinal products by ensuring that they are readily identifiable.

- Appropriate warning or information and instruction must be given with medicines and this includes the labelling of containers and the inclusion of leaflets with medicines.
- In 1994 a European Community directive came into force that covered labelling of medicines and the format and content of user leaflets to be supplied with each medicine.

- Packs that conform to the directives are known as 'patient packs' in the UK. They are ready-to-dispense packs containing a patient information leaflet (PIL) which has been approved by the MHRA (www.gov.uk/mhra).
- All new medicines are required to comply with this directive.
- The packs will usually contain enough medicine for 1 month, but other sized packs are available.
- A summary of product characteristics for UK licensed medicines may be found at https://www.medicines.org.uk/emc. This is the electronic Medicines Compendium (eMC) and contains up-to-date and easily accessible information about medicines licensed for use in the UK.

The Misuse of Drugs Act 1971

- This act relates to drugs that are liable to cause dependence if misused. The act controls the export, import, production, supply and possession of dangerous or otherwise harmful drugs. It is also designed to promote education and research relating to drug dependence and addiction.
- Accurate records of all purchases, amounts of drug issued and dosages given have to be kept. There must be special labels on the containers of these drugs to make them clearly recognizable and to distinguish them.
- The drugs subject to control are referred to as 'controlled drugs' and known as 'CDs'. They are divided into three classes – Class A, Class B and Class C.
- Drugs are included in each of the classes according to the potential for harm they are thought to present to individuals and to society at large.
- The divisions are for the purpose of determining penalties for offences under the act and are not directly relevant to client care.

Penalties for possession

Within each class the highest penalties are for trafficking and the least for possession and maximum penalties can only be imposed by a crown court judge. New drugs can be added at any time to the Misuse of Drugs Act 1971.

Class A drugs are thought to be the most harmful when being misused, then Class B drugs (but if a Class B drug is prepared for injecting it becomes a class A drug) followed by Class C drugs having the least potential for harm.

Class A drugs

- Opiates such as heroin (diamorphine), methadone and morphine, but not codeine and dihydrocodeine.
- Cocaine (including crack and coca leaf).
- Hallucinogens: lysergic acid diethylamide (LSD), mescaline, psilocybin/ psilocin (e.g. magic mushrooms when prepared, deliberately dried, or

otherwise altered by the hand of man in any way) and 3, 4-methyl-enedioxymethamphetamine (MDMA; Ecstasy and virtually all derivatives).
- Methamphetamine (crystal meth, ice, glass), a stimulant. Moved to Class A in 2006.

Class B drugs

- *Amfetamine* and derivatives (other than Ecstasy-type) − if prepared for injection become Class A.
- *Methylphenidate (Ritalin).*
- *Codeine* and *dihydrocodeine* (except medicinal preparations).
- *Temazepam* and most barbiturates.
- Cannabis.
- *Methaqualone* (mandrax/quaaludes).
- *Ketamine* (often in fake Ecstasy tablets, also sold as 'special K').

Class C drugs

- Tranquillizers (benzodiazepines, e.g. *diazepam, nitrazepam*).
- *Buprenorphine.*
- Most anabolic steroids.

Not included in the Misuse of Drugs Act are: *ephedrine* (often in fake Ecstasy tablets, and several 'legal highs'), solvents (including alcohol), nicotine and caffeine.

The misuse of drugs regulations 2001

These regulations allow professionals to possess and supply a controlled drug while performing professional duties. These regulations divide drugs into **five schedules** each with its own requirements governing supply, prescribing and record keeping.

Schedule 1 drugs are the most stringently controlled.

- The drugs are not authorized for medical use and possession and supply require a licence from the Home Office − usually for research purposes.
- This is the closest that British law comes to total prohibition.
- Examples are hallucinogenic drugs such as *lysergic acid diethylamide* (LSD), coca leaf and raw opium.

Schedule 2 includes more than 100 drugs subject to full controlled drug requirements.

- These are Controlled Drugs and are subject to safe custody requirements.
- It is illegal to possess drugs in schedules 2 or 3 without a prescription or other authority.
- A Home Office licence is required to produce, import, export or supply substances in this schedule.
- Examples include opiates such as *diamorphine* (heroin), *fentanyl*, *morphine*, *methadone*, *pethidine*, *dihydrocodeine* injection, *codeine phosphate* injection.
- Major stimulants, for example *amfetamines*.
- *Cocaine*, *ketamine* and cannabis-based products for medicinal use.

Schedule 3 drugs are subject to the same special prescription requirements (except *phenobarbital*) but not to the safe custody requirements (except *buprenorphine* and *diethylpropion*).

- They do not need a special register but invoices must be retained for 2 years.
- Examples include *buprenorphine* and *pentazocine*, *midazolam*, *gaba-pentin*, *tramadol*.
- Less likely to be misused than drugs in schedule 2.

Schedule 4 drugs are subject to minimal control. No prescription or other authority is required to legally possess them, so long as they are in the form of a medicinal product.

- No licence is needed to import or export schedule 4 drugs.
- However, authority is required for production and supply.
- Included in this schedule are 34 benzodiazepines, examples being *diaz-epam, flurazepam and loprazolam.*
- Anabolic steroids are also in this schedule.

Schedule 5 includes those drugs which because of their strength are exempt from virtually all controlled drug regulations other than retention of invoices for 2 years.

- They pose a minimal risk of abuse and are non-injectable small-dose preparations that can be purchased over the counter at a pharmacy without prescription, but once obtained it is illegal for them to be supplied to another person.
- Many of these preparations include well known cough mixtures and pain killers and an example is medicinal opium containing not more than 0.2% morphine.

Drug addiction

There are separate rules relating to supply of certain controlled drugs to drug addicts. A person is regarded as being addicted to a certain drug if he/she has, as a result of repeated administration, become so dependent on a drug that he/she has an overpowering desire for the administration of it to continue. A doctor must supply the Chief Medical Officer at the Home Office with certain details within 7 days of attending the addict. The drugs to which this ruling applies include cocaine, methadone, morphine, diamorphine and pethidine.

Prescribing drugs

Drugs should only be prescribed when necessary and the benefits of administering any medication should be considered in relation to the risk involved (British National Formulary; Joint Formulary Committee, 2019). The patient should always be made aware of the possible adverse effects of any prescribed drugs and treatment options should be discussed. In 2012 a prescribing competency framework was published by NICE to support all prescribers to prescribe effectively. The Royal Pharmaceutical Society (RPS) worked with prescribing professionals in the UK to update this in 2016. The framework is for all prescribers, whoever the prescribing professional is. As the range of professionals trained to prescribe increases, these competencies help to ensure that all healthcare providers are safe and effective prescribers. This is available at: www.rpharms.com/resources/frameworks/prescribers-competency-framework.

The Medicines Act 1968 allowed only doctors and dentists (and veterinary surgeons for animals) to prescribe drugs.

Prescription forms are classified as secure stationery. They are serially numbered and have antiforgery features.

A **patient-specific direction** (**PSD**) is a written instruction by a doctor, dentist or nurse/pharmacist prescriber, for medicines to be supplied or administered to a named patient. The instruction must include the dose, route and frequency of administration. In primary care it could be an instruction in the patient's notes. In secondary care it is likely to be instructions on the patient's medicines administration chart.

Non-medical prescribing

Prescribing has been rapidly changing within the NHS in recent years. In England, from May 2006, certain nurse and pharmacist independent prescribers can prescribe any licensed medicine (apart from most controlled drugs) within their sphere of competence.

Nurse prescribing has been on the professional agenda since 1986 when the Cumberledge Report recommended that community nurses should be able to prescribe from a limited list of items.

- The Advisory Group on Nurse Prescribing was established in 1987 and has led to two *Reviews of prescribing*, known as 'the Crown Reports'. These have led developments in non-medical prescribing in the UK.
- The first report was published in 1989 and recommended that district nurses and health visitors who completed the necessary training should be

allowed to prescribe from a limited list. Nurses were also to be allowed to supply medicines within 'group protocols'.

- The second report was commissioned in 1997 and was part of the *Review of prescribing, supply and administration of medicines.* Following this review 'patient group directions' (PGDs) were introduced in 2000 to replace the group protocols (see below).
- The review also defined two types of non-medical prescribing. These are **independent prescribing** and **supplementary prescribing** (dependent prescribing).

Independent prescribing means that the prescriber takes full responsibility for prescribing a medicine to a patient and for the appropriateness of the prescription. The independent prescriber is responsible and accountable for the assessment of patients with both diagnosed and undiagnosed conditions, and for decisions regarding their clinical management, including prescribing.

Supplementary prescribing is a voluntary partnership between an independent prescriber who must be a doctor or dentist and a supplementary prescriber, to implement an agreed patient-specific clinical management plan (CMP) with the patient's agreement.

Patient group directions (PGD)

A PGD is a specific written instruction for the supply and administration of a licensed named medicine or vaccine in an identified clinical situation. The PGD applies to groups of patients who may not be individually identified before presenting for treatment and is drawn up locally by senior doctors and other healthcare professionals. In general, a PGD is not meant to be a long-term means of managing a patient's clinical condition. This is best achieved by a healthcare professional prescribing for an individual patient on a one-to-one basis.

- PGDs allow a range of specified healthcare professionals to supply and/or administer a medicine directly to a patient with an identified clinical condition without them necessarily seeing a prescriber.
- PGDs are appropriate when the medicines to be given, and the circumstances under which they should be given, can be clearly defined in the written direction, especially if there are 'high volume' groups of patients who present for treatment, such as people needing vaccines. The PGD may include a flexible dose range.
- Professionals work under PGDs as named individuals, and no delegation of the supply or administration of the medicine is permissible. The healthcare professional working within the PGD is responsible for assessing that the patient fits the criteria set out in the PGD.

- A list of individuals named as competent to use PGDs is held locally within each organization. There is no specific national training programme but organizations must ensure competency.
- Guidance for PGDs is published by NICE and was updated in 2017. This is found at: https://www.nice.org.uk/guidance/mpg2.
- Those using PGDs must have undertaken training and have been assessed as competent and authorized to practise by the provider organization. They must also understand the relevant information about the medicine involved. This includes knowing how to administer the drug, how the drug acts within the body, how to calculate dosages, possible adverse reactions to the drug and any interactions. They must also be aware of any necessary follow-up arrangements.

Many branches of health professionals can legally carry out PGD instructions when they have been assessed as competent and if their name is identified within each document. This includes ambulance paramedics, nurses, midwives, health visitors, optometrists, chiropodists/podiatrists, radiographers, physiotherapists, pharmacists, dieticians, occupational therapists, prosthetists and orthoptists, and speech and language therapists.

Independent nurse and pharmacist prescribing

In 1992, the Act of Parliament entitled Medicinal Products: Prescription by Nurses Act 1992 became law.

- This legislation allowed health visitors and district nurses who had recorded their additional qualification on the Nursing and Midwifery Council (NMC) register to prescribe from the *Nurse Prescribers' Formulary.*
- The formulary included such items as laxatives, local anaesthetics, drugs for threadworms, skin preparations, urinary catheters, mild analgesics, drugs for scabies and head lice, stoma care products and fertility and gynaecology products. Specific drugs included aspirin tablets, lactulose solution, magnesium hydroxide mixture, nystatin, paracetamol and senna tablets.
- The formulary is now named the *Nurse Prescribers' Formulary for Community Practitioners (NPFCP)* and is used by community nurses who have successfully completed a programme of study. The formulary can be found on the BNF website at www.bnf.org.
- In 2002, a second form of independent prescribing for nurses was introduced in England. This allowed registered nurses and midwives with additional training to prescribe from the *Nurse Prescribers' Extended Formulary (NPEF)*. The formulary included over 120 prescription of medications (POMs) for specific conditions. Independent prescribing for nurses and pharmacists from a full formulary (excluding most controlled drugs) is permitted by legislation since May 2006.

> Independent prescribers (IPs) are nurses who have successfully completed the NMC Independent Prescribing Course and are registered with the NMC as an IP.

- Independent prescribing is only allowed within the nurse's area of competence. This includes medicines listed in the BNF, unlicensed medicines and all controlled drugs in schedules two to five.
- Qualified nurse and midwife prescribers in the UK must successfully complete an NMC approved post-registration prescribing programme in order to meet the standards of proficiency required to be entered on the NMC register as a nurse or midwife prescriber. This can be read in detail at: https://www.nmc.org.uk/globalassets/sitedocuments/education-standards/programme-standards-prescribing.pdf.
- The NMC programmes deliver outcomes that meet the RPS competency framework for all prescribers. This can be found at: https://www.rpharms.com/resources/frameworks/prescribers-competency-framework.
- Many pharmacists are also Independent Prescribers.

Supplementary prescribing

Supplementary prescribing was first introduced into the UK in 2003 for nurses and pharmacists and was extended in England in 2005 to chiropodists/podiatrists, physiotherapists, radiographers and optometrists. It is a voluntary prescribing partnership between the doctor (independent prescriber) and the supplementary prescriber to implement an agreed patient-specific clinical management plan (CMP), with the patient's agreement.

- A CMP must be in place before supplementary prescribing can begin.
- The plan is drawn up by the independent prescriber, following diagnosis, but with the supplementary prescriber who can then prescribe any medicines specified within the plan.
- The CMP is held within the patient's records.
- There is no formulary and no restrictions on the medical conditions.
- Controlled drugs, schedules 2–5 (except diamorphine, dipipanone and cocaine for treatment of addiction) can be prescribed if specified in the CMP.

The Nursing and Midwifery Council code of practice

For a registered nurse, the administration of medicines is an extremely important aspect of professional practice. In 2000 the United Kingdom Central

Council for Nurses, Midwives and Health Visitors (UKCC) produced *Guidelines on the administration of medicines* to replace the *Standards for the administration of medicines* produced in 1992.

The NMC produced a revised version of the guidelines when they took over in April 2002 and further revised these in 2004. The guidelines were extensively rewritten and updated in 2007 as *Standards for medicines management*.

The standards for medicines management were withdrawn at the end of January 2019 as the NMC felt it was not within their remit to produce this type of clinical practice guidance. However, they have worked alongside the Royal Pharmaceutical Society (RPS) to provide:

- professional guidance on the safe and secure handling of medicines (https://www.rpharms.com/recognition/setting-professional-standards/safe-and-secure-handling-of-medicines/professional-guidance-on-the-safe-and-secure-handling-of-medicines)
- administration of medicines in healthcare settings available at https://www.rpharms.com/Portals/0/RPS%20document%20library/Open%20access/Professional%20standards/SSHM%20and%20Admin/Admin%20of%20Meds%20prof%20guidance.pdf?ver=2019-01-23-145026-567
- advisory guidance on administration of medicines by nursing associates available at https://www.hee.nhs.uk/sites/default/files/documents/Advisory%20guidance%20-%20administration%20of%20medicines%20by%20nursing%20associates.pdf.

1.3 MEDICATION MANAGEMENT

Drug administration

To ensure safe medication management nurses are encouraged to follow the '**five rights**', which serve as a reminder of some of the essential points of drug administration.

- **Right patient** − this is to ensure medications are administered to the correct patient by checking the wristband against the prescription chart and/or asking the patient their full name.
- **Right drug** − the drug prescribed should be clear and legible, the generic name used, drug allergies should be noted on the patients' wristband, as well as on the drug chart. Many drugs have similar names.
- **Right dose** − the drug dosage should be checked against the name of the drug to be administered, any decimal point should be noted, as well as whether the drug dose is within the known dose range.
- **Right time** − the preparation time of the drug should be considered; administration needs to occur at the appropriate time(s) for effective therapeutic level and outcomes, for example antibiotics; ensure correct rate of administration.

- **Right route** − check this is the right route of administration and that the preparation form is right for the route of administration. Some drugs cannot be administered by the oral route.

Since the inception of the five rights there has been little evidence of their effect in reducing drug errors. This has led to a variety of additional rights being included:

- Cabilan et al. (2017) outlined 1 addition − 6 documentation
- Cox (2000) added 2 − 6 action and 7 form
- Bonsall (2011) and Lampert (2016) another 3 − 6 documentation, 7 reason, and 8 response
- Elliott and Lui (2010) included 4 more rights − 6 documentation, 7 action, 8 form and 9 response
- Edwards and Axe (2015) included 5 more rights − 6 to refuse (patient and nurse), 7 knowledge, 8 questions or challenges, 9 advice, 10 response or outcome.

There are now a variety of rights recommended but all include the original five with some modifications and additions. The 5, 6, 7, 8, or 9 rights approaches are used as protocols, policies or checklists for safer drug administration but can restrict professionals' competency and ability to make autonomous decisions.

The approach suggested by Edwards and Axe (2015) considers the full medication trajectory of medication management from before administration to after administration. The 10 Rs (10 Rights) approach also identifies other skills and competencies required for safer medication management and embraces and encourages the use of professional judgement. The approach requires a level of knowledge in order to undertake medications management and competence and values the inclusion of discretion in safe medication management.

Thus the registered nurse must use thought and professional judgement when administering medication, going beyond the mechanistic delivery of the prescribed dose on the treatment sheet. This would involve ensuring the correctness of the prescription and explaining the medication to the client if they did not already understand. The effects of the medication should be assessed and evaluated and any side effects reported to the medical team.

- Drugs are very necessary in the treatment of some clients but if the wrong drug is given it could, on occasion, be lethal and safety is of prime importance in the administration of medicines.
- The nurse should never administer a medication without knowing its action, and there should always be a copy of the BNF available when medicines are given so that any new drugs can be found and their action clarified.
- The nurse must be certain of the identity of the patient to whom the medication is to be administered and should also have knowledge of their planned care.

- The prescription must be very clear and legible. Doctors are asked to print the drug name and in hospital must always use the generic name of the medication and not the trade name.
- If there is any ambiguity or query regarding the drug, the dose or the route of administration, which should all be very clear on the prescription sheet, the nurse must refuse to administer the medication and should contact the prescriber.
- When a medication has been administered this must be recorded at the time in a clear and accurate manner and with a signature which is legible.
- If the patient refuses their medication this should also be recorded and the nurse in charge should assess the situation and contact the prescriber.
- A medicine must never be charted before it is given — when you sign for that drug you are saying that the client has actually taken it.
- Always check that the client understands the medication that they are receiving and is aware of any important side effects. Emphasize the importance of the treatment and explain its mode of action in simple terms.
- If an error is made in the administration of a medicine, this should immediately be reported to the nurse in charge, who will inform the prescriber.
- Evaluate the action of the prescribed medication and record any positive or negative effects, informing the prescriber of these.

Students must be given the opportunity to participate in the administration of medicines but only under the direct supervision of a registered nurse.

The prescription of any medication should:

- be based on the patient's informed consent and awareness of the purpose of the treatment
- be clearly written, typed or computer-generated and be indelible
- clearly identify the patient for whom the medication is intended
- record the weight of the patient if the prescription is based on weight
- clearly specify the substance to be administered using its generic or brand name where appropriate and its stated form, together with the strength, dosage, timing, frequency of administration, start and finish dates and route of administration
- be signed and dated by an authorized prescriber
- not be for a substance to which the patient is known to be allergic or otherwise unable to tolerate
- in the case of controlled drugs, specify the dosage and the number of dosage units or total course.

Drug errors

The risk to patients' who are prescribed drugs will never completely be eliminated but attempts need to be made and approaches updated as new evidence emerges to reduce significant risk and move closer towards safer practices. Despite the different opinions about the various rights they generally relate only to drug administration and not to the whole medication management trajectory and according to Redman (2017) none of them account for human, environmental and system errors.

Elliott and Liu (2010) and Macdonald (2010) argue the quality in medication management and the occurrence of drug errors are not solely a matter of adhering to a recommended approach. More recently Cabilan et al. (2017) recognized that none of these strategies offers a universal remedy. Jones (2009) states that the use of checklists has not put into perspective fully the issues related to the causes of drug errors and the faults and tensions that occur in the system. However, this is not to say that the checklists are not useful but perhaps need to be further developed or expanded in some way that encompasses a broader approach.

Drug errors are an international and national issue, which can lead to harm and death (WHO, 2016). To prevent drug errors nurses need to understand the complex issues of being safe while involved in aspects of medication management (Edwards and Axe, 2018).

A drug error can occur at any stage of the drug's chemical preparation/prescription/outcome journey (Table 1.1). The National Patient Safety Agency (NPSA, 2012) reported that drug errors accounted for about 11% of all patient safety incidents reported. These medication incidents are those that caused harm or potential harm due to the processes of prescribing, dispensing, preparing, administering and monitoring or failing to provide medicine advice.

Elliott and Liu (2010) suggest that only a small proportion (between 26% and 38%) of drug errors are nursing-related. Therefore a large majority (between 62% and 74%) of drug errors are due to other healthcare professional groups. However, just using numerical data to show the incidence of drug errors is not always helpful, as it implies less is better and other factors that contribute to drug errors need to be considered.

Factors that contribute to drug error

- Human or personal factors such as poor calculation competency or violation of double-checking practices, which according to Durham (2015) are unintentional and unpredictable.
- Faulty systems or organizational factors such as heavy workloads, lack of staff, a blame culture when mistakes are made, and complex error reporting systems.
- Environmental factors such as errors can occur due to the conditions of the environment where clinicians work; there are distractions and noise and

TABLE 1.1 Drug errors can occur from preparation to outcome.

A drug journey	Drug error	Due to	Responsibility
Chemical preparation/ drug naming	Similar name given to drugs	Looks like and sounds like other drugs; complicated dosage regimens	Drug companies
Packaging	Pharmacy colour coding; difficult to read medication labels	Tiny print on medication labels; use of less readable fonts; inadequate space between words	Packaging companies/ drug label designers; pharmacists
Prescribing/ transcribing	Wrong drug, wrong dose, quantity, indication for the drug, allergy, and contraindication to the drug	Inadequate abbreviations during prescribing; inadequate labelling	Doctor, nurse, non-medical prescribers, checked by nurse or other
Dispensing	Drug name confusion; failure to clarify ambiguous or illegible prescription	Similar packaging; single checking	Drug company; pharmacist from pharmacy to ward/ community setting
Preparing – ward/ community	Wrong: dosage/ calculation; drug/fluid; patient; time; form of medication; route of medication, solvent	Preparing in a crowded clinical room; overcrowded medication trolley; poor lighting, noisy, interruptions	Formulation prepared by pharmacist liquid form/ tablet form/IV etc.
Omission/ failure to administer	Refusal to administer drug by healthcare professional (HCP) if incorrect in any of the above identified; refusal to take the drug by the patient	Patient not understanding the need to take the drug; lapses and unavailability of medications; evidence-based practice issues	Nurse, allied healthcare professional, pharmacist, doctor, patient
Increase or decrease in period of time between drugs	Administering a dose more than 60 min before or after the prescribed time	Stress, distractions, excessive workload; lapses and unavailability of medications	Nurse, allied healthcare professional, pharmacist, doctor

Continued

TABLE 1.1 Drug errors can occur from preparation to outcome.—cont'd

A drug journey	Drug error	Due to	Responsibility
Administration	Not the drug intended by the prescriber; wrong route than ordered (oral instead of IV or dosage form error (tablets instead of liquid)	Illegible prescriptions; verbal orders; wrong administration rate; equipment failure or malfunction	Nurse/doctor/ allied healthcare professional
Providing medication advice/review	Patient not understanding their drugs; poly-pharmacy; complicated regimen	Inadequate knowledge by HCP of the patient and clinical condition; inadequate knowledge of the drug	Nurse/doctor/ allied healthcare professional
Monitoring/ outcome/ response	Overdose/under dose; high/low blood level concentration	Inadequate knowledge by HCP of the patient and clinical condition; inadequate knowledge of the expected outcome/ side effects of a drug	Nurse/doctor/ allied healthcare professional

poor lighting, which can easily be reduced by improving lighting and minimizing noise levels (Table 1.2).

There are a number of issues related to the causes of drug errors and it is not just one factor, but a combination of failures that lead to a change in drug practice behaviour compounded by intense resource and workforce pressures.

- The majority of drug errors are related to human factor errors, and added to this is that drug administration takes place in a system that is faulty within an environment that is often noisy with compounding factors such as poor lighting.
- The main cause of drug errors is often blamed on nurses' poor numeracy and calculation skills, yet the literature examined by Wright (2010) suggests there are more pressing aspects of nurses' preparation and administration of drugs that require urgent attention.
- The focus on reducing drug errors should be they are more of an interrelationship between the person, system and environment, and the effect this has on the nurses' medication management behaviour.

There is some agreement over the strategies that can be combined and put in place to reduce drug errors.

TABLE 1.2 Factors that contribute to drug errors.

Factors	Due to
Human/personal factors that contribute to errors	Poor calculation competency, lack of confidence Poor adherence to prescription/safety administration protocols; illegible prescriptions Poor/inadequate knowledge of medications, lack of experience, faulty judgement, insufficient supervision Inability to access appropriate resources Complacency leading to false sense of security, too much trust in doctors/colleagues, poor safety attitudes, overdependence on clinical support systems Factors that influence behaviour, misconceptions, incorrect interpretations; misreading and misinterpreting prescriptions Misinterpretation of packaging information (e.g. not for oral use) Fatigue/illness, poor communication Prescribers' poor handwriting, prescriptions unclear, use of abbreviations Poor eyesight, e.g. presbyopia or trouble reading fine print on labels
Faulty system errors	Poor teamwork and communication; lack of staff; excessive workloads, stress; poor management/leadership/organization of nursing work; creating a blaming, punitive, fearful culture; lack of funds Organizational procedures and policies and the environment Unclear error reporting processes providing no clear definitions of medication errors and near-miss events Technology with limited or no easily accessible resources such as electronic databases or a means to research unfamiliar drugs Poor storage of drugs; crowded preparation area and medication trolley, equipment failure or malfunction, lapses and unavailability of medications, single checking Ambiguous protocols/policies and procedure guidelines for prescribing/drug administration Pharmaceutical companies with poor medication packaging leading to vague labelling of medications, design of drug vials or containers Lack of training, no regular updates/courses provided Inefficient pharmacy processes
Environmental errors	Changing the conditions of the environment where clinicians work, not the human condition, need to be introduced if error minimization strategies are to be

Continued

TABLE 1.2 Factors that contribute to drug errors.—cont'd

Factors	Due to
	introduced Distractions from other nurses or patients (which are sometimes hard to ignore) Lack of awareness of circumstances of when and where an error can occur Poor lighting on night shifts Busy ward; noisy environment Time pressures to get the work done Increase in nurses' workload

Strategies to mitigate drug errors

Once we start to understand what constitutes the causes and factors that contribute to a drug error, only then can nurses implement strategies to prevent their occurrence (Table 1.3).

Interruption minimizing strategies

These strategies help nurses to modify their practice to enhance patient safety by reducing drug errors. There are practical suggestions as to how to reduce the causes of drug errors:

- Visual reminders can be used as a means to guide medication management, for example the 10 'Rs' can be displayed to provide a visual reminder for practitioners to be safe during medication management (see Table 1.2).
- Protected time to reduce interruptions during medication preparation and administration: patients and staff are discouraged from disturbing a nurse who is administering medications.
- The quality of team communication by the use of wearing a tabard or putting up reminders to make all team members aware a drug round is being performed and therefore reduce distractions.

Information technology

Attempts to reduce medication errors due to faulty system factors have included the introduction of information technologies such as computer physician order entry (CPOE) with clinical decision support systems (CDSSs), bar coding of drugs (Riaz et al. 2017), automated dispensing devices (Bates, 2000), medication systems and procedures (Johnson et al. 2017). However,

TABLE 1.3 Strategies to mitigate drug errors.

Strategy	Type	What can be done
Interruption minimizing strategies	Visual reminders	A reminder such as the 10 'Rs'. A visual reminder can be displayed as a prompt to provide a visual reminder for safer medication administration.
	Protected time to reduce distractions	The wearing of a bright tabard The use of a notice such as 'do not disturb', whereby patients and staff are discouraged from disturbing a nurse who is administering medications.
Information technology	Reduce medication errors due to faulty system factors	Computer physician order entry (CPOE) with clinical decision support systems (CDSSs) Bar coding of drugs Automated dispensing devices Medication systems and procedures Failure mode effects analysis (FMEA) and comprehensive decision support systems (DSSs) or electronic medical records (EMRs)
Adherence to protocols	Report all drug errors	There is a need to report immediately all drug errors and 'near misses', regardless of whether the patient is harmed, to ensure learning experience. Healthcare providers must be in agreement as to which errors count. The use of medication error reporting systems (MERSs) may make drug error reporting less complicated. Reporting, sharing information about drug errors and near misses, through anonymous uncomplicated reporting.
	Implementation of a recommended approach	Implement the 10 'Rs' approach to drug safety, which is a flexible approach and encompasses the need to include professionals' thinking during medication administration and medication review.

Continued

TABLE 1.3 Strategies to mitigate drug errors.—cont'd

Strategy	Type	What can be done
Implementing an evidence-based approach	When a patient refuses to take a drug	This may be because a patient has difficulty in taking the medicine, e.g. through difficulties in swallowing or when they do not perceive the need for the medication.
	The nurse can refuse to administer a prescribed drug	If the prescription is incorrectly written; the wrong drug name is entered If there is any ambiguity and if there are any doubts about the legitimacy of the prescription, a nurse does not have to give/administer the drug to the patient.
	Omission of a drug	If a nurse omits or fails to administer a drug or does not give it at the correct time; these constitute a medication error, and the nurse is placed in a difficult position.
Improving knowledge and understanding	In-depth knowledge of pharmacology	Nomenclature, pharmaceutics, pharmacokinetics, pharmacodynamics, therapeutics, side effects, drug toxicity, interactions and poisoning, blood tests to check for drug levels, kidney and liver function as essential
	Regular updates	The implementation of regular/yearly updates
	Medication safety courses	Undergraduate nursing students medication safety courses to provide early insight for future nurses to action change in drug administration practice
Questioning practice/challenge	Appropriate drug/route	Is the drug appropriate for the condition/patient? Most nurses working on any typical hospital ward setting only administer medications. A high level of IV drug administration contributes to this; the nurse has the right to request the drug be changed (if appropriate) to help with ease of administration and workload.

TABLE 1.3 Strategies to mitigate drug errors.—cont'd

Strategy	Type	What can be done
	Concordance – improving the frequency of dosing, timings	A slow release preparation may be given less frequently and may also cause fewer side effects. Questioning the formulation chosen for the patient The very young and elderly may require liquid preparations for ease of swallowing Could another group of drugs be considered? Conducting a comprehensive medication review with the potential to reduce polypharmacy
Medication review	Reviewing patients' medications at regular intervals	Is the outcome as expected? Providing monitoring of the drug(s) to establish the continuing effect The safety of the drug for the individual patient; has any harm come to the patient? Public health to inform the Medicines and Healthcare Products Regulatory Agency (MHRA) of significant adverse affects to drugs via the Yellow Card Scheme.
Providing medication advice		A patient should be informed by the nurse and understand the medication and side effects The purpose of the prescribed drug(s) Explain to a patient what to do if things do not progress as expected and what action to take. This information should also be recorded in the patient's notes.
Complacency and attitudes	Safety	There is often an attitude that a drug error will not occur Overconfidence in ability and knowledge The clinical support systems in place will protect nurses from making a drug error.

Crane and Crane (2006) focused on systems improvement drawn from those used successfully in aviation and other industries such as comprehensive decision support systems (DSSs) or electronic medical records (EMRs). Yet, resistance to adopting these technologies include the expense to implement and maintain, and there are issues with patient privacy. Cabilan et al. (2017) thought it worth noting that these technologies are reliant on user input to ensure patient data is accurate and complete.

These technologies may be seen to reduce risk to patients but may create new problems in relation to drug error risk. Cabilan et al. (2017) highlighted 'alert fatigue' stating it is easy to override the safety systems put in place by system improvement technologies, e.g. if alarms begin to irritate the nurse working with the new technology. Goddard et al. (2012) discussed the possibility of professional's over-reliance on technology and the danger of putting too much trust in the ability of systems to provide clinical decision support rather than their own judgement.

Fowler et al. (2009) have provided some evidence to suggest technology can improve patient safety. Yet, according to Durham (2015) more studies need to be undertaken as the impact of these technologies on the reduction of drug errors is unclear. In a press article (*Guardian*, 2018), the Health Secretary highlighted some initiatives that included providing funding to speed up the introduction of implementing medicine-prescribing systems into the NHS.

Drug error reporting

It is important to report all drug errors so these can be collated and the common causes identified and learned from. Learning through the reporting of drug errors is essential to ensure the same errors do not occur again. Drug reporting systems often use numbers of reported errors as a marker of safety, yet this implies that less is better, which in reality is unhelpful. However, if more drug errors are to be reported the process needs to be easy, but utilizing and comparing the data is hard if not impossible. Thus what organizations often do is concentrate on the drug error rather than using the reported data to improve knowledge and use the drug error information as a learning tool. This leads to more attention being given to the drug error and less being given to the situation that should be examined, i.e. why the error occurred.

According to Redman (2017) definitions of a drug error vary between providers and this is reflected in the literature. For example, a drug error can be a sentinel event or an unanticipated event that results in death or serious physical or psychological harm (NHS England, 2014), or a deviation from policies and procedures (Banja, 2010) to near misses (Cabilan et al. 2017). This causes problems with reporting of an error, as processes and procedures for reporting errors may vary, and sometimes it is not always clear if an error has occurred, as perception of importance and severity is not clearly outlined by a proper definition. The differing definitions and beliefs about drug errors can lead to miscommunication, thus leading to non-reporting of the error as it was not clear which errors need reporting and those that do not.

The Agency for Healthcare Research and Quality (AHRQ, 2014) identify that reporting drug errors can have consequences, such as work suspension, disciplinary action or being reported to the NMC for misconduct. However, the barriers to drug error reporting are not just concerns about consequences, even though this can be a deciding factor for some nurses not to report an error. What is needed according to Vrbnjak et al. (2016) is to create a non-punitive, fearless learning culture, which is necessary to enhance patient safety and prevent drug error reoccurrences.

Comparisons in relation to patient safety have been made between aviation and healthcare. Kapur et al. (2016) state that aviation has a more blame free culture in relation to reporting and admitting to safety incidents than healthcare. Safety in healthcare is regarded as the number one priority of some, not an obligation of all; whereas, safety permeates all levels of the business of airlines. Snowden and Barron (2011) identified that when prescribers felt supported they integrated medication management more easily into practice, which can serve as an essential benchmark for managers and leaders introducing ways to reduce drug errors.

The NMC supports an open and multidisciplinary approach to investigating adverse events.

Errors or incidents in the administration of medicines should be reported immediately to the prescriber and line manager. Actions should be documented.

Incidents should receive sensitive management and an assessment of circumstances before management decides on the way forward. Immediate and honest disclosure of errors is essential in the patient's interest and is taken into account by the NMC should they be involved in the case.

Implementing an evidence-based approach

A less identified strategy to mitigate against drug errors is the use of evidence to support medication management. All doctors, prescribing and non-prescribing professionals including nurses must aim to provide safe, evidence-based medication management. Utilizing research studies that provide evidence of the risks of drug errors to patients in hospital such as Roughead et al. (2016) or the work undertaken by Westbrook et al. (2010), which contributed to our understanding of the effects of interruptions on medication administration errors, can contribute to better outcomes in reducing drug errors. In addition, if a nurse has read the literature available on what contributes to the occurrence of a drug error, s/he knows to take more care during medication management episodes on his/her shift, and can use this evidence to support a claim to senior management for additional staff.

Other ways of applying an evidence-based approach to medication management is by applying pathophysiological principles. An example would be a nurse involved in medications management omitting digoxin if the apex and radial pulses were below 60 beats per minute (bpm).

This discussion lends itself to an evidence-based approach that can change and improve practice, and question policies and procedures. Medication management is not just about following orders on a prescription chart, but about being able to put all the evidence together and apply this to medication management at the bedside and in situations that are not safe for it to take place. Medication management without the application of evidence-based practice fails to represent nurses as autonomous knowledgeable practitioners able to use their own clinical judgement without the fear of being accused of a drug error.

Improving knowledge and understanding

Edwards and Axe (2015) identify the need for nurses to have an in-depth knowledge and understanding of pharmacology, which can contribute to reducing the occurrence of drug errors during medication management. Qualified nurses and prescribers whether doctors, nurses, pharmacists or allied health professionals have a duty to ensure the staff delegated to administer medicines have sufficient knowledge to undertake the task safely.

A healthcare practitioner (HCP) or nurse should not administer a drug if they do not know what it is for, are not able to explain it to the patient, do not understand the outcome of its administration or are unable to notice the side effects.

Medication reviews

To reduce drug errors that take place along the medication trajectory, frequent medication reviews of patients' medications needs to be undertaken at regular intervals. Medication review is ultimately the responsibility of all HCPs involved with medicines management. A review of the patient and their response to the medicine is concerned with 'safety netting'. Pharmacists, doctors, nurses and increasingly non-medical prescribers are all in a position to undertake medication reviews to identify potential errors and also to stop medicines when they are no longer required.

Providing better medication advice

All HCPs that prescribe or administer a drug should be able to provide medicine advice about actions, and indications of all medications, side effects, importance of taking a drug at the correct time and the expected outcome of the drug(s). This can serve to prevent the occurrence of drug errors during medication management.

- The NMC (2015) recommends that nurses should follow appropriate guidelines when giving advice about medicines and only if they have enough knowledge about the drug, they understand the persons health and are sure that the treatment or medicine serves the persons' health needs should advice be given.
- In addition, a nurse must make sure that advice given takes into account other care the person is receiving.

Having said all of the above, a quote in the *Guardian* (23 February, 2018) from Dr Helen Stokes-Lampard, the chair of the Royal College of General Practitioners (GPs), stated that the best solution is to 'properly fund the NHS with enough staff to deliver safe patient care'.

1.4 FORMULATION AND ADMINISTRATION

Pharmaceutics is the branch of pharmacology that deals with drug formulation. In-depth knowledge of this area is not needed by those administering drugs but it is useful to understand some of the terminology used.

Drug forms

A medicine is made of one or more active ingredients and various additives that are selected to give the medicine the necessary properties for dissolution and absorption by the selected route of administration. Inactive ingredients are sometimes added to flavour or colour or to improve the drug's chemical stability and allow longer action.

Tablets

When a drug is administered orally it is usually given in this form. The tablet contains one or more medications and is prepared by compressing the powder in a machine.

- The active drug is only a very small amount and may be less than a milligram. This means that an inert filler (diluent) such as lactose needs to be added to give bulk.

- To make disintegration in the gastrointestinal tract easier, a substance that swells on contact with water, for example starch, is added. This is called an excipient and ideally should allow a constant release rate of the medicine.
- Binding agent (e.g. sucrose) is necessary to keep the tablet whole before it is administered.
- Lubricating material such as magnesium stearate is added to prevent the tablet sticking to the machinery.
- Dyes, flavourings (especially to liquids) and preservatives may also be added.
- Disintegrating agents such as starch help the tablet to dissolve.
- Some children and older adults have difficulty in swallowing tablets but these should never be crushed and added to food or drink as this may interfere with the absorption or action of the medication. It is better to see if the medication is available in a liquid form.

Enteric coated (EC) tablets have a hard, waxy coating that allows them to dissolve in the alkaline intestine rather than the acidic stomach. These tablets should certainly never be crushed.

Sustained release or retard preparations are formulated so that absorption and effects are prolonged, thus making it possible to take the medication less frequently. This encourages the patient to adhere to their drug regimen. The more times a drug has to be taken daily, the less likely the patient is to remember it.

Controlled release is a more accurate form of sustained release. The release does not depend on pH as the medication has a semipermeable membrane around it that has a small hole made by a laser and allows the drug to be released over time.

Capsules

Soft gelatine capsules are completely sealed and contain a drug in a liquid form. Hard capsules have a powder inside.

- The drug is liberated when the capsule is digested in the stomach or intestine.
- If the capsule contains beads, some of these may be EC for slow release.
- Capsules are good for disguising the taste of a drug.
- Non-gelatine capsules are now available.

Oral liquid preparations

It is not just children but also many adults who find tablets difficult to swallow. If the patient has difficulty swallowing, many drugs are formulated in liquid form but it may be necessary to check with the pharmacist if this is available.

Flavourings such as raspberry are added to make the medicine more palatable.

Liquids are prescribed with a standard oral syringe that measures up to 5 mL and has 0.5 mL markings. If larger amounts are to be given, a 5 mL plastic spoon may be used.

Many liquid preparations should be shaken before use to ensure the drug is distributed evenly through the mixture.

- **Mixtures** are liquids with ingredients dissolved or diffused in water or another solvent.
- **Elixirs** are clear liquids containing water, alcohol, flavours and sweeteners.
- **Suspensions** are mixtures of solid and liquid particles where the solid particles do not dissolve.
- **Emulsions** are mixtures of two liquids such as oil and water that are not mutually soluble, for example milk of magnesia.
- Stabilizers are added to suspensions and emulsions, but they still tend to separate into two layers on standing and need to be mixed thoroughly before administration as do all liquid medicines. It has been known for an overdose to occur when the mixture has separated and the drug is more concentrated in one layer.
- Some drugs are prepared as **powders** due to their instability. Water is added before use. An example is penicillin.
- **Syrups** are solutions containing sugar and water to which the drug is added. They are usually flavoured and are frequently used in children's medicines. Nowadays other forms of sweetener are often used instead of sugar as they have low calorie content and do not contribute to dental caries. There is still a lot of research into the best way to hide the bitterness of children's medicines without using sugar.
- A **linctus** is a syrup specially formulated for coughs. It may contain a cough suppressant such as *dextromethorphan.*

Topical preparations

These are applied to an area of the body for direct treatment. They include preparations used on the skin but also many other examples such as eye drops, ear drops and antibiotics applied to body cavities in surgery.

Lotions are liquids with a creamy consistency that are applied to the skin, for example calamine lotion.

Gels are semi-solid in consistency with an alcohol base. Evaporation of the alcohol is rapid and very little systemic absorption occurs.

Creams and ointments are used to treat skin conditions and often a drug is available in both forms. Creams have a water base and this evaporates leaving the drug on the skin surface. This means there is little systemic action as very little of the drug is absorbed. Ointments are lipid-based and feel greasy. They are used for dry skin conditions but systemic absorption is more likely to occur.

Pastes are water repellent and have high powder content. They protect the skin from moisture and so are used in nappy rash.

Liniments are rubbed into the skin and contain the drug dissolved in alcohol or oil.

Tinctures are alcoholic extracts of vegetable or animal substance usually administered topically, for example tincture of benzoin.

Eye and nose drops are isotonic. This decreases discomfort or pain when they are administered. Eye drops may be aqueous or oily in nature whereas nose drops should not be oily. This is because they could enter the trachea and be aspirated leading to aspiration pneumonitis. Ear drops are oily and coat the external canal of the ear.

Suppositories and pessaries are solid and bullet-shaped for ease of insertion into the rectum or vagina. They contain the drug and an inert substance, for example cocoa butter, and the active drug is slowly released as the pessary dissolves with the heat of the body.

Transdermal patches are adhesive pads impregnated with the drug which is slowly released and absorbed via the skin into the circulation.

Injection solutions

Solutions for injection must be sterile and are preparations of the drug in liquid form. They contain other chemicals, for example buffers to regulate acidity or alkalinity of the solution or chemicals to increase stability. They are often packaged in sterile disposable syringes.

Inhalers

A solution or suspension of the drug is under pressure in an aerosol inhaler. These are used for administering drugs to the respiratory system and are widely used in asthma.

Drug administration

The aim of drug administration is to administer a dose that will maintain the optimum concentration of the drug at the target site for the required length of time, while minimizing adverse drug reactions (ADRs) that may occur from the drug's general distribution. Most drugs have to be absorbed into the bloodstream in order to reach their site of action.

Pharmacokinetics studies how the body deals with drugs. Its study tells us the best route for administration of a drug and also includes the study of drug absorption into the bloodstream, drug distribution around the body and finally drug elimination. Pharmacokinetics is the topic of Section 1.5.

- Using pharmacokinetic principles, the dose of a drug has to be carefully calculated following experiments with cells, tissues, animals and humans.
- It is necessary to determine the dose of the drug needed for effectiveness as well as the dose of the drug that may be toxic.
- To determine how often the drug has to be given, its rate of metabolism and elimination from the body has to be known.
- All individuals do not respond to a given dose of a drug in the same manner and variables such as age, body fat, genetics and disease are important, especially if the drug can be toxic.
- It may be necessary to monitor the blood levels of some drugs and adjust the dose accordingly. One such example is phenytoin for epilepsy. There may be wide variations in blood level of phenytoin in different patients, even though all are receiving the same dose of the drug.

Routes of administration

The route selected for administration will affect:

- the speed of action of a drug
- the availability of a drug to the tissues
- the length of time the drug is active within the body.

Some drugs are effective only when given by certain routes of administration. An example is glyceryl trinitrate (GTN) which cannot be given orally as the drug is destroyed by the liver before it reaches the tissues.
The routes of administration are:

- topical
- oral
- sublingual or buccal
- transdermal
- rectal
- vaginal
- inhalation
- parenteral — by injection
  - intravenous
  - intramuscular
  - subcutaneous
  - intradermal
  - intrathecal
  - intraosseous.

Most patients would prefer to receive a drug orally but sometimes there are advantages in using other routes. Drugs are often available in different forms so that they may be administered via different routes, for example as tablets or solution for injection.

All routes of administration are briefly described below and illustrated in Fig. 1.1.

Topical administration

These drugs are applied locally to act on the area they are applied to. Any systemic action is usually an undesired side effect. It is easier to control the effects of drugs administered locally and so avoid some side effects.

The largest area for topical administration is the skin. Most of these preparations are used for treating skin disorders such as eczema and psoriasis. They may also be used for treating fungal infections such as athlete's foot.

The products are formulated into lotions, creams, ointments or powders.

They may provide symptom relief such as reducing itching and are easily applied at home.

It must be remembered that there may be **long-term side effects** of some topical preparations and these may be both local and systemic.

One example is steroid creams which are used for the treatment of eczema. They must be used sparingly and not applied thickly to the skin because over a long period of time their use can cause thinning of the skin. This means that the skin tears easily and may make the treatment of lacerations difficult as suturing is not usually possible.

Overuse of steroid creams may also lead to some absorption through the skin, resulting in systemic side effects.

Topically applied creams are more easily absorbed through a baby's skin than an adult's. Care must be taken in young babies to avoid the use of creams that could produce systemic side effects if absorbed through the skin.

Other topical applications include eye drops and ear drops.

- In ophthalmics, **eye drops** may be used for excessive dryness of the eyes, infections, to dilate the pupil for eye examination or to treat a condition such as glaucoma.

Administration	Absorption and distribution	Elimination

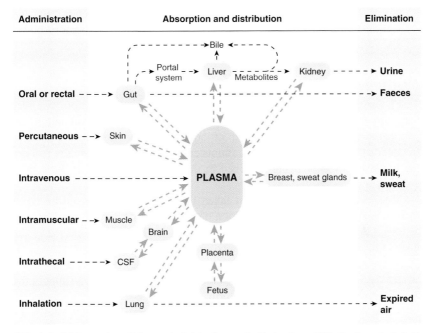

FIG. 1.1 **Main routes of drug administration and elimination.** *CSF,* Cerebrospinal fluid. *Adapted with permission from Rang, H.P., Dale, M.M., Ritter, J.M., et al. 2007. Rang & Dale's Pharmacology, sixth ed. Churchill Livingstone, Edinburgh.*

• Local anaesthetics may be administered in the form of eye drops to make the eye insensitive to pain. Many eye operations are carried out under local anaesthesia, for example cataract removal and lens replacement.

• **Ear drops** are used to treat local conditions of the ear, for example the accumulation of wax in the outer ear or infection of the outer ear (otitis externa).

• The **nasal route** may be used both for local and systemic drug administration. Some medications are well absorbed through the nasal mucosa and one example is antidiuretic hormone given intranasally (desmopressin) in diabetes insipidus or in primary nocturnal enuresis (bed wetting). Drugs given locally as nasal sprays include corticosteroids for the treatment of allergic rhinitis, especially hay fever.

• The **vaginal route** is also used to deliver medications to treat local infection or itching. The drug is usually in the form of suppositories, creams, jellies or foams.

• **Rectal administration** may be used for both local and systemic action and may be in the form of suppositories, foams or microenemas. Examples are the use of glycerol suppositories for constipation (local action) and the administration of corticosteroids in the treatment of inflammatory bowel disease (systemic action).

Oral administration

This is usually the most popular route with the patient as it is simple and non-invasive. It is the most common route for drug administration but in an emergency situation, where speed of action may be essential, it is less frequently used (Box 1.1). When administered orally the drug usually reaches the bloodstream after being absorbed in the small intestine. Very little drug absorption occurs in the stomach.

Most oral medications are best taken with water. Some should be taken before meals to allow better absorption but others are taken with or after food to lessen any irritant effects they may have on the gastrointestinal tract. The instructions should always be provided on the tablet container.

Some patients (especially children and the elderly) have great difficulty swallowing tablets and it is usually possible for the pharmacist to supply the medicine in a liquid or dispersible form.

Some drugs, for example antacids for indigestion, are taken orally for their local action on the stomach. In most cases, however, it must be remembered that after a tablet has been swallowed, it then has to be absorbed

---

BOX 1.1 Advantages and disadvantages of oral administration

Advantages of oral administration
- Convenient for the patient — more likely to take oral medication
- Noninvasive — avoids any fear of needles
- The gastrointestinal tract has a large surface area for absorption
- Usually lower cost
- Safe method of administration

Disadvantages of oral administration
- Variable absorption of the drug into the circulation (bioavailability). This may be low for some drugs
- Onset of action may be slower
- May interact with food
- Reach the liver first via the hepatic portal vein and may be metabolized before they reach the general circulation
- Have to remember to take the drug — important if the patient is at all confused

into the bloodstream before it can start to have a systemic action. Drug absorption is described in Section 1.5.

No tablet should be crushed without pharmacist advice. The crushing may alter the properties of the drug and even make it ineffective.

Sublingual and buccal administration

The drug is administered under the tongue or next to the mucosa of the mouth. Absorption takes place directly through the mucosa and into the small blood vessels and the venous system. This route is used when drugs are metabolized very quickly by the liver. If swallowed, the drugs would pass into the circulation and reach the liver before their target organ, thus being destroyed before they have any action. An example is *glyceryl trinitrate* given for angina.

This route is also useful if the patient is not allowed fluids or feels sick. One example is postoperatively where the analgesic *buprenorphine* may be given sublingually.

Aspirin is also absorbed via the mucosa when it is chewed and is administered by this route in prehospital care to reduce platelet adherence and the risk of myocardial infarction.

Transdermal administration

Drugs are usually given in the form of a sticky patch which releases the drug through a rate-controlling membrane. It is absorbed through the skin and into the blood supply.

Examples are *glyceryl trinitrate*, *estradiol*, nicotine (as an aid to stopping smoking) and *fentanyl* (a strong analgesic).

The skin is less permeable than other epithelial areas of the body due to the presence of keratin. Only drugs that are very lipophilic (fat soluble) and active in small amounts can be given by the application of a patch on the skin surface.

This method is ideal when a low blood level of the drug is needed over a long period.

Rectal administration

Drugs may be given rectally for local (see above) or systemic action.

Drugs are often formulated for rectal use as suppositories. These are torpedo shaped and should not be cut in half as the drug may not be distributed evenly within the suppository.

Normally the rectum is empty and a suppository will melt and be absorbed via the rectal mucosa into the bloodstream, thus making this a good route for systemic drug administration.

This form of drug administration does have some advantages but is more popular in some European countries than in the UK where suppositories tend to be unpopular with patients.

Examples of drugs available as suppositories are *paracetamol, prochlorperazine* (an antiemetic) and *diclofenac* (a nonsteroidal anti-inflammatory drug) (Box 1.2).

Vaginal administration

Usually drugs are given as pessaries (similar to suppositories) or foam and are always for topical treatment. The drug should be inserted as high into the vagina as possible and is best given at night for maximum retention.

Inhalation

This route is used for drugs that are absorbed via the respiratory mucosa for systemic action, for example volatile anaesthetics and for drugs acting locally on the lower respiratory tract.

The drug may be administered as:

● a gas as in anaesthetics

BOX 1.2 Advantages and disadvantages of rectal administration

Advantages of rectal administration
● Many drugs are absorbed well through the rectal mucosa which has a good blood supply
● Safe route if the patient is unconscious (when the oral route cannot be used)
● May be given if the patient is nauseous or vomiting
● Avoids some of the first-pass effect − but if inserted into the upper third of the rectum will be absorbed into the hepatic portal vein and taken to the liver first. This means suppositories should be inserted only just past the anal sphincter
● Useful when a vein may be difficult to locate. Lipid-soluble drugs may have a rapid action when given rectally, for example diazepam given rectally to control convulsion
● Can be given if the patient has difficulty in swallowing due to an oesophageal stricture
● Acidic drugs absorb slowly by this route and this may be useful as in the case of analgesia given at night. Some nonsteroidal anti-inflammatory drugs are available as suppositories, for example *diclofenac.* This also avoids some of the gastric irritation caused by these agents

Disadvantages of rectal administration
● Some patients object to this route of administration
● The patient has to be taught how to self-administer
● The suppository is manufactured to melt at body temperature and may have to be kept refrigerated
● Some suppositories may irritate the rectal mucosa

- an aerosol as in *salbutamol* inhalers used to treat asthma. Metred dose inhalers deliver a set dose of the drug as particles dispersed in an inert gas and small enough to remain suspended for a long time. The patient needs to be taught how to use the inhaler and good hand−breath coordination is needed. Often now a spacer is used in conjunction with the inhaler and acts as a reservoir between the inhaler and the mouthpiece, allowing the dispersed particles to be inhaled over several breaths. This is especially important in small children who have not got the necessary coordination to successfully use an inhaler
- a powder dispensed from a rotary inhaler as in sodium cromoglicate for the treatment of asthma
- a nebulizer − the machine uses air or oxygen to convert a solution of the drug into an aerosol. Nebulizers are used in respiratory conditions such as severe asthma and chronic bronchitis. They can deliver larger doses of medication over a longer timespan.

It is important to check the patient's technique when using the inhaler and to provide careful instruction when necessary.

Parenteral administration

Strictly speaking this is administration avoiding the gastrointestinal tract but the term is usually taken to mean administration by injection. The administration of any injection is an aseptic procedure and must involve good hand washing and drying techniques.

Intradermal injection − into the skin (dermis)

- Drugs are not usually administered for systemic action as absorption is slow.
- Used for allergy testing and some diagnostic tests.
- Less than 0.1 mL may be administered by this route.

Subcutaneous injection − under the skin

This is a widely used route for injection − commonly into the upper arm, the thigh or the abdomen. Sites for subcutaneous injection are shown in Fig. 1.2.

- The subcutaneous tissue does not have a very good blood supply and so absorption is quite slow.

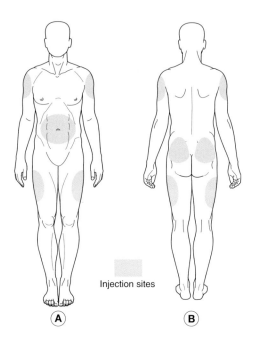

Injection sites

FIG. 1.2 **Sites used for subcutaneous injection.** (A) Anterior aspect. (B) Posterior aspect. *Reproduced with permission from Jamieson, E.M., McCall, J.M., Whyte, L.A. et al. 1996. Clinical Nursing Practices. Churchill Livingstone, Edinburgh.*

- Local blood supplies vary and absorption from the arm or leg may be more rapid when the muscles are active as in exercise.
- This route is used for *insulin* and *heparin* administration.
- Up to 2 mL may be administered.

Intramuscular injection − into a muscle

- Skeletal muscle is vascular and absorption is quicker than with the subcutaneous route.
- Rate of absorption is still variable dependent on the site and the state of the circulatory system.
- Absorption can be increased by increased blood flow as in exercise or by rubbing the site of injection.
- Poor circulation, as in shock, decreases the rate of absorption.
- The main danger is damage to the nerves, especially if the gluteal muscle is used as the sciatic nerve passes through this region.
- May be painful.
- Up to 5 mL may be given into one site.

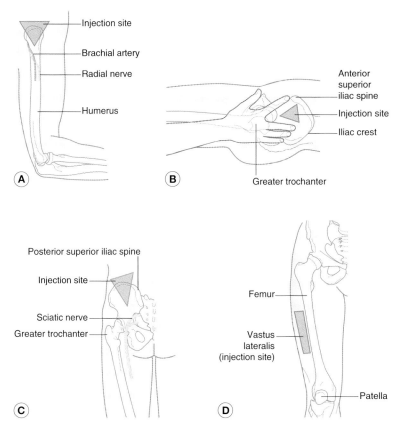

FIG. 1.3 Common sites for intramuscular injection. (A) Deltoid region of arm. (B) Ventrogluteal site. (C) Dorsogluteal site. (D) Vastus lateralis site. *Reproduced with permission from Richards, A., Edwards, S., 2008. A Nurse's Survival Guide to the Ward, second ed. Churchill Livingstone, Edinburgh.*

Intramuscular injection sites are shown in Fig. 1.3. An intramuscular injection should deposit the medication below the subcutaneous fat and in the muscle itself.

- The **mid-deltoid site** is easily accessible but due to the small area available a limited number of injections can be given here. It is the most common site for vaccinations and can only receive small amounts, usually 1 mL or less.
- The **ventrogluteal site** is the site of choice and is used for antibiotics, antiemetics, analgesics and deep intramuscular injections. Up to 2.5 mL may be safely injected. The site is free from penetrating nerves and blood vessels and is where the gluteal muscle is the thickest.
- The **dorsogluteal site** (upper, outer quadrant) for deep intramuscular injections is rarely used nowadays as there is a risk of hitting the sciatic nerve

---

BOX 1.3 Advantages and disadvantages of intravenous administration

Advantages of intravenous administration
- The drug is delivered into the bloodstream and so is able to act immediately
- There is no reliance on absorption and the whole dose of the drug reaches the bloodstream. This enables the amount the patient actually receives to be better calculated
- A continuous infusion allows the rate of administration to be controlled and the action of the drug thus modified

Disadvantages of intravenous administration
- Once the drug is given it cannot be removed from the body
- Any allergic response is likely to be more severe
- There is danger of infection if rigorous asepsis is not applied
- If injected by mistake into an artery tissue damage can result from arterial spasm
- Only those with special training can administer the drug

---

or the superior gluteal arteries. It has the lowest absorption rate and does become atrophied in the elderly or emaciated patient.

- The **vastus lateralis site** can be found by dividing the lateral aspect of the thigh into thirds and using the middle third. There are no major blood vessels or nerves associated with this site and it is easily accessible. This site is commonly used by people who need to self-administer injections.

Intravenous injection – into the venous circulation

- This route avoids the need for absorption, resulting usually in fast action.
- The entire dose is available within the circulatory system.
- It is often used in an emergency where rapid action is needed (Box 1.3).

The Standards for Infusion Therapy updated in 2019 are available on the RCN website at www.rcn.org.uk.

Nurses are not allowed to administer drugs by the intravenous route until they have undergone a training programme and assessment for IV drug administration.

The effects of the route of administration on the plasma concentration of a drug are shown in Fig. 1.4.

Intrathecal injection – through the spinal theca and into the cerebrospinal fluid

- Needle is inserted at the level of the third or fourth lumbar vertebra so that the spinal cord is avoided.

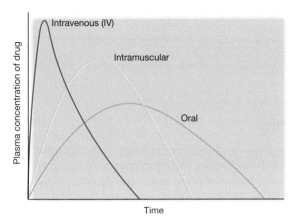

FIG. 1.4   **Effects on plasma concentration of the route of administration following a single dose of a drug.** *Reproduced with permission from Greenstein, B., 2004. Trounce's Clinical Pharmacology for Nurses, seventeenth ed. Churchill Livingstone, Edinburgh.*

- This route may be used to get drugs directly into the central nervous system and avoid the blood—brain barrier (BBB).

   Epidural injection — above the dura mater

- Given at the same position as intrathecal injections but the drug is deposited above the dura mater and so does not enter the cerebrospinal fluid.
- Local anaesthetics are administered via this route in some surgical procedures and in labour.

   Intraosseous infusion — into the bone marrow
- This route is used in a life-threatening situation for vascular access in babies and children when intravenous access is not possible.
- The marrow cavity can be used to administer fluids as it is continuous with the venous circulation.
- Must be an aseptic procedure to avoid osteomyelitis (infection in the bone).

   Some other routes of injection.
   Injections may be given into various body cavities such as the **peritoneum** and the **pleura**.

   Intra-articular injections into a joint may be used especially in inflammatory conditions to give high doses of corticosteroids.

1.5 PHARMACOKINETICS

Pharmacokinetics is literally the movement of a drug through the body. It includes:

- drug absorption — the drug enters the bloodstream following administration

- drug distribution — most drugs leave the bloodstream and enter the tissues
- drug metabolism — the drug is converted by enzymes into a form that can be eliminated from the body
- drug excretion — the drug is removed from the body, usually into the urine or faeces.

Drug absorption

Unless a drug is given intravenously, it has to be absorbed into the bloodstream. This involves **crossing cell membranes**. A drug given orally has to be absorbed from the gastrointestinal tract before it reaches the bloodstream.

- Although some absorption takes place in the **stomach**, the surface area here is much less than the **small intestine**, where most of the absorption takes place.
- The amount and rate of absorption are affected by the **chemical nature** of the drug. Drug absorption usually takes place by **simple diffusion** of **uncharged molecules**. Diffusion is the passage of the drug molecules from an area of high concentration, for example in the intestine following a dose of oral medication, to an area of lower concentration as in the bloodstream.
- For diffusion to occur the drug will have to pass through cell membranes. These are a **lipid bilayer** and so composed mostly of fatty material. This means that drug molecules that are **fat soluble** and uncharged will be able to pass more easily through the membranes. Charged molecules or **ions** are water loving rather than fat loving and do not pass readily through the fatty membrane.
- Drugs do need part of their molecule to have some water solubility so that they can dissolve in the aqueous intestinal juices. Bile salts aid the absorption of fatty drugs.
- The **size** of the drug molecule is important and small molecules diffuse more rapidly.
- A drug that has small molecules but is water loving (hydrophilic) and not fat soluble is likely to **ionize** into positive and negative particles in solution. The drug will only pass across the membrane when it is in its unionized state as ions do not diffuse readily across membranes.

A famous example to illustrate the importance of ionization in drug absorption is the use of the arrow poison, *curare*, by the Macusi people in South America. They used curare to kill animals, which were then eaten. Curare causes death by paralysis when it reaches the bloodstream but because it is a highly ionized molecule it cannot be absorbed through the gastrointestinal tract. This meant that meat from an animal killed with curare could still be eaten without paralysing the Macusis. Muscle relaxants similar to curare are still used to paralyse patients in certain surgical procedures.

Drugs may be **acids** or **bases** and this will also affect their absorption. A drug that is weakly acidic will not ionize in an acid environment such as the stomach but it will ionize in a basic environment such as the small intestine. The reverse is true for a basic drug that will therefore ionize in the stomach but become uncharged in the small intestine.

- A weakly **acidic drug** such as *aspirin* will not ionize in the stomach and so will be absorbed through the stomach mucosa.
- A weakly **basic drug** such as *morphine* will ionize in the stomach and so not be readily absorbed there. In the intestine the environment is basic and the morphine now will be un-ionized and so can be absorbed more rapidly.
- As drugs spend so little time in the stomach and the small intestine has a much larger area for absorption (equivalent to that of a tennis court), in reality even weakly acidic drugs such as aspirin are mostly absorbed from the small intestine. Their absorption here will be slower than in the stomach.

There are a few drugs that are so similar to biological molecules within the body that **carrier systems** are involved in their absorption. Examples are *levothyroxine* (one of the hormones produced in the thyroid gland) and *levodopa* used in Parkinson's disease.

Other factors affecting drug absorption

The drug concentration in the intestine depends on:

- the amount of drug ingested
- the rate at which the drug is released from the formulation
- the volume of gastrointestinal contents with which it is mixed.

Drugs are usually absorbed more quickly if the stomach and small intestine are empty. If there is food in the intestine it may take the drug a long time to actually reach the absorptive surface. In the case of most **antibiotics** the client is instructed to take the medication 1 hour before food for this reason. Drugs which may irritate the stomach should be given with or after food and this instruction will usually be on the container. An example of such a drug is *aspirin*.

- Interactions with other drugs may also be important. For example, drugs that inhibit gastric emptying, for example *atropine*, *amfetamine*, *morphine*, may reduce the rate of absorption of other drugs.
- Diseases of the gastrointestinal tract such as ulcerative colitis may interfere with absorption.
- Transit time is the time taken for passage through the small intestine and this will affect the amount of drug that is absorbed. Gastrointestinal movement aids the dissolution and absorption of a drug and as the drug passes through the intestine it is fragmented and dissolved. The longer the

medication is in the gut, the more of it will usually be absorbed. If there is excessive peristalsis, as in diarrhoea, the drug will not have time to be absorbed.

- Reduced absorption of certain drugs, especially if they are enteric coated (EC), occurs in patients with an ileostomy.
- **Laxatives** decrease absorption.
- Acid in the stomach destroys some drugs such as acid-sensitive **penicillins.** These drugs have to be given by injection.
- **Enzymes** in the gastrointestinal tract may break down proteins and amino acids such as *insulin* which therefore has to be given by injection.
- *Tetracycline* (an antibiotic) forms a complex with metal ions such as **calcium** or **iron.** If either of these are given with tetracycline a large molecule is formed that cannot be absorbed. As there is calcium in milk, tetracycline should not be taken with a drink of milk. Magnesium and aluminium found in some antacids also complex with tetracycline.

Bioavailability

Bioavailability is the percentage of unchanged drug reaching the systemic circulation following administration by any route.

If a drug is given by the intravenous route bioavailability will be 100%.

If a drug is given orally the bioavailability will depend upon:

- the amount of drug absorbed from the gut — many drugs are incompletely absorbed, for example *ampicillin* is approximately 40% absorbed from the gastrointestinal tract but *amoxicillin* is approximately 90% absorbed. *Digoxin* is 70% absorbed
- how much of the drug is destroyed by the liver the first time the drug molecules pass through this organ. This is known as **first-pass elimination** and is described below. The first-pass effect may be largely avoided by using other routes of administration such as rectal, sublingual or transdermal.

Drug distribution

Once absorbed, the drug is in the bloodstream and able to travel to its site of action. Most drugs leave the bloodstream by being filtered through the capillaries into the tissues and their concentration in various tissues is affected by many factors.

Protein binding

Some drugs bind to **plasma proteins** in the blood. Acidic drugs usually bind to **albumin** whereas basic drugs bind to some **globulins.**

- Plasma proteins do not usually leave the bloodstream and so a drug that is **bound** to the albumin does not reach the tissues whereas **unbound** (**free**) drug does.
- As free drug leaves the bloodstream more bound drug will be released from the plasma protein to maintain the equilibrium.
- The more strongly a drug binds to the plasma protein, the less free drug will be available for action and the drug will remain in the plasma longer. This acts rather like a slow release.
- Sometimes there can be competition between drugs that both bind to the same sites on the plasma protein. If two such drugs are administered together this can affect their available concentrations in the tissues. This can occur with *warfarin*, an anticoagulant that is readily protein bound, and *aspirin* which can displace some of the warfarin from its binding sites and so raise the free concentration of warfarin. As warfarin is highly toxic, this could be dangerous.
- If there is a deficiency in plasma proteins, as in severe malnutrition, burns or liver disease, this may raise the concentration of free drug available and enhance its effects.

Hepatic first-pass effect

When a drug is administered orally, it will leave the gastrointestinal tract via the hepatic portal vein and reach the liver before it reaches its target tissues. If the drug is heavily metabolized the first time it passes through the liver, little will be available for systemic action.

- Some drugs cannot be given orally because they are nearly completely metabolized the first time they pass through the liver. An example is *glyceryl trinitrate* which is about 96% destroyed the first time it passes through the liver and is given sublingually or buccally to avoid this effect.
- If there is a high first-pass effect, the dose of a drug when administered orally may need to be higher than when the drug is administered by other routes. *Morphine* is almost completely absorbed in the intestine but about two thirds of the oral dose is metabolized by the liver the first time the drug passes through, making the bioavailability only 33%.
- Drugs with high first-pass elimination will show **varied bioavailability** in different people dependent on their liver function and blood flow as well as genetic differences in their liver enzymes.

Barriers to distribution

Most drugs are small molecules that readily leave the capillaries and pass into other fluid compartments by capillary filtration.

- A few drugs are confined to the plasma because their molecules are too large to cross the capillary wall easily, for example *heparin*.
- Some polar (ionized) compounds only distribute in the extracellular fluid, for example *vecuronium* (a paralytic agent) and *gentamycin* (an antibiotic). This is because they have very low lipid solubility and cannot readily cross cell membranes. They do not usually cross the placenta or reach the brain.

The blood–brain barrier (BBB)

The endothelial cells in the cerebral circulation are packed tightly together and there are also some connective tissue cells that help to create a barrier. This effectively prevents many molecules from entering the brain tissue.

- Only substances that are very lipid soluble (lipophilic) can readily cross the membranes, examples being *ethanol* (alcohol) and **general anaesthetics.**
- Part of the **vomiting centre** is not protected by the BBB. This is a protective mechanism allowing toxic substances to cause vomiting before they reach the brain. It does mean that many drugs do have nausea as a side effect.
- The BBB may be useful and prevent entry of harmful drugs into the brain. One example is the neuromuscular blocking muscle relaxants used in surgery (e.g. *vecuronium*). These drugs inhibit the action of *acetylcholine* and if they were to enter the brain, death could ensue.
- *Penicillin* does not cross the BBB and this is a disadvantage in infections of the central nervous system. In **meningitis** where there is inflammation of the meninges, penicillin can cross.
- Many drugs do cross the BBB and attempts are made to manufacture less lipophilic drugs that cannot cross. Antihistamines such as *chlorphenamine* have drowsiness as a side effect because they cross the BBB but there are some antihistamines now available such as *loratadine* that are less lipid soluble and so unlikely to cause drowsiness.

The placental barrier

This is not an efficient barrier and most drugs will cross the placenta.

- Unless it has been shown otherwise it is assumed that all drugs cross the placenta and enter breast milk.
- As many drugs are **teratogens** and may cause fetal malformations, it is advisable to avoid the administration of any unnecessary drugs in pregnancy.
- The BNF provides warning of drugs that are known to cause adverse effects in pregnancy.

Volume of distribution

This is a measure of the distribution of the drug in the body. The volume of the plasma in a 70 kg man is about 3 L. If the apparent volume of distribution (Vd) of a drug is 3 L then the drug is staying within the bloodstream. The Vd is larger if the drug is more widely distributed in the body. The Vd is useful in estimating the dose needed to reach a given plasma concentration. This can be important when peak plasma concentration is essential for the therapeutic effect of a drug

- The Vd of a drug is higher if the drug binds to certain tissues. The drug may be sequestered outside the circulation and may localize in certain tissues. One example is *amantadine*, an antiviral drug that has a concentration in the liver, lungs and kidneys that is several times that found in the circulation.
- *Digoxin* concentrates in muscle tissue and so the dose needed to produce the correct therapeutic level in the plasma varies according to the patient's muscle mass.

Clinical implications

The most important causes of variations are as follows.

- Vd varies with individual height and weight.
- Accumulation of fat (for lipid-soluble drugs) seen in obese patients.
- Accumulation of fluids (for water-soluble drugs) seen in ascites, oedema or pleural effusion.
- Fluid compartments, and so the Vd for most drugs, vary with age, thus some drugs need to be reduced in the elderly.

Drug metabolism

The majority of drugs are metabolized before they are lost from the body. Drug metabolism involves chemically changing the drug and usually making it more **water soluble** so that it can be eliminated in the urine. Some drugs that are already water soluble are not metabolized and are excreted largely unchanged from the body. Drug metabolism can occur in most body cells but mostly takes place in the **liver**. The process does not always involve detoxification and sometimes the metabolite may be more active than the drug itself. In the case of **prodrugs** the drug as administered is inactive and is only active after it has been chemically changed within the body.

Drug metabolism is divided into two stages called phase 1 and phase 2.

- **Phase 1 reactions** are oxidation, reduction or hydrolysis reactions that usually increase water solubility.
- **Phase 2 reactions** involve the attachment of a chemical group to the molecule and facilitate excretion from the body usually by increasing water solubility.

Drug metabolizing enzymes

Drugs are metabolized by **enzymes**. These drug metabolizing enzymes are nonspecific and one enzyme may metabolize many drugs with similar chemical bonds and groupings. Competition between drugs for these enzymes can lead to **drug interactions**.

- **Enzyme induction** is increased manufacture of an enzyme due to stimulation by a chemical from outside the body. This may lead to an increased rate of metabolism of certain drugs. Induction may be produced by smoking, alcohol, certain foods and some drugs. Alcohol stimulates the production of several liver enzymes. Barbiturates are one group of drugs that may need to be administered in larger doses in heavy drinkers. Examples of drugs that are **enzyme inducers** are *rifampicin, omeprazole* and *phenobarbital.*
- **Enzyme inhibition** may be a problem when some drugs are co-administered. *Cimetidine* inhibits some liver enzymes involved in the metabolism of other drugs such as *propranolol.* Certain foods may also act as **enzyme inhibitors**, an example being the inhibition of certain drug metabolizing enzymes by **grapefruit.**
- With some drugs, the more often the drug is given, the more effective the breakdown process — **tolerance** develops. This occurs with alcohol.
- There are **genetic differences** in the ability to metabolize drugs. Some people metabolize more slowly or rapidly than others depending on their ability to manufacture certain enzymes.

If the liver is damaged, as in liver failure, the inactivation process may be slower than normal. This means that the drug will be active for longer and smaller doses of certain drugs are necessary.

Drug elimination

Some volatile drugs such as general anaesthetics are eliminated via the lungs but most other drugs are excreted in the bile or urine. This means that patients with kidney or liver disease may require reduced doses of certain drugs as their excretion will be delayed and accumulation may occur.

Drugs may also leave the body in the saliva, sweat, breast milk, tears and expired air. It is because alcohol is excreted by the lungs that breath testing detects drivers with over the limit of alcohol in their system although quantitatively the amount of alcohol excreted in this way is unimportant.

In the urine, drugs are eliminated either unchanged or as metabolites.

Renal elimination involves glomerular filtration, tubular secretion and distal tubular reabsorption. Drugs vary greatly in the way they are handled by the kidney. *Penicillin* is virtually all eliminated the first time it passes through the kidneys as it is actively secreted into the nephron. Other drugs may be eliminated extremely slowly but most drugs lie between these two extremes.

- Lipid-soluble drugs are readily reabsorbed from the kidney tubule, so to be effectively eliminated in the urine, a drug or metabolite must be water soluble.
- Some very polar compounds such as *mannitol* are too water soluble to be reabsorbed at all.
- A **basic drug** is more readily excreted in acidic urine where it will ionize and so not be reabsorbed.
- An **acidic drug** will ionize in alkaline urine and so be more rapidly eliminated.
- This principle may be used in some cases of drug overdose. One example is making the urine alkaline to aid the elimination of *aspirin* from the body.
- **Renal impairment** reduces the elimination of drugs that rely on glomerular filtration for their clearance such as *digoxin* and some antibiotics.

The kinetics of drug elimination

Most drugs are eliminated at a rate proportional to their concentration, following **first-order kinetics**. The rate of elimination depends on how much drug is present, being higher when there is more drug in the plasma. A **constant fraction of the drug** is being eliminated in unit time.

Less often, the **rate of elimination of the drug is constant** and is independent of the drug concentration. This is termed **zero-order kinetics** and is often due to the saturation of an enzyme involved in metabolism of the drug.

Some drugs exhibit first-order kinetics at low concentrations and zero-order kinetics at higher concentrations. **Alcohol** (ethanol) is an example of this.

Alcohol elimination
If less than 8 g/h of alcohol is consumed (about half a glass of wine), the alcohol follows first-order kinetics. If consumption is faster, the liver enzyme that metabolizes alcohol is saturated and elimination of the drug follows zero-order kinetics. This explains why a person can still be 'over the limit' of blood alcohol concentration the morning after a night's heavy drinking.

Plasma half-life

- If a drug exhibiting first-order elimination is injected continuously into the arm via a syringe driven by a constant infusion pump, a plot of plasma concentration against time can be constructed.
- The drug is being eliminated as it is infused and drug concentration will rise rapidly at first then more slowly until a steady state is reached whereby

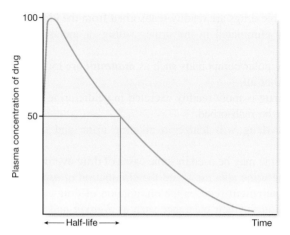

FIG. 1.5 Plasma levels and half-life of a drug after a single intravenous injection. *Reproduced with permission from Greenstein, B., 2004. Trounce's Clinical Pharmacology for Nurses, seventeenth ed. Churchill Livingstone, Edinburgh.*

the rate of input of drug into the body is equal to the rate of elimination of the drug from the body. The plasma concentration at this point is the steady-state concentration.

● When the infusion is stopped, the plasma concentration declines towards zero. The time taken for plasma concentration of the drug to halve is the plasma half-life.

● The plasma half-life following a single intravenous administration is shown in Fig. 1.5. After a second half-life has passed, the concentration of the drug will have again halved and so on.

● Half-life not only determines the time course of the drug's disappearance when the infusion is stopped but also the time course of its accumulation when the infusion is started.

● The faster the elimination of a drug, the less time it will remain in the circulation and be available to the body tissues. This type of drug will need to be given more frequently than a drug with a longer elimination time.

Half-life and drug dosage

If the concentration of a drug is 600 µg/L at a certain time and this level drops to 300 µg/L in 2 hours, the drug's half-life is 2 hours. In another 2 hours the concentration will have halved again to 150 µg/L and so on.

Half-lives are useful when calculating how frequently a drug needs to be given.

● If a drug is given at approximately half-life intervals, it will reach a steady-state concentration after about **five repeat doses** have been given (Fig. 1.6).

● For drugs with long half-lives this could be a long time, for example if the half-life is 48 hours, a steady-state concentration of the drug would not be achieved for 2 weeks.

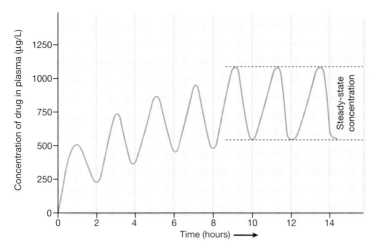

FIG. 1.6 **Development of a steady-state concentration with repetitive doses of a drug at half-life intervals.** In this example the half-life of the drug is 2 hours. A steady-state concentration (97%) is reached after approximately five half-lives.

- A way round this is to give a **'loading dose'** of the drug. This is usually double the normal dose.
- Repeated doses of any drug will result in significant drug accumulation if the drug is ingested at intervals more frequent than twice the plasma half-life.

Missed doses

Patients often ask what to do if they have forgotten to take their medication. This does depend on what the medication is and the disease it is being used to treat. If there is any doubt, a pharmacist should be consulted.

1.6 PHARMACODYNAMICS

It is important to study what drugs actually do and how they do it. This is pharmacodynamics − the study of how drugs work.

Drug action may be studied at the molecular level, the cellular level, tissue and organ level or system level. Although detailed understanding of drug action at the molecular and cellular level is not necessary for drug administration, it aids understanding of possible side effects and drug interactions.

Mechanisms of drug action − drugs with nonspecific action

These drugs often require higher doses than those discussed later that act on specific enzymes or drug receptors.

Simple chemical reaction

Antacids such as *magnesium hydroxide* are an example

- These are taken to relieve indigestion and because they are alkaline they react with the stomach acid and neutralize it.

Chelating agents facilitate elimination of a heavy metal ion from the body

- *Desferrioxamine mesylate* (*Desferal*) used in iron toxicity is an example.
- Called chelating agents because they latch onto the ion firmly like a crab grabs something with its claw (chela).

Simple physical action

Osmosis is the passage of water molecules across a semipermeable membrane from an area of low solute concentration to one of higher solute concentration. Some drugs work by exerting an osmotic effect.

- There are osmotic diuretics such as *mannitol* and osmotic laxatives such as *lactulose.*

Other examples of physical action are **adsorbents** such as *activated charcoal.*

- These have a large surface area and can physically bind to other drugs.
- Activated charcoal is given by mouth in many types of drug overdose to bind the drug molecules and lessen absorption of the drug.

Another example of physical action is a drug called *simeticone* that is an **antifoaming agent** given to lower the surface tension in the intestine and relieve flatulence.

Drugs with more specific action

Drugs usually act by binding with certain proteins on or in cells. These could be:

- receptors
- enzymes
- ion channels
- carrier molecules.

Drugs that act on receptors

Most drugs work by interacting with receptors. Receptors are sensing elements in the system of cellular communication. They are proteins found on the cell surface or intracellularly. They translate extracellular signals into intracellular responses.

The body maintains a state of internal balance called homeostasis. Involved in this are control systems — the nervous system and the endocrine system. Chemical transmission of signals plays a vital part in the communication process between the cells involved. Chemical messengers such as neurotransmitters (e.g. *noradrenaline*) and hormones (e.g. *insulin*) fit into a receptor and stimulate it. This brings about changes within the cell.

Agonists

- Drugs that are agonists fit into a receptor and stimulate it as would the body's natural ligand (a ligand is a substance that fits into a receptor).
- An example is *salbutamol* which fits into the **adrenergic receptor** in the respiratory tract and stimulates it. This leads to smooth muscle relaxation and bronchodilation.
- Some drugs such as steroids bind to a receptor in the cytoplasm and enter the nucleus where they bring about changes in gene transcription and protein manufacture. This takes time and these drugs do not work immediately.

Antagonists

- Drugs that are antagonists decrease the actions of a natural ligand or another drug. They fit into the receptor and block it.
- They may act on the same receptor as does an agonist drug, for example beta blockers block the beta-adrenergic receptor that *salbutamol* and *adrenaline* stimulate.
- They do not stimulate the cell and cause changes to occur. This means they have no action on the cell by themselves.
- They prevent the entry of the natural ligand into the receptor.
- Another example would be antihistamines. These drugs block the receptors for histamine (a chemical released in allergic reactions) and so decrease the actions of histamine. This reduces the itching and rash that accompany an allergic reaction.
- If an agonist and an antagonist bind to the same site on a receptor, they are **competitive**, and when both are present, they compete for receptors to bind to.
- The action of an agonist and an antagonist at a receptor is shown in Fig. 1.7.

Partial agonists

These drugs stimulate the receptor but not fully. They have activity at the receptor but it is less than the full agonist. They prevent the entry of the natural ligand and so although partial agonists they can also act as antagonists at the receptor.

Enzyme inhibition

Enzymes are biological catalysts that speed up chemical reactions within the body. They are needed for every chemical reaction involved in metabolism.

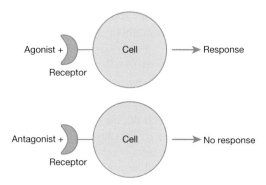

FIG. 1.7   Action of an agonist and an antagonist at a receptor. *Reproduced with permission from Greenstein, B., 2004. Trounce's Clinical Pharmacology for Nurses, seventeenth ed. Churchill Livingstone, Edinburgh.*

The enzyme combines with its substrate which changes to form the product of the reaction. The enzyme is then released unchanged and is available to take part in further reactions. If a drug inhibits the action of an enzyme, the reaction it catalyses will no longer be able to take place.

Competitive inhibition

A drug may be structured in a similar way to the substrate of the enzyme. It will then compete for the enzyme and slow down the normal reaction that the enzyme catalyses. This is called **competitive inhibition** as the drug is competing with the natural substrate. If there is enough natural substrate available it can overcome the inhibition of the drug. This can sometimes enable an antidote to be given for the drug. An example is **vitamin K** which is the antidote for **warfarin**.

Noncompetitive inhibition

These drugs combine with the enzyme and disable it permanently. The cell will have to make new enzyme before the effects of the drug can be overcome. An example here is **aspirin** as an antiplatelet drug. Aspirin prevents the manufacture of thromboxane (needed for platelet adhesion) by platelets for the whole life of the platelet.

Prodrugs

These are drugs that require the action of an enzyme to convert them from an inactive form to the active form.

Ion channels

Ion channels are proteins that regulate the flow of ions across cell membranes.

- Some ion channels open only when an agonist is present.
- Others are voltage gated. They open and close according to the membrane potential. An example is the sodium channel in the nerve cell. When an electrical impulse is received, the sodium gates open and sodium enters the cell. This causes depolarization and the transmission of an impulse along the nerve fibre.
- Ion channels regulate the flow of such ions as sodium, potassium, calcium and chloride in and out of the cells.
- Some drugs may block ion channels. *Lidocaine* is a local anaesthetic that blocks sodium channels and so prevents sensory transmission.
- Other drugs may bind to ion channels and affect their gating.
- They may inhibit the opening of channels. **Calcium channel blockers** such as *amlodipine* that are used as treatment for hypertension and angina work this way.
- Some drugs facilitate the opening of ion channels. Drugs that allow chloride ion channels to open in the brain act as sedatives. *Diazepam* is a benzodiazepine that fits into a receptor called the GABA receptor and facilitates the entry of chloride ions into the cell.

Carrier molecules

Many small molecules are carried across the cell membrane by carrier proteins. This is necessary because the molecules are not sufficiently fat soluble on their own to cross the lipid bilayer of the membrane.

Some drugs may block these transport systems. An example is *ciclosporin* which is an immunosuppressant used to prevent transplant rejection. Ciclosporin is a calcineurin inhibitor.

Desensitization

If a drug is given continuously or repeatedly its effect may gradually diminish. This may even happen in a few minutes and is called **desensitization** or **tachyphylaxis**.

A more gradual decrease in drug responsiveness is referred to as **tolerance** although this may also be used to describe a more rapid loss of responsiveness.

Drug resistance is usually a term used to describe the loss of effectiveness that may occur with the use of some antibiotics as bacteria mutate to become resistant to the drug.

Desensitization may be caused by several different mechanisms:

- loss of receptors (described below)
- extrusion of the drug from the cell actively – important in resistance to cancer chemotherapy

- running out of necessary mediators that take part in a chemical reaction as in tolerance to *amfetamines*
- increased drug metabolism as in tolerance to alcohol. People who are regular drinkers produce more of the liver enzymes needed to degrade the alcohol which is therefore eliminated more rapidly from the body
- change in receptor shape.

Receptor regulation

Receptors are not fixed elements in the cell and can increase or decrease in numbers dependent on the body's long-term needs.

The cell may **internalize receptors** (by a process called *endocytosis*) if it is exposed to a drug over a prolonged period of time. This decreases the number of receptors available for stimulation. One example is the response of cell cultures to a low concentration of *isoprenaline* — a beta-adrenergic agonist. The number of beta-adrenergic receptors can fall to 10% of normal within 8 hours. Recovery takes several days.

Receptors may also increase in numbers if they are blocked by a drug. An example here is beta-adrenergic blockers (beta blockers). The number of adrenergic receptors increases over a period of time. This means the drugs should not be discontinued suddenly or there are more receptors to respond to adrenaline. Hypertension or chest pain may result. The drug should be reduced gradually so that the receptors can decrease.

Drug specificity

The more specific a drug is for a particular cell or tissue, the more useful it usually is therapeutically. Drugs that work on receptors usually have higher specificity.

No drug has complete specificity and while working on one type of receptor may produce side effects due to blocking or stimulation of others, for example tricyclic antidepressants increase the availability of noradrenaline and serotonin in the central nervous system but also produce side effects (for example a dry mouth) due to blocking of other receptors.

Efficacy

This is the ability of the drug, when bound, to produce an effect. A drug with maximal efficacy is a full agonist.

An antagonist may have zero efficacy as it does not produce an effect of its own.

Affinity

This is the tendency of a drug to bind to a receptor.

A drug may have affinity without efficacy if it is an antagonist.

Dose—response relationships

Usually as the concentration of a drug increases, the effect it produces on the body also increases.

The relationship between dose and response is a gradual and continuous one that can be plotted on a graph. There will be a dose at which the drug has maximal effect.

It is possible to study the effects of agonists, partial agonists and antagonists using dose—response curves.

Potency

Describes the amount of drug needed to produce a given effect. The more potent a drug, the smaller the dose needed to produce the same effect.

Therapeutic index

$$Therapeutic\ index = \frac{Maximum\ nontoxic\ dose}{Minimum\ effective\ dose}$$

It is a measure of **drug safety**. The lower the therapeutic index, the smaller the margin between doses that produce an effect and doses that are toxic.

- An example of a drug with a small therapeutic index is ***digoxin.**** Digoxin toxicity can occur at doses not too much above those needed for therapeutic action. It is important that the patient's plasma levels are monitored to ensure they are not receiving too high a dose.
- A drug with a large therapeutic index is ***penicillin.**** It is safe to give doses higher than those actually needed.

1.7 ADVERSE DRUG REACTIONS

Drugs prescribed for disease are themselves the cause of a significant amount of disease ranging from minor inconvenience to permanent disability and even death. ADRs have become increasingly common over the past few years, perhaps because of the increasing range of drugs available and increased use of drugs in prophylaxis, for example to prevent thrombosis and atherosclerosis. ADRs are responsible for approximately 6%—7% of hospital admissions (NICE, 2017). The hospital inpatient is at an even greater risk and about 10% —20% of patients will have at least one ADR while in hospital.

- Virtually all drug use carries a risk.
- It is often said that the only safe drug is the one that remains in its packaging!
- The patient wants the benefits of drug use without the risks, and while successes are taken for granted, failures or drug accidents are remembered and emphasized.

- The patient should be warned of any ill effects that can be expected while taking the drug. The depth of the explanation will be determined by the needs of each patient.
- The harm caused by medication may be minor, for example the hangover effect from a hypnotic, or the sleepiness from an antihistamine used for hay fever (although this may lead to a serious road accident), or it may be life-destroying — as in rare sudden death following an injection of penicillin, usually one of the safest antibiotics.

An adverse reaction is any unintended reaction to a drug that has been administered in the standard dose by the correct route for the purpose of prophylaxis, diagnosis or treatment. This includes both side effects and drug interactions.

Many unwanted effects of drugs on the body are trivial and some retain the term *side effects* for these and reserve the term *adverse reactions* for harmful or seriously unpleasant effects. They call for reduction of dose or withdrawal of the drug.

Some patients, especially with a history of allergy or previous reactions to drugs, are up to four times more likely to suffer from adverse reactions.

The most important risk factors for ADRs are:

- age
- female gender
- number of drugs taken concomitantly — polypharmacy.

Common drugs involved in ADRs are:

- nonsteroidal anti-inflammatory drugs (NSAIDs)
- psychotropic drugs
- antimicrobials
- diuretics
- analgesics
- antihypertensives
- tranquillizers
- antidepressants
- hypoglycaemic agents
- cardiovascular drugs
- warfarin
- digoxin.

For drug safety, it is vital that ADRs are reported.

Classification of adverse drug reactions

Type A reactions

- Due to excessive, normal, predictable, dose-related, pharmacodynamic effects that are greater than would be expected.
- Form approximately 80% of ADRs. Will occur in everyone if enough of the drug is given.
- Examples are bleeding with anticoagulants or the dry mouth experienced with certain antidepressants.
- Skilled management reduces their incidence. If this type of ADR does occur, it may be sufficient to discontinue the drug or even just to reduce the dose.

Some predictable adverse effects are not related to the main pharmacological effect of the drug — examples are an excessive dose of *paracetamol* causing liver toxicity, aspirin-induced tinnitus when high doses are given, and peptic ulceration following the use of NSAIDs.

Type B reactions (idiosyncratic)

- Bizarre and unpredictable.
- Only occur in some people and are not part of the normal pharmacological action of the drug. They are not dose related and are often due to unusual attributes of the patient interacting with the drug.
- They include anaphylaxis and account for most drug fatalities.
- They tend to be commoner in people who suffer from allergies, for example those with asthma.
- Rapid action is essential if anaphylaxis is present. The drug should be stopped immediately and emergency treatment administered (including adrenaline 1:1000; 0.5 mL by intramuscular injection if needed).

Type C (continuous) reactions

Due to long-term use, for example tardive dyskinesia with drugs used to treat schizophrenia.

Type D (delayed) reactions

Include teratogenesis or carcinogenesis. Teratogenesis results in structural malformations during fetal development (Table 1.4). One example is *isotretinoin*, often used to treat severe acne. This is such a strong teratogen that just a single dose taken by a pregnant woman may result in serious birth defects. Because of this effect, most countries have systems in place to ensure that it is not given to pregnant women, and that the patient is aware of how important it is to prevent pregnancy during and at least 1 month after treatment. Medical guidelines also suggest that pregnant women should limit vitamin A intake to about 700 µg/day, as it has teratogenic potential when consumed in excess.

Type E (ending of use) reactions

Often means that a drug should be tailed off rather than stopped suddenly, for example steroids should not be abruptly discontinued after chronic oral administration due to the lost ability to secrete cortisol in an emergency. The drugs need to be gradually reduced to allow the patient's adrenal glands to recover their ability to respond to low levels of steroid.

Chronic drug use

Many drugs interfere with the body's self-regulating physiological systems normally controlled by negative feedback, for example the endocrine and cardiovascular systems.

TABLE 1.4 Some drugs reported to have adverse effects on fetal development in humans.

Drug	Effect
Thalidomide	Phocomelia (seal limbs), heart defects
Warfarin	Saddle nose, retarded growth, limb defects
Corticosteroids	Cleft palate and congenital cataract (rare)
Androgens	Masculinization in female
Oestrogens	Testicular atrophy in male
Phenytoin	Cleft palate, microcephaly, mental retardation
Valproate	Neural tube defects, e.g. spina bifida
Cytotoxic drugs	Hydrocephalus, cleft palate, neural tube defects
Tetracycline	Staining of bones and teeth, impaired bone growth
Ethanol	Fetal alcohol syndrome
Retinoids	Hydrocephalus and neural tube defects
Angiotensin converting enzyme inhibitors	Oligohydramnios, renal failure

Reprinted, with permission, from the Annual Review of Pharmacology and Toxicology, vol 29 ©1989 by Annual Reviews www.annualreviews.org. Adapted from Juchau 1989 Annu Rev Pharmacol Toxicol 29:175.

The control mechanisms respond by trying to minimize the effects of the interference and so restore homeostasis.

Feedback systems

- High doses of administered hormones often cause suppression of natural production of the hormone.
- On withdrawal of the hormone the body takes time, months in the case of the adrenals, to recover completely.
- Sudden withdrawal of administered corticosteroid can result in an acute deficiency state that may be life-threatening.

Regulation of receptors

- The number (density) of receptors for hormones and drugs on cells, the number of receptors occupied (affinity) and the fit of the molecule (sensitivity) can change in response to a binding molecule (see also Section 1.6).
- The cell is always trying to restore cell function to its usual state.
- Prolonged administration of an agonist can cause a **reduction in the number of receptors** available for activation (**downregulation**). This may occur with overuse of a salbutamol inhaler in respiratory disorders and explains the tolerance seen in severe asthmatics no longer responding so well to *salbutamol* (a β₂ agonist).
- Antagonists lead to an **increase in the number of receptors** − **upregulation**. This may occur in the administration of beta blockers. When the drug is abruptly withdrawn, an above normal number of receptors are available for noradrenaline and the increased oxygen demand by the heart that occurs may result in angina in an ischaemic heart.
- This type of action is called a **rebound phenomenon**.

Important consequences of abrupt withdrawal of drugs are known to occur with:

- **cardiovascular system** − antihypertensives and beta blockers
- **nervous system** − all depressants, for example hypnotics, sedatives, opioids and alcohol.

Gradual withdrawal is used in these types of medication.

Resurgence of chronic disease

This occurs when the disease was suppressed by the drug which is now withdrawn, for example following corticosteroid withdrawal in autoimmune disease − may get resurgence and rebound.

Metabolic changes

These may occur with chronic drug therapy over a long period of time:

- thiazide diuretics (e.g. *bendroflumethiazide*) may lead to diabetes mellitus or gout
- adrenocorticoids may lead to osteoporosis
- *phenytoin* may lead to osteomalacia.

Drug interactions

Drugs may interact with other drugs or something in the diet, for example *digoxin* with diuretics, hypnotics with alcohol, *warfarin* with almost anything!

Risk factors for adverse drug reactions

- Pregnancy
- Lactation
- Childhood
- Being elderly
- Renal impairment
- Disordered enzyme systems in the liver
- Polypharmacy
- Drugs with a low therapeutic index. Examples are given in Table 1.5.

The nurse also needs to check if the patient is taking any OTC preparation – some of these may not be thought of as drugs, for example herbal remedies.

The patient may also forget to mention long-term medication, for example oral contraceptive pill, hormone replacement therapy.

Topical preparations may not be thought of as drugs, for example ointment for eczema.

Pharmacogenetics

This is the study of how an individual's genetic make-up affects the body's response to drugs. It is now an important area of study and is leading to a greater understanding of many ADRs.

There are individual differences in drug metabolism and these can be explained in terms of genetic make up.

- **Enzymes** are very much involved in drug metabolism and the presence of enzymes as well as their amounts are **determined genetically.**
- Our ability to inactivate some drugs and facilitate their excretion depends on inherited traits from our parents.

TABLE 1.5 Examples of drugs with a narrow therapeutic index.

Antiarrhythmics, e.g. amiodarone	Cytotoxics, e.g. methotrexate
Anticonvulsants, e.g. phenytoin	Immunosuppressants, e.g. azathioprine
Cardiac glycosides, e.g. digoxin	Theophylline
Aminoglycosides, e.g. gentamicin	Oral anticoagulants, e.g. warfarin

- Pattern of inheritance can be either monogenic, affecting a single gene, or polygenic, affecting many genes.
- For many of the important enzymes involved in drug metabolism, the population can be divided into two categories: **poor and extensive metabolizers.**
- Poor metabolizers are at higher risk of developing ADRs.
- Different ethnic groups may also demonstrate different pharmacokinetics.
- Drugs excreted by the kidneys unchanged are not subjected to metabolic inactivation and so pharmacogenetics is irrelevant here.

Examples include fast and slow acetylators (can be determined by the ratio of caffeine to its metabolites in the urine).

Poor suxamethonium metabolism

- Enzymes called pseudocholinesterases are important in the breakdown of *suxamethonium* — a paralysing agent that is a neuromuscular blocking drug (see Section 2.3).
- Some people genetically produce a less efficient form of the enzyme which leads to a prolonged paralysis.
- About 1 in 2000 of the population are affected — paralysis of up to 24 hours.
- There is no antidote to suxamethonium — the patient has to be artificially ventilated until the effect of the drug wears off.
- The gene is inherited through an autosomal recessive gene.
- The pseudocholinesterase synthesized has less affinity for its substrate.

Pharmacovigilance and postmarketing surveillance

The problem of ADRs has been recognized since earliest times:

- Hippocrates in 400 BCE warned about the dangers of drugs — should not be prescribed unless the patient had been thoroughly examined.
- William Withering in 1785 described the benefits of *digitalis* but also described the vomiting, disturbance of vision, convulsions and death it could cause.
- There have been enquiries since the 1800s into drug safety.
- In 1870 a commission to investigate sudden deaths due to chloroform anaesthesia was set up. We now know this is due to the ability of *chloroform* to sensitize the myocardium to catecholamines, causing an increased incidence of arrhythmias.

The thalidomide tragedy

- *Thalidomide* was a drug used as a sleeping tablet and an antiemetic in the late 1950s and early 1960s. As such it had been given to pregnant women.

- An outbreak of phocomelia (seal limbs) followed where there are abnormally short limbs due to a failure of the long bones in the arms and legs to develop.
- Ten thousand children worldwide were born with defects and approximately 5000 survived.
- In the UK approximately 600 babies were born and around 400 survived.
- The women need only have taken one tablet of *thalidomide* in the first 3—6 weeks of gestation to produce these terrible effects.
- Teratogenicity testing was not routine at the time.

Are drugs safer today?
- Between 2002 and 2011 in the EU, 19 drugs were withdrawn due to safety reasons (McNaughton et al. 2014)
- Nine due to cardiovascular events, and four due to hepatotoxicity
- One example is rofecoxib (Vioxx) taken off the market in 2004. It is estimated that 88,000—139,000 Americans had heart attacks and strokes as a result of taking the drug as an analgesic (Lenzer, 2004).

The Yellow Card Scheme

This is a system of reporting that started over 40 years ago in Britain for reporting new ADRs. It alerts the MHRA to previously unrecognized side effects of medications including herbal remedies. This scheme is discussed more fully in Section 1.1.

Some common adverse drug reactions

Almost any organ system can be affected. Digestive disturbances including loss of appetite, nausea, a bloating sensation, constipation and diarrhoea are probably most common because most drugs are taken orally and so pass through the digestive tract. In older people, cognitive functioning and the brain are often affected, sometimes resulting in drowsiness and confusion. This may lead to an increased incidence of falls.

Constipation

Common causes include narcotic analgesics, antacids containing aluminium or calcium, antimuscarinics and tricyclic antidepressants.

Diarrhoea

Common causes include several antibiotics, antacids containing magnesium, allopurinol, lactulose, laxative abuse and digoxin (high dose).

Nausea

Again, this is a common side effect that may be caused by narcotic analgesics, anticancer drugs, iron − especially ferrous sulphate − levodopa, oral potassium chloride supplements, oestrogens, progestogens, oral contraceptive pills, sulfasalazine and antibiotics.

Vomiting is the expulsion of gastric contents by the mouth. Medications can cause vomiting by irritating the gastric intestinal mucosa or by stimulating the vomiting centre in the medulla oblongata. Narcotic analgesics and some anticancer drugs are notorious.

Flatulence

This is a problem with metformin taken for type 2 diabetes and other preparations that interfere with sugar or fat absorption.

Rash

Drug-induced rashes are the commonest side effect of many drugs. Often the mechanisms are unknown, and only about 10% of such reactions result from true allergic mechanisms. Typical examples of drug-induced rashes include erythematous maculopapular eruptions and exfoliative dermatitis. Common drugs include antibiotics, benzodiazepines, lithium, gold salts, allopurinol and aspirin.

Dizziness

Dizziness is a sensation of imbalance or faintness, which may also be associated with weakness, confusion and blurred or double vision. It may be caused by central nervous system depressants, narcotic analgesics, decongestants, antihistamines, antihypertensives and vasodilators.

Hypertension

Common causes include sympathomimetics, corticosteroids, oral contraceptives, monoamine oxidase inhibitors and central nervous system stimulants.

Hypotension

This is often postural hypotension − a drop in blood pressure on standing. Common causes include calcium channel blockers, antiparkinson drugs, diuretics, antihypertensives, general anaesthetics, narcotic analgesics, monoamine oxidase inhibitors, benzodiazepines, antipsychotic drugs and antidysrhythmics.

Thrush

Common causes include antibiotics, long-term use of corticosteroid inhalers, cytotoxic drugs and radiation therapy.

Dry mouth

Common causes include antimuscarinics, antihistamines, phenothiazines, narcotic analgesics and antidepressants.

Drowsiness

May be due to overdose or overuse of central nervous system depressants, tricyclic antidepressants, antihistamines and combining alcohol with central nervous system depressants.

Respiratory depression

Medications that commonly affect respiration are the central nervous system depressants. They include narcotic analgesics, barbiturates, phenothiazines and general anaesthetics. If alcohol is taken with any of these, this will add to the problem.

Allergic liver disease

Liver damage is usually due to the toxic effects of the drug and its metabolites (as in *paracetamol*) but hypersensitivity can be involved. An example is induced hepatic necrosis.

Haematological reactions

These include drug-induced agranulocytosis. This is associated with *NSAIDs*, *clozapine*, *sulphonamides* and *carbimazole*.

As a nurse it is important always to be observant and to recognize an ADR so that the drug may be discontinued and the patient treated if this is necessary.

Anaphylactic shock

This is a severe systemic life-threatening hypersensitivity response that may lead to difficulty in breathing and circulatory collapse. It results from the release of histamine and other chemical mediators. Other features include an urticarial rash and angioedema. One of the most common drugs causing anaphylaxis is penicillin, which affects approximately 4 in every 10,000 individuals and is responsible for 75% of deaths due to drug allergy. Penicillin allergy is more likely to occur in people with a familial history of atopic allergy.

Other drugs include various enzymes such as streptokinase, other antibiotics, aspirin and other nonsteroidal anti-inflammatory drugs, heparin, radiological contrast agents, ACE inhibitors and angiotensin II receptor blockers.

- Immediate interventions for the treatment of anaphylactic shock is the administration of adrenaline. For anaphylaxis, the adult dose (over 12 years) is 500 µg (0.5 mg), which is equivalent to 0.5 mL of 1:1000 solution given intramuscularly. This is nearly always effective if given early. A second dose may be given in 5—10 minutes if there is no improvement.

- The action of adrenaline is fully described in Section 2 but its action includes:
  - stimulating the beta-adrenergic receptors in the heart, and thus having a positive inotropic and chronotropic effect.
  - stimulating the alpha-adrenergic receptors in the blood vessels and thus reversing vasodilation and capillary leakage. This reduces mucosal and cutaneous oedema as well as helping to counteract shock.
  - improving blood pressure and coronary artery perfusion. It decreases angioedema and urticaria.

Hydrocortisone is also administered intramuscularly or by slow intravenous injection to help avert further release of mediators.

- This is particularly important in those with asthma who are at increased risk of fatal anaphylaxis if they have been treated with steroids previously.
- Steroids such as hydrocortisone block the manufacture of prostaglandin and leukotrienes, which are also important mediators.

Section 2

Autonomic nervous system

Section Outline

2.1 AUTONOMIC NERVOUS SYSTEM − OVERVIEW

The autonomic nervous system (ANS) is the automatic part of our nervous system that maintains homeostasis and balances our internal environment. We are not usually conscious of its functioning.

The ANS regulates:

- contraction and relaxation of smooth muscle
- all exocrine and some endocrine glandular secretions
- the heart beat
- some steps in metabolism.

The ANS has two main branches:

- the sympathetic nervous system (SNS)
- the parasympathetic nervous system (PSNS).

Nervous transmission is electrical, but at synapses transmission is chemically mediated by substances called *neurotransmitters*.

- The **SNS** is stimulated in conditions of **fight** and **flight** and uses the neurotransmitter **noradrenaline** (**NA**). Fibres that release NA are termed **adrenergic**.
- The **PSNS** functions in relatively peaceful conditions such as when **resting** and **digesting**. It uses the neurotransmitter **acetylcholine** (**ACh**). ACh-releasing fibres are termed **cholinergic**.

Both branches of the ANS generally serve the same internal organs but produce opposite effects. If one division stimulates certain muscles to contract or a gland to secrete, the other division usually inhibits that action. Sweat glands and most of the blood vessels have only sympathetic innervation.

A Nurse's Survival Guide to Drugs in Practice. https://doi.org/10.1016/B978-0-7020-7658-9.00002-0
73

The motor unit of the ANS is a two-neurone chain. There is a preganglionic neurone with its cell body in the brain or spinal cord. The axon from this neurone synapses with a postganglionic motor neurone in a ganglion outside the central nervous system (CNS). The postganglionic axon from this neurone extends to the effector organ.

Neurotransmitters released by the ANS:

- All preganglionic fibres are cholinergic (release ACh).
- All postganglionic parasympathetic fibres are cholinergic at their effectors
- Sympathetic postganglionic fibres release NA but those innervating the sweat glands of the skin, some blood vessels and the external genitalia release ACh.
- The adrenal medulla releases adrenaline (epinephrine; 85%) and NA (15%).

ACh and NA may be excitatory or inhibitory, depending on the type of transmitter on the target organ.

Drug action in the ANS may involve:

- agonists or antagonists at adrenergic or cholinergic receptors
- release, storage or synthesis of neurotransmitters
- reuptake pumps or enzymes inactivating neurotransmitters.

2.2 ADRENERGIC PHARMACOLOGY

The noradrenergic neurone is an important target for drug action. Drugs that mimic the effects of the SNS are known as **sympathomimetic drugs**.

A basic plan of the ANS is shown in Fig. 2.1, and a comparison of transmission in the somatic and ANSs is shown in Fig. 2.2.

The effects of sympathetic nervous system stimulation

These effects are many and varied and will affect the whole body. You have to think of yourself when you are very frightened or nervous − before an exam or interview, for example − to imagine what these effects are. Some effects of stimulation of the SNS and the PSNS are shown in Table 2.1. Anatomical differences are shown in Table 2.2.

The body is being prepared for an emergency where it may have to exert much physical activity, and all the results of SNS stimulation are towards these ends.

The heart

- An **increase in heart rate** (positive chronotropic effect).
- An increase in the **force of contraction** (positive inotropic effect).

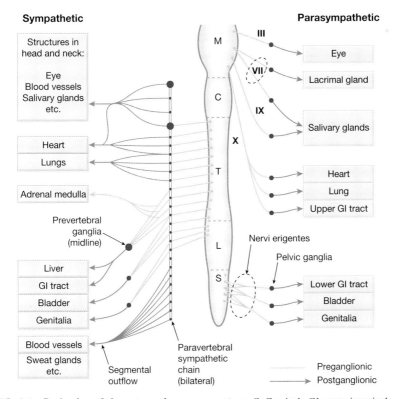

FIG. 2.1 **Basic plan of the autonomic nervous system.** *C*, Cervical; *GI*, gastrointestinal; *L*, lumbar; *M*, medullary; *S*, sacral; *T*, thoracic. *Reproduced with permission from Rang, H.P., Dale, M.M., Ritter, J.M., et al. 2007. Rang & Dale's Pharmacology, sixth ed. Churchill Livingstone, Edinburgh.*

The respiratory system

- Increase in the **rate and depth** of breathing.
- **Dilates** the bronchioles.

The circulation

- **Constriction of some blood vessels** where a good blood supply is not needed − the skin, the gastrointestinal tract and the kidneys.
- **Dilation of blood vessels** where a good blood supply is needed − the coronary vessels, skeletal muscle and the lungs.
- Increase in **blood pressure**.

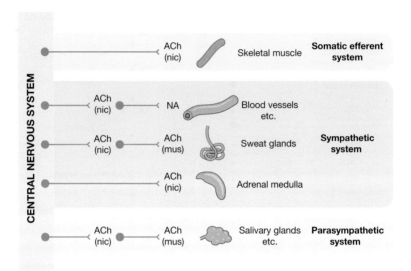

FIG. 2.2 **Transmission in the autonomic and somatic nervous systems.** The main two types of acetylcholine *(ACh)* receptor, nicotinic acid *(nic)* and muscarinic *(mus)* are indicated. *NA, Noradrenaline (norepinephrine). Reproduced with permission from Rang, H.P., Dale, M.M., Ritter, J.M., et al. 2007. Rang & Dale's Pharmacology, sixth ed. Churchill Livingstone, Edinburgh*

The gastrointestinal tract

- A decrease in motility.
- A reduction in secretion of enzymes.

The liver

- An **increase in gluconeogenesis** (manufacture of new glucose).
- Blood glucose levels increase and may result in glycosuria in severe stress.

The kidney

- Renin secretion leads to an increase in blood pressure.
- Vasoconstriction reduces urinary output.

The skin

- Increased **sweating**.
- Piloerection − **goose pimples**.

The eye

- **Dilation** of the pupil.

TABLE 2.1 Some effects of stimulation of the sympathetic and parasympathetic nervous systems

Target organ/ system	Parasympathetic effects	Sympathetic effects
Eye (iris)	Constricts pupil	Dilates pupil
Lens of eye	Accommodation	Slight relaxation of ciliary muscle
Glands (nasal, lacrimal, salivary, gastric, pancreatic)	Mostly stimulates secretory activity	Mostly inhibits secretory activity
Sweat glands	No effect	Stimulates sweating (but via acetylcholine and muscarinic receptor)
Adrenal medulla	No effect	Stimulates secretion of adrenaline (epinephrine) and noradrenaline (norepinephrine)
Arrector pili muscles attached to hair follicles	No effect	Stimulates contraction – hairs stand on end and goose pimples occur
Heart	Decreases rate Decreases force	Increases rate Increases force
Atrioventricular node	Decreases speed of conduction	Increases automaticity
Bladder	Causes contraction of smooth muscle in the bladder wall, relaxes the urethral sphincter and promotes voiding	Causes relaxation of smooth muscle of bladder wall; constricts urethral sphincter and inhibits voiding
Lungs	Constricts the bronchioles	Dilates bronchioles and mildly constricts blood vessels
Digestive tract	Increases peristalsis and secretion by digestive organs Relaxes sphincters and allows movement of food along tract	Decreases activity of glands and muscles of digestive tract Constricts sphincters
Liver	No effect	Stimulates the release of glucose into the bloodstream
Gall bladder	Causes contraction and release of bile	Relaxation and no release of bile
Kidney	No effect	Causes vasoconstriction; decreases urine output Promotes renin secretion

Continued

TABLE 2.1 Some effects of stimulation of the sympathetic and parasympathetic nervous systems—cont'd.

Target organ/ system	Parasympathetic effects	Sympathetic effects
Blood vessels	Little or no effect	Constricts most blood vessels and increases blood pressure Constricts vessels in skin and abdominal viscera to divert blood to the muscles, brain and heart Dilates vessels of skeletal muscle during exercise
Blood coagulation	No effect	Increases coagulation
Cellular metabolism	No effect	Increases metabolic rate
Adipose tissue	No effect	Stimulates fat breakdown
Mental activity	No effect	Increases alertness
Penis	Causes erection	Causes ejaculation

TABLE 2.2 Some anatomical differences between the sympathetic nervous system and the parasympathetic nervous system.

PSNS	SNS
Fibres emerge from the brain (cranial nerves III, VII, IX, X) and sacral spinal cord (S2–S4)	Fibres emerge from thoracolumbar region of SC (3 cervical, 11 thoracic, 4 sacral and 1 coccygeal)
Long preganglionic fibres Short postganglionic fibres Ganglia in effector organs	Short preganglionic fibres Long postganglionic fibres Ganglia close to spinal cord

PSNS, Parasympathetic nervous system; *SNS*, sympathetic nervous system.

Skeletal muscle

- Tone up.
- This may be overdone, so that nervous **tremor** results.

Adrenal gland

- Stimulates secretion of **adrenaline** (epinephrine) and **noradrenaline** (norepinephrine).

Bladder

- Relaxes the muscle and allows the bladder to fill.
- Contracts the urethral sphincter and inhibits voiding.

Other effects

- Increases blood coagulation.
- Stimulates lipolysis (fat breakdown).
- Increases alertness.

It is the neurotransmitter **noradrenaline** that is having all these sympathetic effects on the body.

Body cells have receptors for NA, and when the NA fits into the receptor the cell is turned on and the aforementioned sympathetic effects are produced.

The NA fits the receptor like a key fits a lock. The molecule is just the right shape to fit.

Noradrenaline storage

Mostly stored in vesicles in nerve endings. Release occurs when a nervous impulse arrives at the synapse.

Degradation of noradrenaline

This is not by an enzyme in the synapse but by **uptake** into the cells and degradation by an enzyme in the neuronal mitochondria called *monoamine oxidase* (MAO). Circulating NA is destroyed by the enzyme catechol-O-methyltransferase (COMT).

The adrenergic receptor

- There are two major classes of adrenergic receptor on cell membranes — alpha-adrenergic receptors and beta-adrenergic receptors.
- Organs that respond to adrenaline display one or both types of receptor.

There are subtypes of each receptor — α_1 and α_2, β_1, β_2 and β_3. The effects of stimulation of these different receptor subtypes are shown in Table | 2.3.

- α_1 Receptors are found on blood vessels where stimulation causes vasoconstriction, an increase in total peripheral resistance and an increase in blood pressure. NA is most potent at the α_1 receptor.
- The distinction between β_1 and β_2 receptors is an important one because β_1 receptors are found mostly in the heart, where they are excitatory and are responsible for the positive chronotropic (increased rate) and positive inotropic (increased force) effects of catecholamines. β_1 Receptors have approximately equal affinity for adrenaline and NA.

TABLE 2.3 Summary of action of some drugs affecting noradrenergic transmission

Drug	Main action	Some clinical uses	Adverse effects/side effects	Contraindications
Noradrenaline (norepinephrine)	α/β agonist	Acute hypotension	Hypertension, headache, peripheral ischaemia, bradycardia, arrhythmias	Hypertension, pregnancy
Adrenaline (epinephrine)	α/β agonist	Cardiac arrest, Acute severe asthma, Anaphylaxis	Anxiety, tremor, tachycardia, headache, cold extremities. In overdosage: arrhythmias, cerebral haemorrhage, pulmonary oedema, nausea, sweating, dizziness	Only cautions such as heart disease and glaucoma
Dobutamine	β₁ agonist	Cardiogenic shock	Nausea and vomiting, peripheral vasoconstriction, hypotension, hypertension, tachycardia	Tachyarrhythmias, phaeochromocytoma
Salbutamol	β₂ agonist	Asthma and other reversible airway obstruction, premature labour	Fine tremor, headache, muscle cramps, palpitations, tachycardia	Caution in cardiovascular disease and hypertension

Phenylephrine	α_1 agonist	Acute hypotension, Nasal decongestant	Tachycardia, reflex bradycardia, prolonged rise in blood pressure	Cautions as for NA
Amfetamine	NA release, Uptake 1 inhibitor, MAOI, CNS stimulant	CNS stimulant in narcolepsy, Related drugs used in ADHD, Drug of abuse	Hypertension, tachycardia, insomnia, acute psychosis with overdose, Dependence	Not given if patient taking MAOIs
Ephedrine	NA release, β agonist	Nasal decongestant	As amfetamine but less	
Doxazosin	α_1 antagonist	Hypertension, benign prostatic hypertrophy	Postural hypotension, dizziness, weakness, sleep disturbance, tremor	Cautions only (see British National Formulary)
Propranolol	Nonselective β antagonist	Anxiety, migraine, hyperthyroidism	Should not be stopped suddenly, especially in ischaemic heart disease; Bradycardia, heart failure, hypotension, heart block, bronchospasm, cold hands and feet, fatigue, nightmares, sexual dysfunction	Asthma, uncontrolled heart failure, Prinzmetal's angina, bradycardia, hypotension, heart block
Atenolol	Selective β_1 antagonist	Angina, hypertension	As propranolol but reduced effects of β_2 blockade – less risk of bronchospasm	As propranolol

Continued

TABLE 2.3 Summary of action of some drugs affecting noradrenergic transmission—cont'd.

Drug	Main action	Some clinical uses	Adverse effects/side effects	Contraindications
Labetalol	α₁/β antagonist	Hypertension in pregnancy, hypertension in anaesthesia, hypertensive crisis	Postural hypotension, bronchoconstriction (See also under propranolol)	As propranolol
Carvedilol	α₁/β antagonist	Symptomatic chronic heart failure, hypertension, angina	Postural hypotension, dizziness (See also propranolol)	As propranolol. Avoid in severe heart failure

ADHD, Attention-deficit/hyperactivity disorder; *CNS*, central nervous system; *MAOI*, monoamine oxidase inhibitor; *NA*, noradrenaline.

- β_2 Receptors are responsible for smooth muscle relaxation in many organs, such as bronchiolar muscle relaxation in the respiratory tract and vasodilation in skeletal vascular beds. β_2 Receptors have a higher affinity for adrenaline than NA.

Most organs have a **predominance of one type of receptor**. Blood vessels in skeletal muscle have both α_1 and β_2 receptors, but the latter predominate. Some organs may have one type of receptor almost exclusively — for example, the heart predominantly has β_1 receptors.

The importance of the ANS in the control of such a wide range of the body's vital functions has led to the development of many pharmacological agents, both naturally occurring and synthetic, that may modulate its action.

Catecholamines

You may hear adrenaline and NA referred to as **catecholamines**. This is a term used for chemical compounds derived from the amino acid tyrosine and containing catechol and amine groups. The most abundant catecholamines are adrenaline (epinephrine), NA and dopamine.

Receptor selectivity

Receptor subtypes within the SNS producing specific effects have allowed the development of both agonists to stimulate, and antagonists to block, these effects. Some of the drugs developed show selectivity for certain subtypes of receptor.

Beta$_2$ agonists such as salbutamol are important as bronchodilators. Cardioselective beta blockers are important in ischaemic heart disease.

Adrenaline acts on all adrenergic receptors and so increases heart rate and force while also causing bronchodilation. It can cause peripheral vasoconstriction (alpha receptor) or vasodilation (β_2 receptor). Adrenaline is discussed in more detail later.

Adrenergic agonists

Adrenaline and NA are relatively nonselective. Other drugs have been developed for their ability to be more potent at one type of receptor.

Alpha receptors

There are two main types of alpha receptor, α_1 and α_2.

α_1 Receptors

α_1 **Stimulation produces**

contraction of all types of smooth muscle except the gastrointestinal tract. This affects **vascular smooth muscle** and includes the large arteries and veins as well as the small ones.

This results in:

- reduced vascular compliance
- increased central venous pressure
- increased peripheral resistance
- all leading to an increase in systolic and diastolic blood pressure.

Some vascular beds, for example cerebral, coronary and pulmonary, are little affected.

Baroreceptor reflexes are activated by the increased arterial pressure, and this may cause a reflex bradycardia.

- Dilation of the pupil.
- Contraction of the gastrointestinal sphincters and decreased peristalsis resulting in a **slowing of digestion**.
- Contraction of the external sphincter and relaxation of the detrusor muscle in the bladder leading to **retention of urine**.
- Increased **blood sugar** levels.
- Stimulation of the sweat glands resulting in **generalized sweating**.
- Contraction of the piloerector muscles resulting in 'goose flesh'.

Phenylephrine stimulates the α_1 receptor and is valuable to raise blood pressure in hypotension and circulatory shock. *NA* (see later) may be used for its alpha agonist properties.

α_1 Stimulation of the **nasal blood vessels** will cause vasoconstriction and so decongestion. *Ephedrine nasal drops* may be used but rebound congestion may occur when the drug is stopped.

α_2 Receptors

Not as important clinically. Stimulation of the α_2 receptor causes inhibition of transmitter release (including NA and ACh from autonomic nerves).

A drug such as *clonidine* that stimulates the receptor leads to a decrease in blood pressure. It may also be used to treat hot flushes in the menopause and migraine.

Beta receptors

There are two main subtypes of beta receptor, β_1 and β_2. There is also a β_3 receptor that is not important clinically.

β₁ Receptors

Located on the myocardium, adipocytes (fat cells), sphincters and smooth muscle of the gastrointestinal tract and renal arterioles.

β₁ Stimulation results in:

- increased rate and force of the heartbeat that is **positive inotropic** and **chronotropic** effect. This is the result of an increased influx of calcium into cardiac fibres. Stronger cardiac contractions lead to a more complete ventricular emptying and an increase in cardiac work and oxygen consumption. Overall cardiac efficiency is reduced
- the increased cardiac output may lead to a **rise in systolic blood pressure**
- increased **lipolysis** in adipose tissue leading to increased blood lipids
- **decreased digestion** and intestinal motility
- **release of renin** into the renal blood, resulting in the formation of angiotensin II. This is a powerful vasoconstrictor.

Clinical applications

As positive inotropes in:
- circulatory and cardiogenic shock − *dopamine* and *dobutamine* are cardiac stimulants and act on β₁ receptors in cardiac muscle. They increase the contractility of the heart with little effect on the rate
- cardiac arrest − *adrenaline*.

β₂ Receptors

Located on the smooth muscle of the bronchioles, skeletal muscle, mast cells and the uterus and in liver cells.

β₂ Stimulation leads to relaxation of most kinds of smooth muscle:

- within the respiratory tract producing bronchodilation
- in the vascular system vasodilation, particularly marked in skeletal muscle
- relaxation of uterine smooth muscle
- powerful inhibition of gastrointestinal tract smooth muscle contraction is produced by both α and β receptors
- stabilization of the mast cell, preventing the release of inflammatory mediators.

Clinical applications

- Asthma and chronic airflow limitation as in chronic obstructive pulmonary disease − *salbutamol* is a β₂ agonist.
- Relaxation of the uterus in preterm labour.

Adrenaline (epinephrine)

For medical use adrenaline is prepared synthetically. It is not effective orally as it is destroyed by the acid in the stomach.

Clinical effects

- Increased cardiac output.
- Rise in systolic blood pressure due to the increased output of blood from the heart.
- Low doses may decrease the total peripheral vascular resistance and so decrease blood pressure.
- The **diastolic blood pressure** shows little change as adrenaline (epinephrine) produces an increase in the force and rate of the heartbeat (β_1 effect).
- Vasoconstriction only in the skin and in the splanchnic area (mixed alpha and β_2 effects) and vasodilation in arteries in muscle (β_2 effect).
- Renal artery constriction is greater with adrenaline (epinephrine) than NA.
- Relaxation of smooth muscle, including powerful bronchodilation. Relieves all known allergic and histamine-induced bronchoconstriction.
- Stabilization of the mast cell.
- Rise in blood glucose due to mobilization of glucose from the tissues, increased release of glucagon and decreased release of insulin.

Clinical applications

- Cardiac arrest.
- Anaphylaxis.
- Acute severe asthma.
- Some specialist local anaesthetics may contain 1:100,000 parts of adrenaline (epinephrine) to enable them to remain longer at the site of injection.

Route of administration

Adrenaline cannot be administered orally as it is destroyed in the stomach.

Anaphylaxis − by intramuscular injection. Adrenaline 1:1000, 0.5 mL (500 μg) is given by emergency practitioners to an adult. A self-administered EpiPen has 300 μg of adrenaline (epinephrine). The dose may be repeated in 5 minutes depending on response.

In a cardiac arrest situation adrenaline 1:10,000 (100μg/mL) is used. A dose of 10 mL (1 mg) is usually given by a central line. This dose may be repeated every 3−5 minutes if necessary.

Side effects

These include: anxiety, tremor, tachycardia, arrhythmias, hypertension, pulmonary oedema, nausea, vomiting, sweating and dizziness.

Noradrenaline

Its most important action is to produce widespread vasoconstriction and thus a rise in systolic and diastolic blood pressure (alpha effect).

May **not alter cardiac output** and may **even decrease it slightly**. This is because the strong vasoconstriction increases resistance to the ejection of blood from the heart.

- It may not produce as severe tachycardia as adrenaline. The increased blood pressure and vasoconstriction may actually cause a reflex bradycardia.
- It is rapidly inactivated by the body and thus to produce a continuous effect on the body, needs to be given by infusion.

Clinical applications

Used in the treatment of various kinds of shock associated with a very low blood pressure.

Although a satisfying rise in blood pressure can be obtained by vasoconstriction, this reduces the blood flow to certain organs, particularly the kidneys.

Both adrenaline and NA may produce a spontaneous firing of the Purkinje fibres, causing them to exhibit pacemaker activity and resulting in ventricular extrasystoles which increase the susceptibility of the ventricular muscle to fibrillation.
These effects are more likely with adrenaline than NA.

Adrenoreceptor antagonists

These drugs block the action of the natural ligand − NA − in the SNS. Most are selective for the alpha or beta receptor.

Alpha-adrenoreceptor antagonists

Alpha-adrenoreceptor blockade results in:

- vasodilation and a drop in blood pressure
- relaxation of the bladder neck and capsule of the prostate gland, inhibiting hypertrophy.

Drugs used may be:

- nonselective; for example, *phenoxybenzamine, phentolamine*
- α_1 selective; for example, *prazosin, doxazosin, terazosin. **Tamsulosin*** has some selectivity for the α_{1A} subtype of receptor found in the bladder.

Clinical applications

- Control of hypertension − **doxazosin** − causes vasodilation and a fall in arterial pressure. First dose may cause a profound drop in blood pressure. Some postural hypotension may occur, and impotence may be a side effect.
- Tumours of the adrenal medulla (phaeochromocytoma) − ***phenoxybenzamine***. It is long lasting and binds irreversibly, thus being useful in surgery when manipulation of the tumour may result in the release of a large bolus of adrenaline (epinephrine) into the circulation.
- Urinary retention and prostatic hypertrophy − ***tamsulosin***.

Side effects

- Nasal congestion.
- Postural hypotension.
- Inhibition of ejaculation.
- Lack of energy.

Beta-adrenoreceptor antagonists

First discovered in 1958. They are primarily used for their effects on the cardiovascular system, where it is really the β_1 receptor that we would prefer to block.

Propranolol was the first drug to be used. It blocks β_1 and β_2 receptors equally.

Cardioselective drugs with more potency at the β_1 receptor have since been developed. These include ***atenolol*** and ***bisoprolol,*** with fewer side effects because blockade of the β_2 receptor is reduced.

Some drugs block α_1 receptors as well as beta receptors; for example, ***labetalol, carvedilol***.

Carvedilol and ***bisoprolol*** also cause some vasodilation and can be useful in stable heart failure.

Clinical effects

- At rest they have only a slight effect on heart rate, cardiac output or arterial pressure. They reduce the effect of excitement or exercise on these variables as they reduce the response to the SNS. This reduces the force of cardiac contraction and slows the heart rate.

- Sinoatrial (SA) node automaticity is decreased and atrioventricular (AV) node conduction time is prolonged, leading to a bradycardia. Contractility is reduced.
- Bradycardia lengthens the coronary artery perfusion time (during diastole) which increases oxygen supply to the cardiac muscle while reduced contractility reduces oxygen demand. The improvement in the balance of oxygen supply and demand makes these drugs extremely useful in angina and myocardial infarction.
- Drugs with partial agonist activity — for example *oxprenolol* — increase the heart rate at rest but reduce it during exercise.
- Exercise tolerance is reduced in healthy people — reduced vasodilation in skeletal muscle as well as reduced response of the heart to exercise.
- Antihypertensive effect. This was not an expected effect because they do not vasodilate. They produce a gradual fall in blood pressure over a period of several days. The mechanism is complex and includes a reduction in cardiac output, reduction of renin release and some central action by reduction of sympathetic activity.
- Antidysrhythmic effect.
- Increased airways resistance — this is only slight in normal subjects but does mean that they are dangerous in asthmatics and can produce severe asthma attacks. Cardioselective drugs are less likely to induce asthma, but there are no cardiac-specific drugs yet and so none are free from risk.
- May increase plasma triglycerides and reduce high-density lipoprotein (HDL) levels.

Beta blockers in diabetes

- Beta blockers produce only minor metabolic changes in normal subjects.
- It is better to use cardioselective beta blockers in diabetes.
- They do not affect the onset of hypoglycaemia following insulin injection but do delay the recovery of glucose concentration. They thus delay recovery from hypoglycaemia.
- Nonselective beta blockade may blunt the normal blood glucose response to exercise and hypoglycaemia. This means they make exercise-induced hypoglycaemia in diabetes more likely.
- They may increase the normal resting blood glucose.
- They may mask some of the metabolic and adrenergic symptoms of hypoglycaemia so that the patient is no longer aware that they are becoming hypoglycaemic.

Clinical applications Most of these are for cardiovascular disease and are discussed further in Section 5.

Ischaemic heart disease

- They are used as treatment in angina but are also given following a myocardial infarction.
- Reduce cardiac work and so oxygen consumption.
- Increase exercise tolerance.
- Sudden withdrawal may exacerbate an attack of angina and rebound of myocardial ischaemia. The dose needs to be reduced gradually.
- Several studies have shown therapy with beta blockers reduces the recurrence rate of myocardial infarction.

Heart failure

- Reduce the heart's response to the SNS. May be dangerous in some unstable patients because they can reduce the force of cardiac contraction.
- In chronic stable forms of heart failure, sympathetic activity is counterproductive and beta blockers can actually increase cardiac output and decrease mortality.
- *Carvedilol* or *bisoprolol* are the beta blockers used because their effectiveness is supported by large clinical trials.

Hypertension

- May be combined with other drugs.
- Do not cause postural or exercise-induced hypotension.
- No longer used as first-line treatment.

Cardiac arrhythmias

- Increased sympathetic activity is often a feature of dysrhythmias – including potentially fatal ventricular arrhythmias.
- They reduce the incidence of ventricular fibrillation post myocardial infarction.
- They reduce the automaticity and conductivity of the heart and are used in the treatment of some forms of supraventricular tachycardia.
- They are not safe in all types of arrhythmia (see Section 5.5).

Hyperthyroidism

- *Propranolol* reverses the clinical symptoms of an overactive thyroid within 4 days.
- Can be used with other antithyroid drugs.

Anxiety

- Tremor and palpitations are reduced.
- Have been used illegally by snooker players in the past to make their arm steady.

Glaucoma

- Given as eye drops; for example, *timolol, betaxolol.*
- The production of aqueous is inhibited, and so intraocular pressure is reduced.

- Used to be first choice but prostaglandin analogues (e.g. *latanoprost*) may now be preferred.

Migraine
- Used in prophylaxis, not as treatment for an acute attack. Effective in 60% of patients.
- Affect the cerebral blood vessels, preventing vasodilation.
- *Propranolol* may be used.
- Beta blockers are associated with fatigue, coolness of extremities and sleep disturbances with nightmares.

Side effects
- Smooth muscle spasm may lead to bronchoconstriction and cold extremities.
- Exaggeration of the cardiac effects may occur resulting in bradycardia, heart block or reduced cardiac output (heart failure).
- May get into the CNS if fat soluble and cause nightmares, depression or insomnia. *Atenolol* is one of the most water soluble and therefore less likely to enter the brain. It may cause less sleep disturbance and nightmares.
- Fatigue with exercise.
- Impotence in some men.
- May precipitate diabetes in some patients.
- May cause weight gain by reducing metabolic rate.

Contraindications
- Severe bradycardia, heart block, cardiogenic shock, untreated left ventricular failure.
- Severe asthma. Should also be avoided in those with a history of asthma or chronic obstructive pulmonary disease. All beta blockers given in sufficient dose will precipitate bronchospasm via antagonism of the β_2 receptor.
- Severe depression.
- Raynaud's phenomenon.

Beta blockers are not used in patients with a history of asthma or chronic airflow limitation unless no alternative is available. There is always a risk of inducing bronchospasm. Fatalities have occurred when a history of asthma has not been identified.

Pharmacokinetics

- Variation is mostly due to varying lipid solubility. Water-soluble drugs (poor lipid solubility) include *atenolol* and *sotalol*. Lipid-soluble drugs include *propranolol, labetalol* and *oxprenolol*.
- Those with poor lipid solubility are poorly absorbed from the gut, undergo little hepatic metabolism and are excreted largely unchanged in the urine. This means they should be avoided in renal failure as they may accumulate in the body.
- Those with high lipid solubility are well absorbed from the gut and extensively metabolized in the liver. This means they have a shorter half-life and thus need more frequent administration. In addition, they cross the blood–brain barrier and may result in sedation and nightmares.
- Half-life varies. *Esmolol* has the shortest half-life (<10 minutes). *Propranolol* has a half-life of approximately 3 hours, but with chronic administration this increases.

Some examples of beta blockers you may meet in practice

- *Atenolol* is a relatively cardioselective drug. It is frequently used in angina, post myocardial infarction and as an antihypertensive. The drug is available as tablets and syrup as well as intravenous solution. Atenolol is water soluble and excreted unchanged in urine – so dose should be reduced in renal impairment. Its half-life is approximately 7 hours, but actions appear to persist for longer than this suggests.
- *Bisoprolol* is a highly cardioselective drug (more so than atenolol). It may be used in angina and hypertension but is sometimes given in stable chronic heart failure.
- *Carvedilol* is a nonselective β- and α₁-adrenoreceptor antagonist, with vasodilatory effects. You may see this drug used in the treatment of chronic stable heart failure. Produces less negative chronotropic and negative inotropic effects than some. Rapidly absorbed following oral administration-reaches peak plasma concentration within 1–2 hours. Its elimination half-life ranges from 7 to 10 hours.
- *Esmolol* is a relatively cardioselective beta blocker with high lipid solubility and a very short duration of action (10 minutes). It has a rapid onset of action and is used intravenously for the short term, particularly perioperative management of supraventricular tachycardia, sinus tachycardia or hypertension.
- *Labetalol* is a nonselective beta blocker with some α₁ blocking effects. Ratio of alpha to beta effects is 1:3 when given orally and 1:7 when given intravenously. It is used to treat a hypertensive crisis and to facilitate hypotension in anaesthesia. It lowers blood pressure acutely, unlike drugs that are just beta blockers. Even oral labetalol leads to a rapid fall in blood

pressure. It is well tested in pregnancy and may be used for blood pressure control in eclampsia. The α_1 blockade causes peripheral vasodilation and the beta blockade prevents reflex tachycardia.

- *Metoprolol* is a cardioselective beta blocker that has been shown to reduce infarct size and incidence of ventricular fibrillation when used early following a myocardial infarction. It is also used in the management of hypertension. Absorption following oral administration is rapid and complete. High first-pass metabolism means bioavailability following oral dose is only 50%, but this increases to 70% with continuous use and is increased if taken with food.
- *Propranolol* is not cardioselective and is also lipid soluble, penetrating the brain. It is used when cardioselectivity is not wanted as in anxiety, essential tremor, migraine and hyperthyroidism. If used for hypertension or angina it has more side effects than cardioselective drugs due to blockade of the β_2 receptor. It has to be given twice daily due to its short half-life.
- *Sotalol* is a noncardioselective beta blocker with additional antiarrhythmic properties.

Drugs acting on noradrenergic nerve terminals

Methyldopa

- An early drug used for hypertension but is still used for hypertension in pregnancy due to a lack of documented ill effects on mother and baby.
- Methyldopa is taken up by the noradrenergic neurones where it is converted to a false transmitter that is less effective than NA at the α_1 receptors, resulting in less vasoconstriction.
- It is not used outside of pregnancy because other drugs have fewer side effects.

Indirectly acting sympathomimetic drugs

Include *amfetamine* and *ephedrine* and enhance the effects of NA to which they are structurally related.

- These drugs are taken up into the nerve terminals where they displace NA from its storage vesicles, causing its release from the nerve endings.
- They also inhibit the action of MAO.
- Marked tolerance develops to their actions, perhaps due to depletion of NA.
- Peripheral effects include bronchodilation, increased rate and force of heart beat, increased peripheral vasoconstriction and blood pressure, inhibition of secretions and reduced gut motility.

- The only drug used for its peripheral effect is *ephedrine*. It has fewer central effects and is used as a nasal decongestant.

  Tyramine is a chemical found in various foods that also has this action. Foods with tyramine can cause a hypertensive crisis if taken with MAO inhibitors (see later).

  Amfetamine has potent stimulatory and euphoric effects on the CNS due to the release of NA and other transmitters including 5-HT (5-hydroxytryptamine) and dopamine.

- These effects have led to it being a popular drug of abuse that is dependency producing.
- It can cause restlessness, anxiety, insomnia and a tremor. In high doses it can induce a paranoid state similar to that seen in schizophrenia.
- **Amfetamines** have been used in the past as appetite suppressants, but this is certainly inappropriate.
- *Dexamfetamine* may be used in narcolepsy and some hyperkinetic disorders in children.
- Other drugs that act similarly are *atomoxetine* and *methylphenidate.* They are used sometimes by specialists in the treatment of attention-deficit/hyperactivity disorder (ADHD).

Inhibitors of noradrenaline reuptake and enzymic destruction

Reuptake into the nerve terminal (uptake 1) is the main way that NA is removed from the synapse. Some drugs inhibit uptake 1 and so prolong the action of NA.

The main drugs that inhibit uptake 1 are **tricyclic antidepressants** such as *amitriptyline* (see Section 4.5). They are given for their effects on the CNS but do have side effects such as tachycardia and cardiac dysrhythmias, especially if an overdose is taken (see Section 9.5).

Cocaine enhances sympathetic activity by inhibiting uptake 1 and is a commonly abused drug for its effects on the CNS. It is also a local anaesthetic.

Inhibitors of noradrenaline breakdown

Monoamine oxidase inhibitors (MAOIs) such as *phenelzine* inhibit one of the enzymes responsible for destroying NA. This drug inhibits the enzyme irreversibly and has fallen out of favour due to the limitations it imposes when eating a tyramine-free diet (see Section 4.5). There are newer drugs now that are reversible inhibitors such as *moclobemide* and may be used in major depression. Foods containing tyramine are less dangerous but still need some restriction.

A summary of some of the drugs discussed in this section is shown in Table 2.3.

2.3 CHOLINERGIC PHARMACOLOGY

ACh is a neurotransmitter that has actions in both the CNS and the peripheral nervous system. The receptors that bind ACh are cholinergic receptors. **These receptors are found**:

- in the CNS
- on voluntary muscle at the neuromuscular junction, where ACh causes skeletal muscle to contract
- at all autonomic ganglia, including the adrenal gland, where ACh stimulates the release of adrenaline (epinephrine) and NA (norepinephrine)
- on all effector organs of the PSNS
- on some effectors of the SNS; for example, sweat glands.

Synthesis and inactivation of acetylcholine

- The ACh is synthesized in the nerve terminal.
- When a cholinergic nerve is stimulated, the action potential triggers the release of ACh. The ACh diffuses across the synapse.
- There are postsynaptic receptors for ACh on the effector or postganglionic cell body.
- If the ACh does not attach to a receptor, it is rapidly inactivated by the enzyme acetylcholinesterase (AChE) in 1 or 2 ms. This rapid destruction means that the action of ACh is short lasting.

Cholinergic receptors

Two main types of receptor for ACh have been identified: muscarinic and nicotinic.

Muscarinic receptors

Produce an effect that can be mimicked by the injection of muscarine, the active chemical in the poisonous mushroom *Amanita muscaria.* The actions are those of the PSNS. They can be abolished by a small dose of atropine.

Atropine is an antagonist at the muscarinic cholinergic receptor.

Nicotinic receptors

Produce an effect similar to that of nicotine. They are found at autonomic ganglia and at the neuromuscular junction. Activity at this type of receptor is involved in stimulation of all autonomic ganglia, secretion of adrenaline (epinephrine) and NA (norepinephrine) from the adrenal gland and stimulation of voluntary muscle.

Drugs and cholinergic transmission

Drugs may have an action by affecting:

- muscarinic receptors − may be agonists or antagonists
- nicotinic receptors on skeletal muscle − may be agonists or antagonists
- ganglia − may be ganglion blocking or ganglion stimulating
- ACh synthesis or release − may inhibit or stimulate
- ACh destruction by cholinesterase − may inhibit or stimulate.

Drugs acting on muscarinic receptors

Muscarinic agonists

Effects resemble those of stimulation of the PSNS.

Cardiovascular effects

- Slowing of heart rate.
- Decrease in cardiac output − due mainly to a decreased force of contraction of the atria because there is little parasympathetic innervation of the ventricles.
- Generalized vasodilation. This is an indirect effect due to the release of nitric oxide (NO) by the endothelium of the blood vessels.
- Fall in blood pressure.

Other effects

- Smooth muscle contraction (except vascular). This increases peristalsis in the gut and contraction of muscle in the bladder.
- Increased secretions − lacrimal (tears), salivary (drooling) and bronchial.
- Bronchoconstriction and increased secretions can cause difficulty in breathing − this effect is reversed by *ipratropium (Atrovent)* which is a muscarinic antagonist.
- Pupillary constriction and lowering of intraocular pressure − this is useful in glaucoma. *Pilocarpine* is a muscarinic agonist.

Clinical applications These drugs are not very useful clinically.

Pilocarpine is administered to constrict the pupil and allow drainage of aqueous humour in glaucoma. It is administered up to four times daily.

Bethanechol increases detrusor muscle contraction in the bladder and has been used to assist bladder emptying. In retention of urine, catheterization is the preferred treatment.

Contraindications Heart disease, intestinal or urinary obstruction, asthma and parkinsonism.

Side effects Parasympathomimetic including nausea, vomiting, intestinal colic, bradycardia, blurred vision and sweating. More likely to occur in the elderly.

Muscarinic antagonists

Atropine comes from the plant *Atropa belladonna* (deadly nightshade), and **hyoscine** comes from the thorn apple. Both these are **reversible competitive antagonists**.

They are lipid soluble and so penetrate the blood−brain barrier.

Clinical effects

- Cardiovascular effects − modest tachycardia due to removal of para-sympathetic control on the SA node − *atropine* is used to treat bradycardia.
- Inhibition of secretions − dry mouth, eyes.
- Inhibition of sweating.
- Dilation of pupils − *homatropine* is used to dilate the pupil in ophthalmology.
- Reduction in gastrointestinal motility.
- Bronchial smooth muscle relaxation − *ipratropium* is used in chronic obstructive pulmonary disease.
- Biliary and urinary smooth muscle relaxation. *Hyoscine (Buscopan)* is used to reduce smooth muscle contraction in renal colic and other disorders. It is a muscarinic antagonist.
- Reduction of mucociliary clearance in the bronchi (not *ipratropium* though).
- Antiemetic action.
- Antiparkinsonian action.
- Excitatory effect on the CNS.

Clinical applications
Cardiac
Atropine is used in sinus bradycardia, especially if hypotension is present.

- There is a transient bradycardia first at low doses due to stimulation centrally of the nucleus of the vagus nerve. The tachycardia produced is modest: 80–90 bpm usually.
- This is because atropine only inhibits the cholinergic system.
- It does not stimulate the SNS but **removes the 'vagal break'** that is normally applied to the SA node, allowing a pacemaker to stimulate cardiac contraction uninhibited by the parasympathetic system.

Respiratory

Ipratropium reduces bronchospasm and secretions in chronic obstructive pulmonary disease and asthma (see Section 6.1).

Atropine is used in anaesthesia to reduce secretions from the respiratory tract and to reduce reflex bronchoconstriction. It also prevents bradycardia and hypotension associated with some anaesthetic drugs.

Hyoscine (scopolamine) is occasionally used as an alternative for premedication.

Gastrointestinal and urinary tracts

- Antimuscarinics **relax smooth muscle** and are used as antispasmodics in the gastrointestinal tract and the urinary tract. *Hyoscine butylbromide (Buscopan)* and *dicycloverine (Merbentyl)* are examples.

The MHRA (Medicines and Healthcare Regulatory Agency) warn there is a risk of serious adverse effects following *hyoscine butylbromide* injection *(Buscopan)*, especially in those with cardiac disease. Tachycardia, hypotension and anaphylaxis may occur, and those with cardiac disease should be monitored with resuscitation equipment available, if the drug is used.

In **urinary incontinence,** antimuscarinics reduce involuntary contractions of the detrusor muscle, which can cause urgency and incontinence. They also increase bladder capacity. *Oxybutynin* and *tolterodine* are examples of drugs used.

Motion sickness

- *Hyoscine hydrobromide (Scopolamine)* is an effective drug for prevention of motion sickness. *Kwells* are an example.
- A transdermal patch may be used and needs to be applied several hours before travelling.

Parkinsonism

- These drugs reduce the effects of too much ACh in the brain, which occurs as a result of the deficiency in dopamine. *Orphenadrine* and *procyclidine* are examples. They are more useful in drug-induced parkinsonism (due to antipsychotics; see Section 4.4).
- In Parkinson's disease they may lead to cognitive impairment, and dopaminergic drugs (such as *Sinemet*) are better.

- They are still used as additive therapy and reduce the tremor and rigidity seen in this disease but have little effect on the bradykinesia.

The eye
- Dilate the pupil, and paralyse the ciliary muscle.
- They may be used as eye drops to aid ophthalmic examination of the fundus and also in uveitis (inflammation of the pigmented part of the eye such as the iris or ciliary muscle).
- *Homatropine* and *cyclopentolate* are examples.

Atropine is also used to counteract the muscarinic effects of organophosphate poisoning (see later).

Contraindications
- Glaucoma and myasthenia gravis.
- Increased risk of side effects in children and the elderly.
- Caution in myocardial infarction and hypertension.

Side effects Constipation, dry mouth, transient bradycardia, reduced bronchial secretions, dilation of the pupils and blurred vision, flushing and dryness of the skin, retention of urine. Occasionally confusion.

Drugs acting on nicotinic receptors
The neuromuscular junction and neuromuscular-blocking drugs
Both agonists and antagonists can produce neuromuscular block. This means that impulses cannot be passed from the motor nerves to skeletal muscle, resulting in paralysis.

- Nondepolarizing agents block the ACh receptors. They are competitive antagonists and block the nicotinic receptor.
- Depolarizing agents stimulate the receptor but then remain in the receptor so that it is not free to be stimulated again. This results in twitching first, then paralysis.
- They are used as **paralytic agents** as an adjunct to anaesthesia in surgery or when intubation is required in some severe head injuries.
- Some form of **artificial ventilation** must be available because the patient's respiratory muscles will be paralysed.
- They do not have a therapeutic use.

Caution in anaesthesia – muscle relaxants have no sedative or analgesic properties, but the patient will not be able to respond to pain because they are paralysed.

Nicotinic agonists – depolarizing agents

ACh and nicotine are agonists but are not of use clinically.

Suxamethonium is an agonist at the nicotinic receptor.

- It is known as a **depolarizing muscle relaxant** and **stimulates** the ACh receptor producing **muscular contractions** with some twitching and skeletal muscle movement at first.
- *Suxamethonium* is not destroyed by AChE, and so its action is sustained. This **prevents repolarization at the end plate** and **paralysis** follows.
- When *suxamethonium* is given the muscles from scalp to toe go into spasm briefly; these spasms are called *muscle fasciculations*. They last only approximately a second before flaccid paralysis occurs.
- It has a **rapid onset** and a **short duration** of action.
- It is destroyed in approximately 4–5 minutes by an enzyme in the plasma called **pseudocholinesterase**. If sustained paralysis is needed, longer-acting agents are usually used. Duration of action for suxamethonium is normally less than ten minutes when given intravenously in doses of 1 mg/kg.
- It is used to allow intubation to be done speedily because it rapidly suppresses the gag reflex. It is also used in electroconvulsive therapy.
- There is **no antidote** to suxamethonium because its action cannot be reversed. Anticholinesterases will act to potentiate its action.

Side effects

- Bradycardia and excessive salivation may occur and can be reduced by atropine.
- Painful muscular contractions occur during induction, and so the patient should be anaesthetized before its administration.
- Hyperkalaemia may occur due to loss of potassium from the muscle into the plasma. Not usually important but may be in trauma and burns, where it can result in ventricular dysrhythmia and even cardiac arrest.
- Prolonged paralysis occurs in approximately 1 in 2000 people due to a genetic abnormality of the cholinesterase needed to destroy the drug. Severe deficiency may mean the action lasts for up to 2 hours. If the enzyme is completely absent the paralysis lasts many hours.

Malignant hyperthermia with suxamethonium. This is a rare inherited condition that results in intense muscular contraction and a **dramatic rise in temperature** when certain drugs are given. The condition carries 65% mortality. Suxamethonium and halothane are the two agents most frequently implicated.

Dantrolene is given. This drug inhibits muscle contraction by interfering with calcium release.

Nicotinic antagonists — nondepolarizing agents

Curare is a nicotinic antagonist that was used by South American Indians as a poison on their arrowheads. It is found in various South American plants, and *tubocurarine* became the first paralytic agent to be used in medicine. Several synthetic agents have been developed with a similar action.

- All act as **competitive antagonists** at the nicotinic receptor of the end plate.
- It is necessary to block 70%—80% of receptors at the end plate to produce a failure of transmission.
- Muscle cannot contract without stimulation of the receptors, and paralysis follows sequentially.
- The eye muscles are affected first, causing double vision, then the facial, limb and pharyngeal muscles. The respiratory muscles are the last to be affected and also the first to recover.
- Because they are competitive antagonists they can be reversed by giving a drug (an anticholinesterase) that inhibits the enzyme breaking down ACh, thus allowing the latter to accumulate and overcome the antagonist. *Neostigmine* is used and acts within 1 minute of intravenous administration. Action lasts for 20—30 minutes.

Some competitive antagonists

Drugs differ in their rates of onset and recovery. They are given **intravenously** and most have a slower onset of action than suxamethonium.

Rocuronium has similar onset times to suxamethonium but fewer side effects.

Most are metabolized in the liver and excreted in the urine. Their duration of action varies from approximately 5 minutes to 1—2 hours. The patient can then breathe spontaneously and cough but may have some muscle weakness for much longer (Table 2.4).

Ganglion-blocking agents

These block transmission at both sympathetic and parasympathetic ganglia. This means their effects are many and complex. They include:

- fall in blood pressure from block of sympathetic ganglia
- postural hypotension and fainting.

Hexamethonium was the first antihypertensive drug, but these agents are no longer used because of their many side effects.

TABLE 2.4 Neuromuscular blocking drugs.

Drug	Onset	Duration	Special points
Pancuronium	Intermediate (2−3 min)	Long	Slight tachycardia. No hypotension. Used in long operations.
Vecuronium	Intermediate	Intermediate (30 −40 min)	Widely used. No histamine release. Occasionally prolonged action.
Atracurium	Intermediate	Intermediate (<30 min)	Transient hypotension due to histamine release. Spontaneously degraded in plasma. This is independent of liver and kidney function. Widely used.
Cisatracurium	Intermediate	Intermediate	Greater cardiovascular stability than atracurium. Does not cause histamine release.
Mivacurium	Fast (~2 min)	Short (~15 min)	New drug. Metabolized by plasma cholinesterase.
Rocuronium	Fast	Short (<10 min)	Similar to vecuronium − faster onset. Can be used when rapid effect needed in place of suxamethonium − fewer side effects.

Drugs affecting acetylcholine synthesis and release

- Drugs that **inhibit ACh synthesis** are only used experimentally.
- Drugs that **inhibit ACh release** include *β-bungarotoxin* found in snake venom from some members of the cobra family. The venom also contains *α-bungarotoxin,* which blocks the ACh receptors, so paralysis of victims is absolutely ensured!
- *Botulinum toxin* from the anaerobic bacterium *Clostridium botulinum* also inhibits ACh release. The organism multiplies in preserved food, and the toxin is extremely potent, causing **botulism**, a lethal type of food poisoning. Progressive parasympathetic and motor paralysis occur − dry mouth, blurred vision, difficulty in swallowing and eventually respiratory paralysis occur. Mortality is high and anticholinesterases do not work.
- The toxin is used medically in certain types of muscle spasticity.
- *Botox* is botulinum toxin injected into the little muscles that cause the skin to pucker. It paralyses them and is used to remove wrinkles from the forehead, etc.

Drugs enhancing acetylcholine transmission

These mostly act by **inhibiting acetylcholinesterase** and so preventing destruction of ACh and allowing its accumulation in the synapse. In the CNS this type of drug is used to treat Alzheimer's disease (AD) and other forms of dementia (see Section 4.7).

They have effects at peripheral and central synapses.

- **ACh activity in the parasympathetic nervous system** is enhanced, and this leads to increased secretions from salivary, lacrimal, bronchial and gastrointestinal glands, increased peristalsis, bronchoconstriction, brady-cardia and hypotension, constriction of the pupil and blurred vision.
- **Effects at the neuromuscular junction** lead to repetitive firing of muscle fibres. This is able to counteract blocking agents such as curare and restore movement and is also useful to increase transmission in myasthenia gravis (see later). However, overstimulation, as in organophosphate poisoning, can lead to paralysis.
- **Effects on the CNS** occur if the drug is lipid soluble. They are partly due to stimulation of muscarinic receptors and so can be blocked by atropine. There is initial excitement and sometimes convulsions but later depression of the CNS that may cause unconsciousness and respiratory failure.

Drugs that inhibit acetylcholinesterase

Mechanism of action

Prevent the action of AChE, the enzyme that destroys ACh at the synapse. This leads to an accumulation of ACh in the synapse.

Clinical applications

1. *To treat myasthenia gravis*
    - Myasthenia gravis is an autoimmune condition where there is destruction of the ACh receptor on **skeletal muscle** leading to pro-gressive weakness and extreme muscle fatigue. The selected muscles are **temporarily paralysed**. There may be drooping of the upper eyelid (ptosis), double vision and dysarthria (difficulty in speaking).
    - Anticholinesterases allow the buildup of ACh at the neuromuscular junction and cause an increased rate of firing of the muscle fibres, so restoring movement.
2. *To improve memory in Alzheimer's disease*
    - AD is a common age-related dementia where there are amyloid pla-ques, neurofibrillary tangles and loss of cholinergic neurones in the brain.
    - The loss of cholinergic neurones is believed to lead to cognitive impairment and memory loss.

- Cholinesterase inhibitors have resulted in improved cognitive functioning in approximately 40% of patients.
- Drugs include **donepezil, rivastigmine** and **galantamine**. They do produce measurable improvement.

There are three groups of anticholinesterase drug depending on how they interact with the active site of the enzyme.

Types of anticholinesterase

1. *Short acting*

The reversible reaction is very brief.

Edrophonium is occasionally used in the **diagnosis** of myasthenia gravis when other tests are inconclusive. A single test dose usually results in substantial improvement in muscle power lasting approximately 5 minutes.

2. *Medium duration*

Neostigmine produces an effect lasting approximately 4 hours in myasthenia. In severe cases it may even be given every 2 hours. It has side effects caused by the effect of the ACh on the muscarinic receptor. These include increased sweating, salivation, peristalsis and diarrhoea as well as bradycardia.

It may be used as a **reversal agent** for the competitive neuromuscular blocking drugs.

Contraindications and cautions

- Should not be given in asthma, because it may cause bronchoconstriction.
- Not used in intestinal or urinary obstruction.
- Care if there is bradycardia, recent myocardial infarction, hypotension, epilepsy or parkinsonism.
- The **antidote** to the **muscarinic effects** of the drug is *atropine*.

Pyridostigmine is less powerful than neostigmine and has a longer duration of action. It is preferred in the treatment of myasthenia.

3. *Irreversible anticholinesterases*

Inhibit the action of AChE, often for the life of the enzyme. Most of these are **organophosphate** compounds and have been developed for use as **pesticides** and **war gases**. The effect of some of these drugs, for example *Dyflos*, lasts for weeks because there has to be new synthesis of the enzyme before recovery can occur. The effect of other drugs such as *ethociopate* is shorter and the enzyme slowly reactivates over a period of a few days, so they are not completely irreversible.

The drugs are **highly lipid soluble** and are **rapidly absorbed** through mucous membranes. They even pass through the **cuticle of an insect** and also

unbroken skin — properties which allow them to be used as **war gases** and **insecticides**.

Effects of organophosphate poisoning

ACh accumulates at synapses in both the central and peripheral nervous systems. This leads to overstimulation at both neuromuscular and autonomic synapses.

The clinical picture produced by stimulation of the **muscarinic receptors** can be remembered by the mnemonic **DUMBBELS** (Chomchai, 2001):

- **D**iarrhoea
- **U**rinary incontinence
- **M**iosis
- **B**radycardia
- **B**ronchospasm and bronchorrhoea
- **E**mesis
- **L**acrimation
- **S**alivation.

Stimulation of the **nicotinic receptors** at the **neuromuscular junction** causes muscle weakness, fasciculations and paralysis.

Early symptoms are due to stimulation of nicotinic receptors at ganglia and include sweating, tachycardia (but later this becomes bradycardia) and hypertension.

Effects on the CNS include confusion, restlessness, anxiety and seizures.

Death may occur secondary to respiratory failure and cardiovascular collapse.

Treatment of organophosphate poisoning

- All those in contact should **wear protection** — latex or vinyl gloves offer insufficient protection, and neoprene or nitrile gloves must be used until the patient is decontaminated.
- All contaminated clothing should be regarded as **toxic waste.** Skin should be cleaned with plenty of soap and water. Activated charcoal (see Section 9.5) may be given for decontamination of the gastrointestinal tract.
- *Atropine* is given as a muscarinic antagonist. It dries secretions and will increase the heart rate, if bradycardic. In organophosphate poisoning, it is still given even if the patient is tachycardic. A much larger dose than normal is used and an initial dose of 1—2 mg may be given intravenously to adults. This dose may need to be doubled every 5—10 minutes until the symptoms are relieved and further boluses or an infusion may be needed for 24 hours or longer. Atropine has **no effect at the neuromuscular junction**, where the receptors are nicotinic and not muscarinic.

TABLE 2.5 Some cholinergic and anticholinergic drugs.

Cholinergic	Anticholinergic
Muscarinic agonists	**Muscarinic antagonists**
Pilocarpine	Atropine, ipratropium and hyoscine
Nicotinic agonists	**Nicotinic antagonists**
Suxamethonium	Atracurium, pancuronium
Inhibit ACh destruction – acetylcholinesterases	**Ganglion blocking**
Donepezil for dementia	Trimetaphan
Neostigmine used in myasthenia and as an antidote to	**Inhibit ACh release**
competitive nicotinic antagonists	Botulinum toxin –
Organophosphates – war gases and pesticides	*Botox*

ACh, Acetylcholine.

● *Pralidoxime* is the only available antidote to organophosphate poisoning and must be given as soon as possible. It can regenerate AChE as long as 'ageing' has not occurred. This is a process whereby the enzyme loses a chemical group and can no longer regenerate. Ageing occurs in **24–48 hours** after which new enzyme molecules must be produced before ACh can be destroyed.

Delayed complications

May start to develop approximately 1–3 weeks after exposure. They may be due to inhibition of a neuronal enzyme involved in myelin formation. There is slowly developing **sensory loss** and **muscle weakness**, often beginning with leg cramps, numbness and tingling in the feet.

A summary of the action of some of the drugs discussed in this chapter is shown in Table 2.5.

Pain, analgesia and anaesthesia

Chapter Outline

3.1 PAIN, ANALGESIA AND ANAESTHESIA – OVERVIEW

Pain is a complex sensation that is felt in very many conditions and may be the most distressing component of a disease for the patient. It is often the prime reason for seeking medical help but is also frequently medically induced, as in surgery. The presence of pain can interfere with obtaining accurate and reliable measurements; therefore pain should be treated at an early stage. Pain is feared and may hinder the healing process but although pain control has vastly improved over recent years it is still difficult to ensure that the patient receives adequate pain relief.

Drugs that provide pain relief are called *analgesics*. Ideally analgesics should relieve pain without affecting other sensations or consciousness. Following the administration of any analgesic it is important to reassess the pain felt by the patient and evaluate the effect of the drug.

Anaesthesia is a loss of feeling in a part or all of the body. In pharmacology it is the reduction of pain that allows otherwise painful procedures to be carried out. General anaesthesia renders the patient unconscious whereas local anaesthesia blocks sensory nerve transmission in one area.

Pain

Pain is an unpleasant sensory and emotional experience that is also a protective mechanism and as such gives warning of the presence of injury or disease.

- Pain alerts us to damaging forces in and around our bodies and arises if there is:
  - local ischaemia, for example angina
  - chemical damage, for example leakage of enzymes in the pancreas as in pancreatitis

- spasm of smooth muscle, for example colic
- overdistension of a hollow organ, for example retention of urine
- irritation, for example of the peritoneum, pleura or pericardium
- stimulation of the inflammatory immune response and release of mediators
- physical trauma.
- The sensation of pain is evoked by the excitation of nerve cells in the brain but pain intensity is difficult to measure objectively.
- It is associated with emotion such as anxiety, fear, depression and alarm. These and many other sensations can be inseparable from pain and can alter the intensity and response to pain.
- Pain is an unpleasant sensory experience that relies on the nervous system to conduct impulses to the brain where sensation is interpreted. Should anything interfere with this pathway, such as damage to the spinal cord, pain will not be felt no matter how much damage is occurring to the body.
- Pain felt is not just determined by the intensity of the painful stimulus but is also a subjective experience with strong central and emotional components. This means that intense pain may sometimes be felt when the brain's interpretation of a harmless stimulus is deranged. An example of this is seen in trigeminal neuralgia when a minimal mechanical stimulus to the face triggers brief but excruciating pain in one of the branches of the trigeminal nerve in the face.

Types of pain

- **Acute pain** is a common symptom that frequently aids diagnosis, as in acute appendicitis or myocardial infarction. Usually it may be effectively dealt with by analgesia and the cause can be found and treated.
- **Chronic pain** causes much suffering and often appears to serve little purpose. It may be debilitating for the patient and is often the most difficult type of pain to treat, often not responding to standard analgesic drugs.
- **Chronic pain syndrome** is a term used to describe the situation when disease appears to have disappeared but pain persists.
- **Neuropathic pain** can occur as a result of injury or disease to the nerve tissue itself. This can disrupt the ability of the sensory nerves to transmit correct information to the brain which may then interpret painful stimuli as present even though there is no obvious or known physiological cause for the pain. Neuropathic pain is very difficult to treat and does not respond well to opioids or nonsteroidal anti-inflammatory drugs (NSAIDs).
  - Damage to the peripheral sensory nerves as in neuropathy can result in a distortion or amplification of naturally generated signals leading to intense pain usually described as burning or shooting pains, observed in:
    - neuralgia — intense, intermittent pain occurring along a nerve
    - fibromyalgia — pain all over the body

- peripheral neuropathy — nerves in the body's extremities are damaged
- complex regional pain syndrome — severe and persistent debilitating pain; a slight pain, bump or change in temperature can cause intense pain.
- Pain can sometimes appear to come from where an amputated limb used to be. This is known as **phantom limb pain** and may be excruciating and difficult to treat.

Pain assessment

Prior to the administration of pain relief, assessment of pain is essential and contributes to the treatment and monitoring of pain levels. Steps to pain assessment include obtaining a pain story from the patient.

- Assessment of the physical component of the pain:
  - initial assessment — pain assessment tools
  - ongoing assessment
  - response to treatment.
- Assessment of the nonphysical aspects of pain:
  - anxiety — about treatment and meaning of pain
  - helplessness and depression
  - social worries.

It is important that the same pain assessment tool be used throughout and that the tool used is the most appropriate for the patient's needs at that particular time. Also, when assessing patient's pain it is vital to listen to what the patient is saying about their pain. Assess the location, type and intensity of patient's pain in order to select the appropriate treatment. There are many simple pain assessment tools:

- The visual analogue scale — a straight line, usually 10 cm in length, with one extreme marked 'no pain at all' and the other end marked 'worst possible pain'; descriptive words may be added.
- Numerical rating scales are marked between 0 and 10, with 0 signifying 'no pain' and 10 meaning 'unbearable pain'.
- Verbal rating scales or verbal descriptors use four or five pre-set categories and consist of a list of adjectives that describe levels of pain intensity by extremes ('no pain', 'mild pain', 'discomfort', 'severe/distressing pain', 'excruciating/very severe pain').
- The Bourbonnais pain assessment tool — two pain assessment tools designed to complement each other. The tool, a 'pain ruler', consists of two parts: a scale ranging from 0 (reflecting no pain) to 10 (reflecting excruciating pain), and a list of adjectives, which describe different perceptions of pain. The person experiencing pain is then asked to match the word or

words that describe his or her pain to the number, which corresponds to the intensity of the pain.

- The London Pain Chart – the chart includes a body chart to record the site(s) of pain, a verbal descriptor scale for intensity and measures to relieve pain.
- The Abbey Pain Scale is used for the measurement of pain in individuals with dementia who cannot verbalize and gives a score using six questions on vocalization, facial expression, change in body language, behavioural change, physiological change or physical changes.
- The pain and function assessment tool combines the verbal descriptor scale using a scale of 1–10 being no pain and 10 worst possible pain, with the Wong-Baker Facial Grimace Scale.

If one of these pain assessment tools is deemed to be unsuitable to meet the individual needs of a patient, then special pain assessment tools may be available through an online search for:

- the unconscious patient
- the elderly
- those with intellectual difficulties
- patients with delirium
- pregnancy
- burns
- chronic pain
- dementia.

Pain can affect physiological measures and the bedside nurse must be adequately equipped to take into account and interpret the patient's physiological parameters as an early indicator of pain – for example elevated blood pressure, tachycardia and sweating are all recognized signs of pain.

Once assessed, it is imperative that the pain is treated; a failure to relieve pain is morally and ethically unacceptable, as under-treatment can lead to poor outcomes.

Under-management of pain

Pain can have a detrimental effect on a patient's condition and can significantly slow recovery. The under-treatment of pain can lead to:

- decreased tidal volumes and alveolar ventilation, leading to decreased oxygen delivery to organs

- preventing the patient from coughing, resulting in an increase in the collection of secretions contributing to atelectasis and chest infections
- avoidance of movement, leading to an increase risk of deep vein thrombosis and pulmonary embolism
- increased stress response and sympathetic stimulation, resulting in vasoconstriction and tachycardia, raising blood pressure, increasing the workload of the heart
- stress, which:
  - interferes with intestinal smooth muscle leading to an increase in stomach acid leading to the formation of ulcers
  - increases metabolic rate, leading to difficulties in meeting nutritional needs and may lead to loss of weight.

There is no doubt that pain management is the role of the nurse to organize and co-ordinate with the multidisciplinary team. Pain can be avoided, leading to better patient satisfaction and quality of life. Medication management must move towards effective care in this important area of clinical practice.

Pain relief

Drugs that relieve pain are chosen according to the cause and severity of the pain (see above). They fall into the following categories:

- Narcotic or opioid analgesics such as *morphine*. These act on the central nervous system (CNS) reducing the appreciation of pain but sometimes causing drowsiness and respiratory depression.
- *Paracetamol* and NSAIDs such as *aspirin* which act peripherally to reduce pain and inflammation, especially of musculoskeletal origin. They also have some central action.
- Local anaesthetics (LAs) such as *lidocaine* that suppress conduction along sensory nerve fibres from the painful area.
- **Adjuvant drugs** that are used alongside analgesics in pain management. These include various centrally acting nonopioid drugs such as *amitriptyline*, an antidepressant, and *gabapentin*, an antiepilepsy drug.
- Drugs for specific conditions − *carbamazepine* for trigeminal neuralgia, *ergotamine* for migraine.

The **World Health Organization (WHO)** produced an analgesic ladder in 1986 as a guide to prescribing pain relief. The ladder forms the basis of many approaches to the use of analgesic drugs and essentially has three steps. If the patient does not experience pain relief on one step of the ladder, they should move onto the next.

Step 1: nonopioids − *paracetamol* and NSAIDs.
Step 2: mild opioids − *codeine, dihydrocodeine* − may be combined with paracetamol or an NSAID.

Step 3: strong opioids — for example *morphine* — larger doses give more pain relief — no ceiling effect.

Pain relief using one prescribed analgesia can be less than effective, as pain reoccurs as the effects of the drug begins to wear off; users can then not have another of the same until the appropriate amount of hours have passed. Thus in many instances two analgesics should be prescribed and given prior to the reduction of the effects of the first. The second analgesic will take effect before the first has completely worn off. This explains the need for combinations of analgesia types from:

- steps 1 and 2
- steps 1 and 3.

Do not combine paracetamol with other painkillers containing paracetamol, anti-sickness medications. Paracetamol is often an ingredient in cold and flu remedies.

In the last few years there is some concern that opioids may be being overused in chronic pain.

Drugs used in analgesia and anaesthesia are described below.

3.2 OPIOID ANALGESIA

Opium is the natural extract derived from the dried juice of the seed head of the opium poppy *Papaver somniferum*. It has been used since prehistoric times and derivatives from the poppy still play a large role in pain relief. Opium contains over 20 different alkaloids but the most important are morphine and codeine.

- Opioids are used to relieve moderate to severe pain, particularly of viscous origin.
- Nearly all opioids are potentially drugs of dependence.
- Side effects include nausea, vomiting, constipation and drowsiness. With larger doses, respiratory depression and hypotension may occur.

It has been known since 1975 that opioid peptides are actually produced by our own bodies. These include endorphins, enkephalins and dynorphins that are sometimes called 'the brain's own morphine'. These **endogenous opioids** are neurotransmitters in the pain inhibitory pathway and attach to opioid receptors in the CNS. Their presence explains why the brain actually has opioid receptors.

Opioid receptors

All opioids, whether produced by our own bodies, naturally occurring in the opium poppy or chemically synthesized, interact with specific opioid receptors and thus produce their effects.

- There are three major subtypes of opioid receptor named mu (μ), kappa (κ) and delta (δ). *Morphine* is an agonist at all three types of receptor.
  - μ Receptors are responsible for most of the analgesic effects of opioids and some of the major unwanted effects for example respiratory depression, euphoria and dependence.
  - κ Receptors do contribute to analgesia at the spinal level but produce fewer side effects and do not cause dependence.
  - δ Receptors are more important in the peripheries but do contribute to analgesia.
- Drugs may be agonists, antagonists, partial agonists or mixed agonists–antagonists at opioid receptors.
- Some drugs are pure agonists. They may be typical morphine-like drugs such as *fentanyl* that have a high affinity for the μ receptor but also include weak agonists such as *codeine*.
- A weak analgesic like *codeine* will compete for receptors with a strong drug like *morphine* and so reduce the efficacy of the latter.
- Some opioid drugs may be an agonist at one type of receptor and an antagonist at another.
- The effects of opioids are blocked by antagonists such as *naloxone*, an antidote to opioids.

An opioid is any substance that produces morphine-like effects that are antagonized by naloxone.

Morphine

Morphine is described here in full and other opioids such as *diamorphine*, *pethidine* and *fentanyl* are briefly discussed.

Mechanism of action

Morphine acts on all opioid receptors but has a higher affinity for the μ receptor sites. It inhibits the transmission of pain via the spinal cord to the brain.

Clinical effects

- *Morphine* is still the most valuable opioid for severe acute and chronic pain and is the standard to which all other opioids are compared. It is not just an analgesic but also relieves anxiety and produces mental detachment and euphoria.
- *Morphine* causes both depression and excitation of the CNS and causes the development of both tolerance and dependence to its central effects (Box 3.1).
- Its effect on the peripheral nervous system include constipation, histamine release, urinary retention and increased smooth muscle tone.

Central effects

Analgesia

- Morphine both eliminates pain and allows tolerance to pain.
- If the pain is still present, it is no longer unpleasant.
- It is effective in most kinds of acute and chronic pain.
- It remains the drug of choice in terminal cancer care.

Euphoria

- Induces a state of relaxation, tranquillity, detachment and well being that is referred to as euphoria. This is an important component of its analgesic effect.
- Occasionally it can cause dysphoria (a feeling of unpleasantness).
- Different opioids produce different amounts of euphoria. This is mediated by the μ receptor and does not occur with *codeine*.
- Euphoria depends on the circumstances. In distressed patients it is marked but in those accustomed to chronic pain it is not present although the pain is relieved.
- It also causes sleepiness, lethargy and inability to concentrate but this may be destroyed by nausea and vomiting.

BOX 3.1 Central nervous system depressant and stimulant effects of morphine

CNS depressant effects	CNS stimulant effects
Analgesia	CTZ − vomiting
Respiratory depression	Constriction of the pupil
Suppression of cough reflex	Increased spinal reflexes
Drowsiness and sleep	Stimulates the vagus nerve
Occasionally convulsions	

CNS, *Central nervous system;* CTZ, *chemoreceptor trigger zone.*

Respiratory depression

- Dose related.
- Decreases the sensitivity of the respiratory centre to a rise in blood carbon dioxide tension.
- This results in increased arterial partial pressure of carbon dioxide (pCO_2) with a normal analgesic dose of morphine.
- Hypoxic drive that is mediated through the peripheral chemoreceptors is not affected.
- Respiration slows to a measurable degree after a normal dose.
- This may be partly counteracted by the stimulatory effect of nociceptor input in severe pain.
- Respiratory arrest is usually the cause of death after an overdose.

Depression of the cough reflex

- This does not correlate closely with the analgesic action and respiratory depressant action − may be a different receptor.
- *Codeine* suppresses the cough in sub-analgesic doses.

Pupillary constriction

- Due to a stimulatory effect on the nucleus of the third cranial nerve.
- Important diagnostically in overdosage.

Nausea and vomiting

- Chemoreceptor trigger zone (CTZ) of the vomiting centre is stimulated and nausea occurs in approximately 40% of those receiving morphine, vomiting in approximately 15%.
- Worse if ambulant.
- Does not appear separable from the analgesic action.
- Tolerance to this effect occurs with prolonged use.
- May be reduced by the administration on an antiemetic such as *cyclizine.*

Stimulation of the vagus nerve

- This may cause bradycardia and lowering of blood pressure. May be important when used as an analgesic in acute myocardial infarction.
- Reduced output from the hypothalamus to the sympathetic nervous system contributes to vasodilation and hypotension.

Peripheral effects

Gastrointestinal tract

- Increase in tone and reduced motility lead to constipation, which may be severe.
- There is also a delay in gastric emptying which may retard the absorption of other drugs.
- Increased biliary tone may mean that morphine can actually increase the pain in biliary colic.
- May interfere with bladder function and lead to urinary retention, especially postoperatively.

Other actions

- Releases histamine from mast cells, which may lead to urticaria and itching as well as occasionally bronchoconstriction and hypotension. May be serious in asthmatics.
- Long-term use depresses the immune system.
- *Morphine* crosses the placenta and may depress the baby's respiration at birth.

Tolerance to morphine

- Tolerance is present when an increase in dose is needed to produce the same effect.
- Tolerance develops rapidly and may be detected within 12–24 hours of commencement of administration.
- The duration of tolerance after the cessation of drug taking varies from a few days to weeks.
- Tolerance and withdrawal effects are less common when used for analgesia (Ritter et al. 2019) but may be a problem in long-term administration for chronic pain.

Dependence

- Both physical and psychological in nature.
- Some physical dependence may be detected within 24 hours of regular administration.
- Dependence appears to be less when the drug is given for analgesia rather than taken for pleasure.
- If physical dependence occurs, there are definite withdrawal symptoms when the drug is stopped.

Indications for use

Moderate to severe pain, especially of visceral origin:

- acute pain
- following injury
- perioperative analgesia
- postoperative pain
- myocardial infarction
- acute left ventricular failure with pulmonary oedema
- on a regular basis for terminal related pain both cancer and non-cancer patients.

Routes of administration

Oral

- Oral absorption is incomplete and 70% of the dose is removed by first-pass metabolism, necessitating a larger dose by this route.
- Immediate-release tablets may be given every 4 hours.
- Modified-release preparations are taken twice daily for long-term pain control.
- Oral morphine solutions are also available.

Rectal

- Suppositories of morphine 10 mg.

Injection

- May be given by subcutaneous, intramuscular or intravenous route for acute pain, 10−15 mg every 4 hours if necessary.
- Analgesia starts within 20 minutes of subcutaneous injection and within 10 minutes of intravenous. The effect peaks after about 1 hour and lasts up to 3−4 hours.
- By slow intravenous injection a quarter to half the intramuscular dose may be given.
- Produces analgesia rapidly by this route and the effect peaks in about an hour.
- May also be administered as patient-controlled analgesia (PCA) according to hospital protocols.

Contraindications

- Acute respiratory depression.
- Phaeochromocytoma – rare tumour of the adrenal gland tissue.
- Asthma attack.

- Acute alcoholism.
- Paralytic ileus.
- Head injury (Box 3.2).

Cautions

- Hypotension.
- Asthma (avoid during attack).
- Enlarged prostate.
- Pregnancy and breast feeding. Opioids cross the placental barrier and so can produce respiratory depression in the newborn.
- Care in liver failure but sometimes tolerated well.
- Reduce dose in renal impairment or avoid as accumulation occurs causing prolonged action. Morphine is excreted as a metabolite in the urine.

In palliative/end-of-life care these cautions will not always be a deterrent.

Adverse/side effects

Many of these have been described earlier under clinical effects. They often limit the size of the dose that can be given. The most serious side effect is respiratory depression. Others include:

- nausea and vomiting
- constipation
- sedation/drowsiness
- tolerance and dependence
- euphoria
- itching (histamine release).

Larger doses produce:

- respiratory depression, hypotension, muscle rigidity.

Other side effects include:

- difficulty passing urine
- dry mouth, sweating, headache, facial flushing, vertigo

BOX 3.2 Head injuries

Morphine is not given to patients with a head injury
- It interferes with **pupillary responses**
- Carbon dioxide retention caused by **respiratory depression** results in cerebral vaso-dilation – in patients with **raised intracranial pressure** this can lead to alterations in brain function

- bradycardia, tachycardia, postural hypotension, palpitations
- hallucinations, mood changes
- decreased libido
- rashes.

Interactions

- Alcohol enhances the sedative and the hypotensive effects of morphine.
- Hypnotics also enhance the sedative and the hypotensive effects of morphine.
- Possible hypotension or hypertension when given with the antidepressant monoamine oxidase inhibitors (MAOIs).

Cyclimorph is morphine combined with the antiemetic *cyclizine*. This may be given for moderate to severe pain but is not recommended in myocardial infarction as it may aggravate heart failure.

Effects of overdosage

- Respiratory depression is the main danger.
- The patient may be drowsy or unconscious and the pupils are pinpoint.
- Cyanosis may be present.

The antidote is *naloxone*, the opioid antagonist, which may be given intravenously.

Acute withdrawal in opioid dependency

Fear does play a part. After missing only one injection an opioid addict senses mild withdrawal distress.

- First 8−16 hours − increasingly nervous, restless and anxious.
- Within 14 hours frequent yawns, sweating profusely, running eyes and nose.
- All increase in intensity then 'goose flesh' occurs and the pupils dilate.
- Severe twitching of the muscles occurs within 36 hours and painful cramps in both the legs and the abdomen.
- All body fluids are released copiously and vomiting and diarrhoea are acute.
- There is very little appetite for food.
- Insomnia is present.
- The respiratory rate increases.
- Blood pressure increases moderately.
- Temperature increases by about 0.5 degrees on average and subsides after the third day.
- Basal metabolic rate rises steeply in the first 48 hours.

- Peaks within 48—72 hours after the last injection of the drug and subsides over the next 5—10 days.
  If an addict chooses acute withdrawal, this is known as '**cold turkey**' and is possible but is unnecessarily cruel.
- *Methadone* is a great help in these situations. It is given orally and has a long half-life of 48 hours.
  Chlorpromazine and **benzodiazepines** may be given as well to help.

Opioid antagonists

- Produce little effect on their own but block the effects of opioids.
- *Naloxone* is a full antagonist of morphine. It reverses the action of opioids at all three subtypes of receptor. It has greatest affinity for the μ receptor sites.
- The sedative effects, respiratory depression and adverse cardiovascular effects are **blocked** within **1—2 minutes**.
- The duration of the antagonist effect is dose dependent but is shorter than morphine so that one dose may be insufficient and an infusion is sometimes required.
- If it is administered to opioid addicts, an acute withdrawal occurs.
- It may cause hypertension, pulmonary oedema and cardiac arrhythmias.

Diamorphine (heroin)

Diamorphine is obtained by chemical modification of morphine.

Mechanism of action

- When administered is rapidly metabolized to morphine.
- Highly lipid soluble and enters the brain more rapidly than morphine so its action starts a little sooner.
- Twice as potent as morphine, but rapidly metabolized to morphine.
- Greater solubility than morphine so requires a smaller volume for injection. This is important in palliative care when the patient may be emaciated.

Clinical effects

- Causes more euphoria but relatively less nausea, constipation and hypotension than morphine.
- It exerts the same amount of respiratory depressant effect as morphine, and when used intravenously is more likely to cause dependence.
- Is the opioid most frequently used by drug addicts.

An addict may take 300 mg of heroin several times a day and some may take as much as 600 mg in one dose. A non-addicted person would die of respiratory depression after such a dose. Addicts who return to the habit after a longish break may inadvertently overdose themselves by using the old dose when tolerance has gone.

Indications

● Acute pain, especially myocardial infarction.
● Chronic pain in end-of-life/palliative care. Used in some centres as an alternative to pethidine for analgesia in labour. The usual dose is 7.5 mg intramuscularly.

Route of administration

● By injection.
● 5 mg intramuscularly and up to 10 mg in heavier patients.
● May be given intravenously at a quarter to half the intramuscular dose by slow intravenous injection.
  If given orally it is subject to first-pass metabolism and is immediately converted by the liver into morphine.

Pethidine

Pethidine is a synthetic narcotic that is similar in action to morphine. It has a rapid onset of action (15 minutes) due to high lipid solubility and a shorter duration of action (2–4 hours) than morphine.

Mechanism of action

● Binds to μ and κ receptors.
● Less potent analgesic than morphine, even at high doses.

Pharmacokinetics

● Absorbed from gastrointestinal tract but availability is less with oral rather than parenteral routes.
● Metabolized by the liver to norpethidine – active and toxic.
● Eliminated in the urine.
● Crosses the placenta and appears in breast milk.
● Half-life 2.4–4 hours.

Clinical effects

- Little hypnotic action and may cause restlessness rather than sedation.
- Does produce a euphoric effect similar to that of morphine and it gives rise to dependency.
- Shorter duration of action than morphine, especially in the neonate. This is because morphine is not easily metabolized by neonates.
- Equal analgesic doses of morphine and pethidine depress respiration equally (10 mg morphine is approximately equal analgesic to 100 mg pethidine; O'Connor et al. 2000).
- Does not increase smooth muscle tone in the small intestine, biliary tract and ureters. Some antispasmodic action and is useful in colic.

Indications for use

- Moderate to severe pain especially renal colic, biliary colic and acute pancreatitis.
- Obstetric analgesia.
- Perioperative analgesia.
- Not suitable for severe, continuing pain.

Pethidine is often used in labour because of its shorter duration of action, less pronounced adverse effects on the baby and because it does not inhibit uterine contractions. It may cause respiratory depression in the neonate if given too late in labour.

Administration

- Oral: 50–150 mg not more often than every 4 hours.
- Subcutaneous or intramuscular injection 25–100 mg. May be repeated in 4 hours.
- By slow intravenous injection 25–50 mg. May be repeated in 4 hours.

Cautions

Accumulation of some of the metabolites of pethidine (see below) may result in neurotoxicity and cardiac arrhythmias.

- Severe renal impairment.
- Respiratory failure.
- Acute alcoholism.
- Concomitant use of MAOIs or within 14 days of ceasing therapy.

- Severe liver disease.
- Raised intracranial pressure.
- Convulsive states.
- Supraventricular tachycardias.

  Adverse effects are as morphine but convulsions can occur in overdosage.

Drug interactions

- Pethidine interacts seriously with MAOIs and severe reactions have been reported.
- Excitement, delirium, hyperthermia and convulsions may occur. This is due to an accumulation of the metabolite norpethidine.

Acute toxicity

- Respiratory depression may occur.
- Metabolized differently to morphine. Is converted to norpethidine which is hallucinogenic and can cause convulsions.
- It does not cause pupillary constriction.
- Is antagonized by ***naloxone***.

Tramadol

Produces analgesia by two mechanisms. It stimulates opioid receptors but also enhances serotonergic and adrenergic pathways. It has similar contraindications to morphine.

- Fewer opioid side effects, such as respiratory depression and constipation, and a lower addiction potential (note that it still produces dependency).
- Used for moderate to severe/acute or chronic pain including musculo-skeletal and pain associated with diabetic neuropathy.
- May be given orally or by intramuscular or intravenous injection.
- Psychiatric reactions have been reported following its use, including confusion and hallucinations.
- Withdrawal symptoms of anxiety and agitation have been reported when the drug is stopped.

Methadone

This is a synthetic drug with a much longer half-life than morphine, which can be greater than 24 hours — it does not give the same euphoria but does have powerful analgesic power.

- It should not be given more than twice daily as accumulation and over-dosage may occur.
- Orally it is used in a daily maintenance dose to aid opioid withdrawal in those dependent on heroin. It occupies the opioid receptors and reduces the desire for heroin. Should the latter be taken there is less 'buzz' from the intravenous heroin.
- Dependence does occur but this is less severe than with heroin.
- It may also be used as a cough suppressant in terminal illness.
- Less sedative action than morphine.

Fentanyl

A potent synthetic opioid that is an agonist at the μ receptor and so has similar effects to morphine but has a rapid onset of action due to its high lipid sol-ubility (600 times more lipid soluble than morphine). It has minimal cardio-vascular effects and is less likely to cause the release of histamine.

- It is widely used for intraoperative analgesia, to enhance anaesthesia and also as a respiratory depressant sometimes in assisted respiration. It may be given by intravenous injection or infusion.
- Available as a transdermal self-adhesive patch which is renewed every 72 hours and is used in chronic pain. When the first patch is applied it takes 12 hours to be fully effective.
- Lozenges may be given for breakthrough pain in those already receiving opioids for chronic cancer/non-cancer pain.
- The dose of fentanyl varies according to the use and the amount and duration of analgesia and sedation required.

Remifentanil is a μ receptor agonist with a shorter duration of action. It is administered by intravenous infusion in anaesthesia for perioperative analgesia.

Alfentanil is also a μ receptor agonist that is used in anaesthesia. It has a more rapid onset of action than fentanyl.

Fentanyl and other analogues have become drugs of abuse; they are easily synthesized without the need to harvest the poppy.

Meptazinol

- Claimed to have a low incidence of morphine side effects causing neither euphoria dysphoria or respiratory depression.
- Length of action 2−7 hours with onset within 15 minutes.

- Some nausea and vomiting, sedation and dizziness may occur.
- May be given orally or by intramuscular or slow intravenous injection.
- Due to short duration of action may be useful as an obstetric analgesia.

Oxycodone

- Used mostly for acute or chronic pain relief in non-cancer/palliative care.
- Is available as suppositories for rectal administration but may also be given orally, subcutaneously or intravenously.
- It is sometimes used as PCA postoperatively.

Opioid partial agonists

Buprenorphine is a partial agonist at the μ receptor but other drugs are mixed agonist/antagonists at the three opioid receptors.

Buprenorphine

Has a long duration of action and may be administered sublingually when it provides pain relief for 6—8 hours. It may also be administered by transdermal patch where length of effect is variable due to the gradual increase in plasma buprenorphine concentration (two patches may be occasionally used early in administration).

- The drug has both agonist and antagonist actions. As a high-affinity partial agonist on μ receptors it may precipitate withdrawal symptoms when given to patients dependent on other opioids. It may also antagonize the analgesic effect of any opioids previously administered.
- It is used in moderate to severe pain, perioperative analgesia and in opioid dependence to reduce withdrawal symptoms.
- May cause prolonged vomiting.
- If respiratory depression occurs, it is difficult to reverse with naloxone as the buprenorphine has a high affinity for the μ receptor and only dissociates slowly.

Administration

- Sublingual 200—400 micrograms every 8 hours.
- Intramuscular or slow intravenous injection 300—600 micrograms every 6—8 hours.
- Patches — release 5, 10 or 20 micrograms per hour for 7 days or 35 micrograms per hour for 72 hours.

Pentazocine is a mixed agonist—antagonist at opioid receptors and so may precipitate withdrawal in patients taking other opioids. It does produce analgesia with little respiratory depression but has unpleasant side effects, producing hallucinations and thought disturbances, and so is little used.

Mild opioids

Codeine, codeine phosphate, dihydrocodeine

- Effective for mild to moderate pain relief. About one-twelfth the analgesic action of morphine.
- Too constipating for long-term use.
- **Codeine phosphate** is used as an antidiarrhoeal agent.
- **Codeine** requires metabolism by the liver before it works as an analgesic. It is less effective as a painkiller in about 10% of the population as they lack the necessary enzyme in the liver.
  May be combined with paracetamol as:
- **Co-codamol**— codeine phosphate and paracetamol
- **Co-dydramol** — dihydrocodeine and paracetamol.

Dextropropoxyphene and paracetamol, as **co-proxamol**, was a popular analgesic but has been withdrawn in the UK due to the high mortality following overdoses of this medication.

3.3 NONSTEROIDAL ANTI-INFLAMMATORY DRUGS AND PARACETAMOL

Almost one-quarter of patients visiting their general practitioner (GP) in Britain have rheumatic type complaints. NSAIDs are analgesic, antipyretic and anti-inflammatory to varying degrees and are extensively used in the UK for bone and joint pain such as that found in rheumatoid and osteoarthritis. In addition, millions are bought over the counter as minor analgesics for self-treatment of headaches, dental problems, musculoskeletal disorders, etc.

They are called nonsteroidal to differentiate them from steroids such as **prednisolone** which are also anti-inflammatory but have a very different chemical structure. In a single dose NSAIDs have an analgesic effect similar to paracetamol but in regular dosage also have an anti-inflammatory effect.

There are more than 50 different NSAIDs on the market — none is ideal and all have side effects. Different NSAIDs may penetrate certain body tissues more effectively — for example, some drugs are more able to enter joints.

Mode of action

NSAIDs are a diverse group of drugs chemically but all reduce the synthesis of chemicals called **prostaglandins** (PGs) by inhibiting the enzyme **cyclo-**

oxygenase (COX) needed to make PGs from a chemical called *arachidonic acid*. PGs are significant in the inflammatory immune response, needed for glomerular filtration and clotting.

It is the inhibition of PGs that provides the therapeutic action of these drugs.

There are many different PGs — all are given their own letter and number — and not everything is understood about them all, but some of their functions are:

- act as mediators of inflammation — prostaglandin E_2 (PGE_2)
- inhibit gastric acid secretion and are also needed for the production of the thick mucous lining of the stomach (PGE_2)
- reset the body's thermostat in the hypothalamus in infections and so cause pyrexia
- vasodilation — especially important in the renal artery — prostaglandin I_2 (PGI_2) (prostacyclin)
- inhibition of platelet aggregation — PGI_2
- responsible for contraction of the pregnant uterus and the onset of labour at term (PGE_2 and prostaglandin F_2 [$PGF_2\alpha$])
- involved in the synthesis of thromboxane A_2, a vasoconstrictor that stimulates platelet aggregation.

The enzyme cyclo-oxygenase

There are three subtypes of the enzyme COX — **COX-1**, **COX-2** and **COX-3**.

- **COX-1** is present in most tissues including platelets.
- **COX-2** is induced in inflammatory cells when they are activated.
- Most NSAIDs inhibit both isoenzymes but vary in their degree of inhibition of the two.
- Anti-inflammatory, antipyretic and analgesic action is related to inhibition of **COX-2** and pathological PG production.
- Most of the **unwanted effects** are due to inhibition of **COX-1**.
- Another isoenzyme, **COX-3**, was identified in 2002 and it is thought that the action of paracetamol (analgesic and antipyretic) may be due to inhibition of this variant. However, COX-3 does not appear to be a form found naturally in humans.
- Drugs were developed with a greater selectivity for **COX-2** — **Coxibs** or **COX-2 inhibitors**. These produce anti-inflammatory action and pain relief without the gastrointestinal side effects but will not be effective as anti-platelet drugs to reduce the incidence of cardiovascular disease. Research showed that some actually **increased the incidence of cardiovascular disease** in certain client groups. Some drugs in this category have been withdrawn.

Adverse/side effects of nonsteroidal anti-inflammatory drugs

Nearly one-quarter of adverse drug reactions in the UK have been ascribed to the original NSAIDs − partly because they are heavily prescribed to the elderly.

All NSAIDs can cause gastric problems − gastrointestinal ulceration and intolerance − due to both their systemic and their local action.

- As PGs are needed for mucus production in the stomach, when they are inhibited the stomach lining gets thinner and thus users are more susceptible to ulceration. Hydrochloric acid and pepsin secretion is increased.
  - Most of the drugs are also acidic in nature and cause local irritation. Some produce more profound gastric irritation than others.
  - Occasionally can cause a massive haematemesis − bleeding or perforation from the use of these drugs is estimated to be responsible for around 700−900 deaths in the UK each year.
- There is also an effect on the kidney and glomerular filtration rate may be decreased. This is due to the inhibition of PG-mediated vasodilation and can lead to salt and water retention and hypertension. Rarely renal failure can occur. This is important in those with reduced cardiac output where the effect of PGs counter the vasoconstrictive compensatory mechanisms that are mediated by noradrenaline (norepinephrine) and angiotensin II.
  - NSAIDs have little effect on renal perfusion in individuals with normal cardiac output.
  - They should not be given to patients with renal problems.
- They inhibit uterine motility and so may prolong gestation. This may be useful as a short-term measure in premature onset of labour.
- PGs also are released during inflammation and integral to platelet aggregation, thus users can complain of nosebleeds, bleeding from the gums following brushing and women may have heavier than normal periods. Users should be advised to stop NSAIDs if any type of bleeding occurs.

Hypersensitivity reactions occasionally occur.

Approximately 20% of asthmatics are aspirin sensitive, and administration of NSAIDs can provoke an asthma attack.

Cautions and contraindications

- Hypersensitivity to aspirin or any other NSAID.
- Coagulation defects.
- Severe heart failure.

- Previous or active peptic ulceration.
- Caution is needed if there is any renal, hepatic or cardiac impairment.

Paracetamol is not an NSAID and is a better drug in the elderly where there is an increased risk of side effects. Fatalities have occurred especially from haematemesis following peptic ulceration.

No one NSAID drug is superior and differences in analgesic effect are small so about 60% of patients will respond to any of these drugs. However, patients do vary in their response to different NSAIDs and if after 2 weeks there is poor relief then a different drug should be tried. There is no benefit in giving two drugs of this type concurrently.

- The full analgesic effect is usually felt within a week but the full anti-inflammatory effect may not be achieved for up to 3 weeks.
- When there is a satisfactory response use the lowest dose possible.
  All can cause gastric irritation and should be taken with or after meals.

Classification of nonsteroidal anti-inflammatory drugs

NSAIDs may be classified according to their chemical nature.

Salicylates

Aspirin – acetylsalicylic acid

This is the oldest anti-inflammatory derived originally from the willow bark. It has good anti-inflammatory and antipyretic properties.

- It remains the **drug of choice** in many sorts of mild pain and bone pain.
- Not good in the treatment of visceral pain (myocardial infarction, renal colic, acute abdomen, etc.).
- Good in inflammatory joint disease but up to 50% of patients cannot tolerate the side effects.
- Reduces platelet cohesiveness and therefore reduces the occurrence of myocardial infarction and cerebrovascular accident in those with increased tendency to thrombosis (see Section 5.7).
- A single dose approximately **doubles the bleeding time** in a normal person for a period of **4–7 days**.

Pharmacokinetics

- Rapidly absorbed from the stomach and upper small intestine yielding a peak plasma salicylate level in 1–2 hours. Acid environment in the stomach keeps a large proportion of the salicylate in the non-ionized form, promoting absorption.

- When high concentrations enter the mucosal cell, the drug may damage the mucosal barrier.
- Aspirin is absorbed as such and hydrolysed to acetic acid and salicylate by esterases in the tissues and blood.
- Does bind to plasma albumin.
- May be excreted as unchanged salicylate but most is converted to water-soluble conjugates that are rapidly cleared by the kidney.
- Excretion of aspirin may be increased by making the urine alkaline. This increases the ionization of the salicylate in the renal tubules and thus hinders reabsorption from the tubule, increasing elimination.

Formulations

Available in many forms – fast-release soluble aspirin to work quickly and enteric-coated and slow-release forms to reduce gastric complications.

Liniments are also available to rub in the skin and are useful in sports injuries.

Side effects

- Include tinnitus, nausea, vomiting and epigastric pain.
- Adverse effects increase with higher doses.
- 70% of patients taking aspirin bleed although this may be hidden (occult blood).
- Long-term use can result in renal damage – especially when large doses are used – this is known as analgesic nephropathy and may result in terminal renal failure.
- Not given to children under 12 years due to its association with an increased incidence of **Reye's syndrome**. This is a rare form of encephalopathy with concomitant liver damage.
- There is some epidemiological evidence that points towards an inverse relationship between aspirin use and the risk of **colorectal cancer but others did not observe any association**.
- May also be associated with prevention or relief of symptoms in **Alzheimer's disease**. A study led by Pahan (2018) produced some evidence that aspirin may stimulate lysosomes in mice to clear away amyloid plaque (deposited in Alzheimer's).

Aspirin should never be taken on an empty stomach as this increases the risk of gastric side effects.

Antipyretic effect

- Does not decrease normal body temperature or temperature elevated in heat stroke which is due to hypothalamic dysfunction.
- During fever, endogenous pyrogens are released from leucocytes and reset the hypothalamus at a higher level.
  These are PGs and aspirin inhibits them causing vasodilatation and sweating.

Administration

Orally − dose: 300−600 mg.
Excreted rapidly and may need to be repeated in 4 hours for pain control.
To suppress inflammation larger doses may be needed: 900 mg 4 hourly.
Fatal dose is 10−30 g resulting in plasma concentrations exceeding 450 μg/mL.
Dose to reduce risk of thrombosis is 75−150 mg daily. Usually taken in the form of an enteric-coated tablet.
Soluble aspirin − mixed with calcium carbonate and citrate − is less irritant to the stomach but can still cause bleeding.

Some patients with a tendency to asthma may have an attack induced by the administration of an NSAID. These drugs should be avoided in these patients.
  Thought to be due to increased production of leukotrienes when PG synthesis is blocked.
  Leukotrienes are important mediators in asthma, causing bronchoconstriction.

Propionic acid derivatives

Ibuprofen, fenbufen, fenoprofen, flurbiprofen, ketoprofen, dexibuprofen, naproxen, tiaprofenic acid

Ibuprofen has the lowest incidence of gastric complications and is similar in effectiveness to aspirin. It has fewer side effects than other NSAIDs but the anti-inflammatory effects are weaker. This makes it unsuitable in such conditions as gout where inflammation is prominent.

- It is available over the counter and is also useful in dysmenorrhoea.
- It is not associated with Reye's syndrome and is available in an oral suspension for paediatric use.

- *Naproxen* is useful because of its long half-life. Some others are available in sustained-release forms. It has a low incidence of side effects but greater than ibuprofen.

Indoleacetic acids
Indometacin, sulindac, ketorolac trometamol

- Very effective as anti-inflammatory agents. More potent than aspirin but less well tolerated and have a high incidence of side effects including gastrointestinal bleeding and irritation, headaches and dizziness.
- Some are available as **suppositories** to prolong their action and are given at night.
- Should always be taken with food.
- *Ketorolac trometamol* is only used for short-term postoperative analgesia and is given intramuscularly. It has precipitated acute renal failure in some patients.

Fenamates
Diclofenac, mefenamic acid

Diclofenac is used widely in accident and emergency units for pain associated with muscles and joints as well as other acute pain such as renal colic. It is used in acute gout and also for postoperative pain.

- Moderate risk of gastrointestinal complications.
- It may be administered orally, as a suppository, by deep intramuscular injection or intravenously.
- It has been combined with *misoprostol*, a PG analogue. This helps to reduce the incidence of peptic ulcers in those with a history of previous gastric problems.

Mefenamic acid is very good for toothache and dysmenorrhoea. It can cause a fall in haemoglobin levels with long-term use.

- Most NSAIDs can cause constipation but mefenamic acid can cause diarrhoea and this may limit long-term use.

Oxicams
Piroxicam, tenoxicam

- Potent anti-inflammatories — main advantage is their long half-life — only daily administration is required.
- They do have more gastrointestinal side effects than Brufen, especially in the elderly. They can also cause serious skin reactions. These side effects have led to the use of *piroxicam* being restricted and only prescribed by specialist physicians in rheumatology. It is not used as first-line treatment.

COX-2 inhibitors (coxibs)

Celecoxib, etoricoxib

These drugs were developed in the hope that they would be effective anti-inflammatory agents with few side effects as they preferentially inhibit COX-2 that is involved in inflammation.

- Appear to be as effective as other NSAIDs in relieving pain and inflammation.
- Slightly less gastrointestinal ulceration in short-term studies (2 years).
- No antithrombotic activity.
- Do not increase bleeding time.
- May cause allergic reactions in those with allergies to other NSAIDs.
- May increase the risk of myocardial infarction and stroke.
- Several have been withdrawn following increased risk of myocardial infarction in those using these drugs.

The National Institute for Health and Clinical Excellence recommends COX-2 inhibitors only for those at high risk of developing serious gastrointestinal adverse effects and not if there is cardiovascular disease present. At present there are few, if any, situations where a coxib is unequivocally indicated.

Paracetamol (acetaminophen in the USA)

Useful analgesic and antipyretic agent with no anti-inflammatory action. It was first made in 1877 and is widely used as an OTC analgesic — yet we still do not understand how this drug actually works!

Paracetamol is thought to inhibit PGs and COXs, perhaps centrally rather than peripherally but there are several theories as to the actual site of action.

Paracetamol may have an impact on COX-3 inhibition, as mentioned earlier. It has also been shown to result in the activation of cannabinoid (CB1) receptors. Its analgesic action is removed if an antagonist blocks CB receptors. It is thought to inhibit the destruction of the body's endogenous CBs and so make them more available to reduce pain.

- Rapidly absorbed from gastrointestinal tract and reaches peak plasma level in 30–60 minutes.
- Best taken on an empty stomach for speed of action.
- Half-life approximately 2 hours.
- Does not decrease platelet adhesion.
- Does not have the same gastric complications.

- Is not associated with Reye's syndrome and so is widely used in paediatrics as an antipyretic and analgesic.
- No depressant effect on respiration.
- It is also the analgesic of choice in the elderly.

Adult dose: 500 mg–1 g orally up to four times daily.

Adverse/side effects

- Unwanted effects with therapeutic doses are rare.
- Chronic use may increase the risk of kidney damage.
- An overdose (10–15 g) can cause acute liver failure due to formation of a highly reactive intermediate when metabolized (see Section 9.5, Emergency treatment of poisoning). This is neutralized by the antidote to paracetamol poisoning, *N*-acetylcysteine (*Parvolex*).

Paracetamol is contained in many over-the-counter preparations and great caution is required in checking the content of these medications and the dose of paracetamol they contain.
Two medications containing paracetamol should not be taken concurrently.

3.4 ANAESTHESIA

This section describes drugs that are used to eliminate pain and sensation while unpleasant procedures such as surgery are carried out. Some of these drugs may also be used for pain relief, especially local anaesthetics (LAs). One example is their use by epidural injection in childbirth.

Local anaesthetics

LAs are used to block sensation in part of the body without affecting consciousness. *Cocaine* was the first LA used in surgery in 1884 but its potential for abuse limits it to very occasional use by ear, nose and throat (ENT) specialists. *Lidocaine* and *bupivacaine* are the LAs most widely used in the UK today.

Mechanism of action

LAs inhibit conduction along nerves. The fine unmyelinated nerve fibres that transmit pain and temperature are more easily blocked than the thicker myelinated motor fibres that supply muscle but if sufficient LA were given the drug would reversibly inhibit all motor as well as sensory fibres.

Electrical conduction along the nerve fibre is dependent on the movement of ions, especially sodium ions. LAs block sodium channels and so inhibit transmission along the nerve.

Some drugs that block sodium channels are also used as anticonvulsant drugs, for example *phenytoin*, and antidysrhythmics, for example *lidocaine*.

The drugs vary in their potency, lipid solubility, duration of action and toxicity (Table 3.1). These factors affect the routes of administration for which they are suitable.

The aim is to administer them in such a way as to minimize spread to other areas of the body.

Routes of administration

- **Topical** – applied directly to the skin to 'numb' the area. May also be applied to mucous membranes.
- **Local infiltration of tissue.** An example is prior to suturing a laceration. Soft tissues including subcutaneous tissue and muscle may be infiltrated. LAs should not be injected into inflamed or infected tissue.
- **Infiltration around local nerves** to provide an area devoid of sensation as in dentistry.
- **Extradural injection** – may be epidural as in labour or caudal (the lowest part of the epidural system) as used for pain relief in surgery, especially in children.
- **Spinal** – injection into the subarachnoid space.
- **Regional anaesthesia** – intravenous injection of prilocaine with the use of a tourniquet. This is commonly used in the arm when a fracture needs to be manipulated and is called a **Bier's block**. The tourniquet has to be left in position for at least 20 minutes to prevent the LA getting into the circulation and reaching the heart or brain.

Most of these drugs are vasodilators. Sometimes a vasoconstrictor such as *adrenaline (epinephrine)* is combined with the LA to slow its rate of absorption and prolong its effects on the surrounding tissues. The adrenaline

TABLE 3.1 Properties of some local anaesthetics.

Drug	Onset	Duration	Penetration of tissues
Lidocaine	Rapid	Medium	Good
Bupivacaine	Slow	Long	Moderate
Prilocaine	Medium	Medium	Moderate
Ropivacaine	Slow	Long	Less motor block
Tetracaine	Very slow	Long	Moderate

(epinephrine) is in a very low concentration and is commonly used in dentistry but should never be used in digits as necrosis due to ischaemia may result and the digit could be lost.

Cocaine has no vasodilatory action and vasoconstricts at all concentrations because it blocks the destruction of noradrenaline. This used to make it useful in ear, nose and throat surgery where it was used as an anaesthetic spray. Nowadays the vasoconstrictor of choice is phenylephrine.

Unwanted effects of local anaesthetics

- Most toxic effects result from absorption of the drug into the systemic circulation.
- The effect after local infiltration is usually greatest 10−25 minutes following administration and the patient should be observed for toxic effects for 30 minutes.
- Absorption varies depending on the LA, the site of administration and the presence of vasoconstrictors.
- In toxicity, the drugs stimulate the CNS causing numbness and tingling around the mouth, restlessness, tremor and confusion. A feeling of inebriation and light-headedness may occur, followed by sedation and twitching. This may progress to generalized convulsions. Further increasing the dose causes CNS depression including respiratory depression and can cause death.
- Cardiovascular effects are due to myocardial depression and vasodilation. They lead to bradycardia, hypotension and even cardiac arrest.
- Hypersensitivity reactions occasionally occur and may take the form of allergic dermatitis or rarely anaphylaxis.

Great care must be taken not to inject LA into a blood vessel by mistake. Convulsions and cardiovascular collapse may occur should the drug be administered intravenously.

Lidocaine

- Available as a solution for injection in various strengths (0.5%−2.0%), a gel or an ointment for local application, a spray for topical use on mucous membranes and combined with a steroid in suppositories for use in haemorrhoids.
- Quick to work and when given with adrenaline lasts about 90 minutes.

Emla, *Denela* and *Nulbia* contain a mixture of lidocaine and prilocaine in an oily cream. They are used to anaesthetize the skin prior to insertion of a venous canula or removing skin for grafting. They are not used on mucous membranes due to rapid systemic absorption.

Bupivacaine and levobupivacaine

- Used when a longer duration of action is required and takes up to 30 minutes to be fully effective.
- Used especially for continuous epidural blockade in labour and for spinal anaesthesia.
- Cardiac toxicity and myocardial depression are greater than with lidocaine.
- *Levobupivacaine* is an isomer thought to have fewer cardiac side effects.

Prilocaine

- Similar to lidocaine but used for Bier's block (intravenous regional anaesthesia) more. It is rapidly metabolized.
- May precipitate methaemoglobinaemia (oxidation of iron in haemoglobin leading to inability to bind with oxygen), requiring treatment with ascorbic acid or methylthioninium chloride (methylene blue).

Tetracaine (amethocaine)

- Supplied as eye drops for topical anaesthesia. May lead to a burning sensation when first instilled. Used to anaesthetize the eye for cataract extraction.
- Also available as a cream for application to the skin. Has a faster action than *Emla* cream. Takes 30 minutes and anaesthesia lasts 4−6 hours. The local vasodilation produced may be helpful when the cannula is inserted.
- Rapidly absorbed from mucous membranes so never applied to inflamed or traumatized surface.

Cocaine

- Has a high potential for abuse and is a profound vasoconstrictor. It is never given by injection due to toxicity.
- Rarely used today except occasionally as a spray for the mucous membrane in ear, nose and throat procedures. It is only administered by experienced personnel due to the risk of arrhythmias from systemic absorption even when used locally.

Epidural anaesthesia in surgery

Epidural anaesthesia is a form of regional anaesthesia that is often combined with a general anaesthetic when good postoperative pain relief is required such as following major bowel surgery or aortic aneurism surgery.

The epidural space is inside the spinal canal but outside the dura mater (Fig. 3.1).

A low dose of anaesthetic is used in labour to give sensory block without motor block or loss of movement. If an emergency caesarean section is needed the epidural will be topped up with a higher concentration of the drug to give motor block as well.

Spinal anaesthesia

The LA is introduced into the cerebrospinal fluid in the subarachnoid space (see Fig. 3.1). This is used for an elective caesarean section, urological operations and hip or lower limb surgery. It is not used for abdominal surgery. Smaller doses of anaesthetic are given than in an epidural but the onset of action is faster. The anaesthesia will last for approximately 2 hours.

- *Fentanyl* is often added to increase the duration of action.
- Main risk is hypotension due to block of sympathetic nerves. With higher doses and as the block rises, bradycardia and respiratory depression may occur due to effects on the phrenic nerve and respiratory centre.
- Postoperative retention of urine may occur due to block of the autonomic nerves in the pelvis.

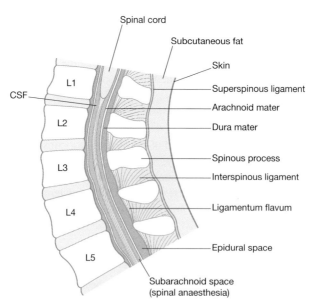

FIG. 3.1 **The vertebral column showing the epidural and subarachnoid spaces.** *CSF,* Cerebrospinal fluid.

General anaesthetics

General anaesthetics act on the brain to induce reversible loss of consciousness. This allows surgery and other painful procedures to be carried out without the patient being aware.

Nitrous oxide was first used for a tooth extraction in 1844 and vapours such as ether and chloroform were used for general anaesthesia. It took some time to lose consciousness and recovery was slow. Cardiac and hepatic toxicity limited the use of chloroform and these agents carried the risk of explosion.

In the 20th century muscle relaxants were developed along with new apparatus and increased clinical expertise, all making the administration of prolonged anaesthesia much safer.

Muscle relaxants are used to paralyse skeletal muscle during abdominal and thoracic surgery. The patient cannot breathe alone and must be intubated and ventilated.

Stages of anaesthesia

When only a volatile agent is given, anaesthesia is usually divided into four stages of increasing depression of the CNS. The stages were first described in ether anaesthesia with an unpremedicated patient. Total intravenous anaesthesia (TIVA) is increasingly being used in anaesthetics now and these stages are only given here for reference.

Stage 1 − analgesia

- Only partial analgesia until stage 2.
- Consciousness and sense of touch are retained.
- At first no amnesia but later in stage 1 amnesia and analgesia occur.

Stage 2 − delirium

Amnesic but appears excited. Respirations may be irregular and vomiting may occur. This stage should be as short as possible and ends with regular breathing being re-established.

Stage 3 − surgical anaesthesia

Begins with re-establishment of regular breathing and extends to cessation of breathing. The required depth depends on the procedure being followed. Depth is determined by the characteristic changes in respiration, pupils, spontaneous eye movements, reflexes and muscle tone.

Stage 4 − medullary paralysis

Arrival at this stage constitutes an overdose. Severe depression of the medullary vasomotor and respiratory centres occurs. The stage begins with respiratory failure and can lead to circulatory collapse.

- In the modern induction of anaesthesia these phases are so quickly merged into each other that they are not apparent.
- Unconsciousness, analgesia and muscle relaxation are produced with separate drugs.
- All anaesthetics are given intravenously or by inhalation because this allows closest control over blood levels and so of brain concentrations.

Modern steps in anaesthesia

The use of intravenously administered anaesthesia (TIVA) has revolutionized the induction of anaesthesia. Speed of action is extremely rapid and induction can take place in 10 seconds without the patient being aware of the onset of unconsciousness.

Today, the steps in anaesthesia would be as follows:

- Premedication is only used in special circumstances such as cardiac surgery, children, patient request.
- Induction with a fast-acting intravenous induction agent for example *propofol, thiopental*, given with a fast-acting opioid such as *fentanyl*. Loss of muscle tone occurs immediately after injection as does a short period of hypoventilation and usually apnoea. There must be facilities for ventilation and oxygen administration at hand.
- Muscle relaxation and intubation using a competitive nicotinic receptor antagonist or *suxamethonium*. These agents also paralyse the respiratory muscles.
- Maintenance may be by inhalational agents, for example *sevoflurane*. Frequently TIVA is used, for example *propofol*, without any inhalation agents.
- Analgesia, for example *remifentanil* or *morphine*.
- 'Wake-up'. Muscle relaxants are reversed using anticholinesterases or *sugammadex*. Maintenance anaesthetic is switched off and the patient wakes up as the effects wear off.

Mechanism of action of anaesthetic agents

General anaesthetics act on the brain, primarily the midbrain reticular activating system and the cortex, but their mechanism of action is still not entirely understood. Some drugs inhibit the excitatory transmitter glutamate and others stimulate the inhibitory neurotransmitter γ-aminobutyric acid (GABA) (Section 4.2).

Anaesthetics are fat soluble and so enter the brain readily. There is good correlation between this and anaesthetic potency.

Different parts of the nervous system have different sensitivities and, luckily, the respiratory centre is less sensitive.

Induction agents

These are intravenous drugs. They are usually used to start anaesthesia although a gas induction is sometimes used, especially for children. *Propofol* is the usual agent but barbiturates such as *thiopental* may be used occasionally.

Induction agents are short acting and anaesthesia may be continued using inhalation anaesthetics. TIVA is increasingly used with *propofol*.

Total intravenous anaesthesia

This has developed alongside improving syringe pump technology. The newer agent, *propofol*, can be used for both induction and maintenance and has allowed TIVA to develop beyond its use in cardiac and neurosurgery. TIVA is now used in a wide range of surgical procedures including day surgery. It has the added advantage of avoiding environmental pollution from volatile agents.

Propofol

First used in 1977 but not released for general use until 1986. It is used for induction and maintenance of anaesthesia and sedation of ventilated patients receiving intensive care. It is notable for quick induction (20−30 seconds) and quick recovery (4 minutes) from a single dose.

- Mechanism of action was thought to be a reduction in the time of opening of sodium channels and potentiation of the GABA-A receptor by slowing channel closing time. The CB receptor may also be involved in its action.
- Very rapidly redistributed into peripheral tissues and the effects wear off within a few minutes.
- It can be used as a continuous intravenous infusion to provide longer periods of anaesthesia or low dose to sedate patients for hours or days in intensive care.
- Recovery from its effects is more rapid and complete than from any of the other induction agents. It is therefore used for short procedures and in day surgery.
- Does not cause sickness and so an antiemetic is not required.
- It is not analgesic.
- It causes more hypoventilation, apnoea and hypotension than any other induction agent.

Unwanted effects

- Fall in blood pressure and bradycardia.
- Occasionally bradycardia is profound and administration of an anti-muscarinic may be necessary to prevent this.
- Respiratory depression leading to apnoea is common.
- Excitation of the CNS with dystonic movements in about 10% of patients.

Not recommended for sedation in a child under 17 as it has been associated with potentially fatal bradycardia and metabolic acidosis.

Etomidate

Imidazole derivative that is metabolized more rapidly than *thiopental* or *methohexitone*. It also causes no pain on injection and involuntary movements.

It has minimal effect on blood pressure and for this reason may be used in patients with cardiac problems. It is not commonly used as it inhibits the production of glucocorticoids and has been associated with increased mortality in septic patients in intensive care.

Ketamine

This is unique among the induction agents as it stimulates rather than depresses the cardiovascular and respiratory systems. It also provides profound analgesia at sub-anaesthetic doses. It is used as a recreational drug as it produces dissociation anaesthesia with a dreamlike state and hallucinations.

Mechanism of action

It is antagonistic at the excitatory *N*-methyl-*D*-aspartate (NMDA) receptor in the CNS and does not appear to have an effect on the GABA receptor.

Interacts with opioids and blocks the μ receptor but is an agonist at the κ and δ receptors.

Effects

- Cardiovascular — stimulates the sympathetic nervous system and increases levels of adrenaline (epinephrine) and noradrenaline (norepinephrine) in the bloodstream. Heart rate, cardiac output and blood pressure all increase but without precipitating arrhythmias.
- Respiratory — rate may be increased and muscle tone is maintained. Often able to maintain own airway despite being unconscious but sometimes increased muscle tone in the jaw may obstruct the airway. Is also a bronchodilator which is useful in those with asthma.
- CNS — has potent analgesic activity and produces dissociation anaesthesia. The patient looks dreamy and is half awake but is unaware of surroundings and is free from pain.
- During recovery nightmares and hallucinations, referred to as emergence phenomena, are common. These limit its use but are less in children and the elderly and if the patient is left to recover quietly.
- Nausea and vomiting are more common than with *propofol* or *thiopental*.
- Can be given intramuscularly as well as intravenously.

Barbiturates — thiopental

First used in 1934 and still in widespread use. *Thiopental* increases the opening of GABA-mediated chloride channels inducing hyperpolarization and neuronal inhibition.

Unconsciousness occurs about 20 seconds after injection and continues for 5–10 minutes. Termination of action occurs as the drug is redistributed away from the brain into other tissues, especially muscle or fat.

- Although it only has a half-life of 2–3 minutes in the plasma its residual effects can be prolonged due to redistribution in the tissues from where it can slowly re-enter the blood and make the patient drowsy.
- After equilibration its half-life is about 8 hours.
- This means that it is metabolized very slowly, over several hours, and so cannot be used as a continuous intravenous infusion as it would accumulate and lead to prolonged sleepiness or unconsciousness when discontinued.
- It causes a drop in blood pressure mainly due to a reduction in peripheral resistance but a marked fall in blood pressure may occur if the dose is too large or the patient has cardiovascular system (CVS) comorbidities.
- Extravasation causes sloughing of the dermis and epidermis.

Inhalational anaesthetics

Nitrous oxide, isoflurane, sevoflurane, desflurane

These are gases or volatile liquids given with oxygen to prevent hypoxia during anaesthesia. They can be used for induction and maintenance of anaesthesia.

Nitrous oxide is not potent enough to be used alone following induction but is used in combination as it produces analgesia and allows lower doses of other drugs to be used.

Mechanism of action

Although forms of inhalation anaesthesia have been used for over 150 years their mode of action is still only partially understood.

- Over a century ago a link between potency and lipid solubility was demonstrated and there appears to be a link between the ability of the drug to dissolve in the neuronal cell membrane and anaesthesia.
- Theories linked this action to an effect on ion channels – perhaps sodium or potassium channels.
- Recent research links anaesthetic agents to interference with neurotransmitters such as glutamate and GABA, either decreasing excitatory transmission or increasing inhibitory transmission.

Entonox

Consists of a 50:50 mixture of nitrous oxide and oxygen. It is used for analgesia in prehospital care, painful procedures and in labour. Can be controlled by the patient using a demand valve.

It is dangerous if there is a pneumothorax as it diffuses into the space, increasing the pneumothorax and compromising respiration.

The ideal inhalational anaesthetic

Should be stable to heat and light, inert in the anaesthetic machine, not explosive or flammable and have a pleasant odour. It needs to be nontoxic, to affect only the CNS, not cause seizures and have some analgesic properties. Modern agents do have many, but not all, of these properties.

Muscle relaxants

These are neuromuscular blocking drugs and block the effects of acetylcholine at the neuromuscular junction. This causes paralysis of skeletal muscle.

- They also relax the vocal cords allowing an endotracheal tube to be passed.
- Assisted respiration is needed as the respiratory muscles are also paralysed.
- Great care must be taken that the patient is fully anaesthetized and so is unaware of the ongoing surgery. They cannot move or communicate even if they are awake and able to feel pain.
- The effects of competitive, non-depolarizing muscle relaxants may be allowed to wear off spontaneously but this can be made to occur more rapidly by the use of anticholinesterases such as *neostigmine*. *Glycopyrronium bromide* is used with *neostigmine* to prevent other anticholinesterase (antimuscarinic) effects such as bradycardia.
- *Sugammadex* is a newer reversal agent that makes possible full reversal but does not inhibit acetylcholinesterase so cholinergic effects are not produced and it is not necessary to give glycopyrronium. It renders *rocuronium* and *vecuronium* inactive by encapsulating the molecules but is short acting.
- Depolarizing muscle relaxants (*suxamethonium*) cannot be overcome with drugs.

The mechanism of action of individual drugs is discussed in Section 2.3.

Sedative drugs used pre- or perioperatively

Drugs may be used to allay anxiety preoperatively and may also provide preoperative amnesia. *Benzodiazepines* are commonly used for these purposes but it must be remembered that they are not analgesic and an opioid analgesic may be required for pain relief.

Benzodiazepines are also used in intensive care for sedation, especially *midazolam*.

Lorazepam or *temazepam* may be used occasionally as premedication prior to theatre.

Opioid analgesics

These are often administered at induction of anaesthesia and may be given in small doses throughout the procedure, especially for painful procedures. They may be continued as postoperative analgesia. The drugs are described in Section 3.2.

Alfentanil and *fentanyl* act within 1−2 minutes and have a short duration of action if used as a single dose. *Remifentanil* is often used as an infusion to provide analgesia intraoperatively.

Section 4

Central nervous system

Section Outline

4.1 CENTRAL NERVOUS SYSTEM — OVERVIEW

This is an important and complex section of the book and includes sections on:

- chemical transmission in the brain
- epilepsy
- Parkinson's disease (PD)
- Alzheimer's disease (AD)
- anxiolytics and hypnotics
- antidepressants
- antipsychotics — schizophrenia and mania.

Our complex nervous system differentiates us from other species on the planet. Drugs that affect the central nervous system (CNS) are important not only therapeutically but also because they are frequently taken for nonmedical reasons; for example, caffeine, alcohol, cannabis, nicotine, opiates. Understanding how the brain functions is more difficult than other organs in the body and not so easily researched. Many drugs have been used for their effects without understanding how they actually achieved these. Translating action at the cellular level to effects on whole-brain function is difficult and often unpredictable; many diseases that affect the brain are still not understood in terms of their biochemical origins. Diagnosis is difficult when a disorder affects the mind; depression is one example where diagnosis is based on symptoms rather than causative factors or laboratory tests.

Section 4.2 describes chemical transmission in the brain and is the foundation for your increased understanding of the action of all drugs on the CNS.

A Nurse's Survival Guide to Drugs in Practice. https://doi.org/10.1016/B978-0-7020-7658-9.00004-4

4.2 CHEMICAL TRANSMISSION IN THE BRAIN

Chemicals released within the brain produce many diverse effects.

- Some neurotransmitters are excitatory and increase activity; others are inhibitory.
- Effects may be immediate or may result in slow changes and neuromodulation.
- The 'wiring' within the brain is extremely complex and this means that the effects of increasing or decreasing certain neurotransmitters are unpredictable.
- If we increase the levels of a neurotransmitter this often results in decreased synthesis of the transmitter or a decrease in receptors for the transmitter, but this takes time.
- The full effects of some antidepressants take weeks to develop and are likely to involve an adaptive response of some kind. However, side effects often occur immediately. This means there is a primary response to the drug and a secondary one that takes much longer. It is often the secondary response that is the therapeutic one.
- Dependence on opiates or alcohol is also a gradual process.

Psychotropic drugs

These are drugs that affect mood and behaviour. Some have been covered elsewhere in this book. They are classified in many different ways and include:

- anaesthetic agents (see Section 3.4)
- anxiolytics and sedatives, including hypnotics and minor tranquilizers; cause sleep and reduce anxiety (e.g. *diazepam*)
- antipsychotic drugs sometimes called *neuroleptics* or *major tranquilizers;* used to relieve symptoms of schizophrenia (e.g. *chlorpromazine*)
- antidepressant drugs that relieve symptoms of depression (e.g. *fluoxetine*)
- analgesic drugs used to relieve pain (e.g. *morphine*) (see Section 3.2)
- psychostimulants that cause wakefulness and euphoria (e.g. **amfetamines**)
- hallucinogens (psychotomimetic drugs) that cause a disturbance in perception (often visual hallucinations) and behaviour (e.g. *lysergic acid diethylamide [LSD]*)
- cognition enhancers that improve memory (e.g. *rivastigmine*).

Neurotransmitters in the central nervous system

The binding of transmitter activates changes in the postsynaptic membrane. At some synapses this encourages the production of impulses in the postsynaptic axon and this is *excitation*. In others the binding may discourage the production of impulses and this is *inhibition*.

- Glutamate is the main excitatory amino acid (EAA) transmitter and is found throughout the CNS in higher concentrations than in other tissues.
- Gamma-aminobutyric acid (GABA) and glycine are the main inhibitory neurotransmitters.
- All are synthesized from glucose in the Kreb's cycle using pathways that are interlinked.
- Other important transmitters include acetylcholine, dopamine, serotonin and noradrenaline.

Glutamate and N-methyl-D-aspartate receptors

EAAs were only discovered in the 1970s and our understanding of them is still not complete.

There are four main subtypes of EAA receptor: (1) *N*-methyl-D-aspartate (NMDA); (2) alpha-amino-3-hydroxy-5-methyl-4-isoxazolepropionic acid (AMPA); (3) kainite; and (4) metabotropic.

The NMDA receptor has been studied in much detail and actually requires glycine as well as glutamate to stimulate it.

- Stimulation promotes Ca^{2+} entry.
- Receptors blocked by Mg^{2+}.
- Some anaesthetic and hallucinogenic substances (e.g. *ketamine*) block the ion channel of the NMDA receptor.

Possible clinical uses

- *Ketamine* (see Section 3.4) as an analgesic and anaesthetic and *memantine* in AD are in clinical use.
- It is thought that blocking glutamate receptors would reduce brain damage following strokes and head injuries; this is disappointing so far and drugs tend to be hallucinatory.
- Control of epilepsy.
- Investigated for treatment of drug dependence and schizophrenia.

Inhibitory neurotransmission

GABA is the main inhibitory neurotransmitter in the brain. Glycine is important in the brain stem and spinal cord.

- GABA is found in the brain but not in other tissues.
- Synthesized from glutamate by the action of an enzyme.

- Destroyed by chemical breakdown using the enzyme *GABA transaminase*. This enzyme is inhibited by **vigabatrin** (used in epilepsy), thus allowing inhibitory GABA to accumulate.
- Acts on two types of receptor: $GABA_A$ and $GABA_B$
- $GABA_A$ increases Cl^- permeability and this hyperpolarizes the cell, reducing its excitability.
- $GABA_B$ inhibits calcium channels and opens potassium channels, reducing excitability.
- **Baclofen** is a selective inhibitor at the $GABA_B$ receptor and is a muscle relaxant that inhibits spasticity.
- **Strychnine** is a convulsant that is a glycine antagonist.
- Tetanus toxin causes hyperexcitability of the nervous system by interfering with glycine release.

$GABA_A$ receptors

Drugs may act at more than one site on the receptor including the GABA binding site, the ion channel and several modulatory sites.

Drugs acting on this receptor include benzodiazepines, barbiturates, alcohol and some anaesthetics.

Benzodiazepines (e.g. **diazepam**) increase the effects of GABA by binding to a site on the receptor and making GABA binding easier. They have powerful anxiolytic and sedatory actions.

Amine transmitters

These include noradrenaline (norepinephrine), dopamine, 5-hydroxytryptamine (5-HT, serotonin) and acetylcholine.

Noradrenaline (norepinephrine)
- Mostly released from an area in the pons (part of the brain stem) called the *locus coeruleus.*
- Neurones here are silent during sleep and activity increases with arousal.
- Drugs that increase noradrenaline (norepinephrine) release in the brain (e.g. **amfetamines**) increase wakefulness and alertness.
- Mood and state of arousal are linked. In depression there is usually reduced response to surroundings.
- Early theories were that depression is due to reduced adrenergic activity but now serotonin levels are thought to be more important in governing mood.
- Many early antidepressants interfered with the re-uptake (tricyclic anti-depressants [TCAs]) or breakdown (monoamine oxidase inhibitors [MAOIs]) of noradrenaline (norepinephrine).

Dopamine

- An important neurotransmitter within the brain that is mostly involved in reward-motivated behaviour and motor control. Dysfunction of the dopamine system is involved in important disorders such as PD, schizophrenia, drug dependency and attention deficit disorder.
- Synthesized, like noradrenaline (norepinephrine), from the amino acid tyrosine. It is produced by dopaminergic neurons in the mid-brain in the substantia nigra and ventral tegmental area and in the hypothalamus; it is metabolized using enzymes.
- There are several distinct dopamine pathways within the brain, one of which plays a large role in the motivation for reward-motivated behaviour.
- Found in the *corpus striatum* in the brain, part of the basal ganglia, and concerned with coordination of movement; it is found in the *limbic system* and the *hypothalamus.*
- Different dopamine pathways are involved in motor control (nigrostriatal pathway), behaviour (mesolimbic system) and endocrine control (hypothalamic).
- Dopamine is important in emotion formation and processing, learning and memory. It is released in pleasurable situations and associated with arousal. It is involved in the detection of pleasurable smells too and plays a role in addiction. The anticipation of most types of reward increases the release of dopamine. Many addictive drugs increase dopamine release or block its reuptake. Dopamine binds to five different subtypes of receptor in the brain, known as: D_1, D_2, D_3, D_4 and D_5.
- Different subtypes are found in different areas; for example, D_3 and D_4 are found in the limbic system where overactivity is important in schizophrenia; D_1 and D_2 are found in the corpus striatum where reduced activity results in PD.
- Often the effects of drugs on the subgroups of the receptor cannot be separated, so drugs used to antagonize dopamine receptors in schizophrenia produce parkinsonian side effects.
- Effects of excess dopamine on behaviour are stereotyped behaviour patterns, and induced by dopamine agonists such as ***apomorphine*** and drugs causing dopamine release (e.g. ***amfetamines***).
- Dopamine acts on the chemoreceptor trigger zone (CTZ) to cause nausea and vomiting.

Serotonin (5-HT)

In 1953 it was found that LSD, a powerful hallucinogen, was a serotonin antagonist in the peripheries, and serotonin was found in the brain a few years later.

- Synthesis, release and metabolism are similar to noradrenaline (norepinephrine). It is made from tryptophan, an amino acid found in the diet, and following release is taken back up into the neurone by re-uptake. Metabolism is by monoamine oxidase.

- Re-uptake can be inhibited by some of the same drugs that block re-uptake of noradrenaline (norepinephrine) (e.g. TCAs).
- There are also **selective serotonin re-uptake inhibitors (SSRIs)** (e.g. *fluoxetine*), which only block the re-uptake of serotonin and not noradrenaline (norepinephrine) and are antidepressants.
- There are many subtypes of serotonin receptor identified so this is a very complex system.
- The neurones containing serotonin have a similar distribution in the brain to noradrenergic neurones.

Functions related to serotonin include:

- behavioural changes and hallucinations; some hallucinogens are agonists and many antipsychotics are antagonists
- mood
- sleep and wakefulness; depletion of serotonin experimentally in animals abolishes sleep whereas its injection into areas of the brain stem induces sleep
- eating behaviour: SSRIs reduce appetite and some antipsychotic antagonists cause increased appetite and weight gain; however, stimulation of some serotonin receptors in animals increases eating and weight gain
- control of sensory transmission, especially pain pathways. The ability to ignore irrelevant sensory input appears dependent upon serotonin pathways in the brain. Drugs that are hallucinogens may block this and so heighten sensory perception. Serotonin appears to inhibit pain transmission and drugs that inhibit re-uptake are used alongside other forms of analgesia in pain control
- a possible role in the regulation of blood pressure, body temperature and sexual function.

Clinical uses
- Serotonin re-uptake inhibitors (e.g. *fluoxetine*) are used to treat depression.
- Antagonists at the 5-HT$_3$ receptors are antiemetics (e.g. **ondansetron**).
- **Buspirone** is an agonist at the 5-HT$_{1A}$ receptor and is used to treat anxiety.
- Treatment of migraine: **sumatriptan** is a 5-HT$_{1D}$ agonist.
- Some antipsychotic drugs (e.g. **clozapine**) act on 5-HT as well as dopamine receptors.

Acetylcholine
Mainly excitatory effects in the CNS mediated by both nicotinic and muscarinic receptors (see Section 2.3).

Functions of cholinergic pathways are related to memory, learning, arousal and motor control. Muscarinic antagonists (e.g. *scopolamine*) cause amnesia. Dementia and PD are associated with abnormalities in cholinergic transmission.

Other transmitters in the central nervous system

Include adenosine, adenosine triphosphate (ATP) and histamine.

Adenosine is mainly inhibitory, causing drowsiness. Caffeine, an antagonist at the adenosine (A_2) receptor, is a CNS stimulant.

In future, adenosine agonists may be useful in epilepsy, sleep disorders and pain. They inhibit excitability of neurones and may reduce ischaemic damage in the brain.

Some antihistamines (H_1 receptor antagonists) cross the blood–brain barrier (BBB) and cause sleepiness (e.g. *chlorpheniramine*).

4.3 EPILEPSY

Epilepsy itself is not a disease but a tendency to have recurrent seizures (also known as fits) with little or no provocation. Even today, with all our advanced technology, it is still not completely understood.

- A seizure is caused by bursts of excessive electrical activity within the brain triggered by abnormal neuronal discharges. It occurs suddenly and may range from a brief lapse of attention to a full-blown convulsive fit lasting for several minutes.
- The site of primary neuronal discharge and the extent of spread within the brain determine the symptoms produced.
- Abnormal electrical activity can be detected by an electroencephalogram (EEG).
- Epilepsy affects more than 500,000 people in the UK. Often there is no recognizable cause and the origin may be complex.

Some causes of seizures

- Head injury.
- CNS infection (e.g. meningitis, encephalitis).
- Brain tumour.
- Brain damage: could be birth trauma or hypoxia.
- Cerebral palsy.
- Stroke.
- Drugs and alcohol.
- Metabolic disturbance (e.g. hypoglycaemia).
- Hormonal changes.

- No known cause in about 50% of cases of epilepsy. There is probably a genetic component in many cases.

Types of seizure

- May be partial (focal) or generalized.
- Partial seizures start in one area of the brain and may either remain there or spread throughout the brain, becoming generalized.
- Generalized seizures affect the whole brain resulting in loss of consciousness.
- There are also febrile convulsions in children with a high temperature.
- Pseudoseizures are seizures of behavioural or psychological origin.
- Status epilepticus is a medical emergency where a prolonged seizure or repeated seizures without recovery of consciousness occurs (Table 4.1).

In someone with epilepsy, individual seizures may be caused by:

- forgotten or incorrect medication
- lack of sleep
- stress or excitement
- boredom
- alcohol
- flashing lights (only 3%—5% of people with epilepsy are photosensitive)
- drugs.

TABLE 4.1 Common types of seizure.

Seizure type	Characteristics
Partial (focal)	
Simple	Consciousness not impaired. May be motor or sensory
Complex	Temporal lobe, psychomotor. Some impairment of consciousness
Secondary generalized	Begin as partial and spread
Generalized	Affects the whole brain with loss of consciousness
Tonic—clonic (grand mal)	Tonic phase: fall to ground with a sudden rigid extensor spasm of muscles, breathing stops (cyanosis occurs), pass urine and salivate; followed by clonic phase with violent jerking
Atonic	Fall to ground with loss of muscle strength
Myoclonic	Sudden jerking of limbs
Absence (petit mal)	Mainly in children. Cause vacant staring for a few seconds without movement disorder. May happen many times a day

Aim of drug therapy in epilepsy

- To keep the patient free from seizures.
- To give a drug as free from side effects as possible.
- To use only one antiepileptic drug if possible, but approximately 30% of patients will continue to have seizures on monotherapy.
- To encourage compliance by giving once-daily drugs where possible.

Drug therapy in epilepsy is highly specific, and different types of seizures respond to different drugs. A drug used to control one type of seizure may potentiate another; for example, *carbamazepine* used in generalized seizures can exacerbate absence seizures.

All anticonvulsants have a low therapeutic index, so the dose has to be the lowest that will keep the patient seizure free. It is usual to start on a low dose and increase if necessary.

Mechanism of action of antiepileptic (anticonvulsant) drugs

The mechanism of action of all anticonvulsants is not clearly understood but seizures are likely to be due to an increase in an excitatory neurotransmitter or a decrease in an inhibitory transmitter (see Section 4.2). Drugs that inhibit the inhibitory neurotransmitter GABA cause convulsions to occur when used experimentally, and antagonists of the EAA, glutamate, suppress the propagation of seizure activity.

Drugs in use today have three main mechanisms of action, described below.

Enhancement of gamma-aminobutyric acid action

- May bind to GABA receptors (e.g. benzodiazepines and barbiturates). This facilitates the opening of chloride ion channels and therefore hyperpolarizes the membrane, making the neurone less excitable. *Diazepam* is used in emergencies and may be given intravenously.
- May increase GABA release or decrease removal (*gabapentin*).
- May inhibit the destruction of GABA by the enzyme *GABA transaminase* (*vigabatrin*).

Blockade of sodium channels

- Sodium entry is needed for an action potential to occur.
- The drugs block sodium channels of cells that are firing too frequently but do not affect normal cells.
- Many early drugs, and some new ones, block sodium entry (e.g. *carbamazepine, sodium valproate, phenytoin, lamotrigine*).

Blockade of calcium channels

- Calcium will also increase excitability in the neurone; thus blockade of calcium channels will reduce neuronal firing.
- The only drug that works by this method is *ethosuximide*, which is used in absence seizures.

At present there are over 20 different medications for epilepsy licensed in the UK (Table 4.2). They are divided into first-generation drugs (e.g. *phenytoin, carbamazepine, phenobarbital* and *valproate*) and second-generation drugs (e.g. *lamotrigine, vigabatrin, felbamate* and *topiramate*).

Drug interactions

Antiepileptic drugs often have an effect on the liver enzymes that metabolize other drugs and may increase enzyme activity, thus increasing metabolism of the drug, or may inhibit the activity, thus potentiating the action of the drug. They may also interact with other antiepileptics and the interaction is often unpredictable and varies between patients. Details of these interactions are given in the British National Formulary (BNF).

Withdrawal of drugs

Antiepileptic drugs should not be stopped suddenly or there may be rebound seizures. The dose needs to be reduced gradually, and if a new drug is to be started, the old drug should only be withdrawn when the new regimen is established.

TABLE 4.2 Drugs commonly used in epilepsy.

Seizure type	First-line drugs
Tonic–clonic	Carbamazepine
	Lamotrigine
	Sodium valproate
	Topiramate
Absence	Ethosuximide
	Sodium valproate
	Lamotrigine
Myoclonic	Sodium valproate
Atonic	Lamotrigine
	Sodium valproate

Some patients do successfully have their medication withdrawn and remain free from seizures but if the patient is taking several drugs, they should be withdrawn one drug at a time.

This is a difficult decision if the patient wants to drive as they must be seizure free for a period of 1 year to drive a car. Specific guidance is available from the Driver and Vehicle Licensing Agency (DVLA).

Medicines and Healthcare Products Regulatory Agency guidance on generic prescribing

In 2017 the Medicines and Healthcare products Regulatory Agency (MHRA) reviewed spontaneous adverse reactions and reported possible harm from switching patients stabilized on a specific branded drug to a generic. There appeared to be loss of seizure control around the switching between products in some patients. This may be linked to the switch. Advice on this issue is available in the BNF.

Antiepileptic hypersensitivity syndrome

This is a rare but potentially fatal syndrome associated with some antiepileptic drugs (e.g. carbamazepine, lamotrigine, phenytoin; please refer to the BNF for a full list). Symptoms usually occur 1−8 weeks after starting the drug and include fever, a rash and swollen lymph glands. The drug should be stopped immediately and expert advice sought as liver dysfunction, vasculitis and multiorgan failure may follow.

Pregnancy

There is an increased risk of congenital malformations with many anticonvulsants.

- Risk is less if only one drug is used.
- The doctor will decide if the risk of convulsions is greater than the potential risks of therapy.
- The woman should be informed of any increased risks and offered extra antenatal screening.
- Guidance for the use of valproate was published by the National Institute for Health and Care Excellence (NICE) in 2019. This drug should not be used in pregnancy due to the risk of birth defects, including spina bifida and face and skull malformations. It should be avoided in women of childbearing age.
- Guidance on the diagnosis and management of epilepsy is published by NICE (updated in 2020). This is available on their website at www.nice.org.uk.

Some individual drugs

Carbamazepine

Derived from the tricyclic antidepressant drugs when found in routine screening to reduce convulsions.

- Action is similar to phenytoin and blocks the sodium channels so reducing excitability of the neurones. It is particularly effective in complex partial seizures (e.g. psychomotor epilepsy).
- Used in partial and generalized seizures (except absence seizures).
- Used also in trigeminal neuralgia and other neuropathic pain.
- May be used to control mood swings in bipolar disorder unresponsive to lithium.

Side effects

- Drowsiness, dizziness and ataxia in about 50% of patients.
- May cause fluid retention and a variety of gastrointestinal and cardiovascular effects.
- Occasionally severe hypersensitivity − suppression of the bone marrow.
- Accelerates metabolism of many other drugs.

Ethosuximide

- Used in absence seizures but has little or no effect against most other types of epilepsy and can precipitate tonic−clonic seizures in susceptible individuals.
- Blocks calcium channels and inhibits neuronal firing in absence seizures.
- Given as syrup.
- Side effects include nausea, vomiting, anorexia and drowsiness.

Gabapentin

- Structurally related to GABA but does not work by acting on GABA receptors. May inhibit calcium channels.
- Is add-on therapy and not so effective on its own.
- Used for neuropathic pain as well.
- Does not bind to plasma proteins or induce liver enzymes, and does not interact with other antiepileptic drugs or reduce the efficacy of oral contraceptives.
- Does not appear to be teratogenic in animal studies.
- Has been associated with a rare risk of severe respiratory depression.
- Patients with impaired renal function should have a smaller dose, and patients with diabetes may notice their blood sugar levels fluctuating.

- May cause drowsiness, dizziness, fatigue and tremor.
  Needs to be given three times daily and this is a disadvantage.

Lamotrigine

Inhibits the release of glutamate and EAAs by inhibiting sodium channels. Aims to restore the balance between excitatory and inhibitory neurotransmitters in the brain.

- Wide spectrum of activity and is effective in partial and tonic–clonic seizures.
- Licensed for monotherapy but can be used with other drugs.
- Not teratogenic in animal studies and does not interact with oral contraceptives.
- May be less sedating than other anticonvulsants.

Side effects

- Occasionally blurred vision, nausea, dizziness and ataxia.
- Has been associated with severe skin reactions and hypersensitivity syndrome (see above). Usually occur in first 8 weeks, and patients should be warned to go to the doctor if they develop a rash.
- Occasionally bone marrow failure is reported.
- Does interact with other anticonvulsants, including *valproate, phenytoin* and *carbamazepine.*

Levetiracetam

Used as adjunctive treatment of partial seizures. Mechanism of action unsure but may increase GABA activity or suppress NMDA receptors from firing in response to glutamate.
   Side effects include nausea, diarrhoea, drowsiness, fatigue and dizziness.

Phenobarbital (phenobarbitone)

A barbiturate drug that has greater anticonvulsant action than other barbiturates and causes less drowsiness.
   It was first used as an anticonvulsant in 1912 and, even today, its mechanism of action is not fully understood.

- It enhances the effect of GABA by binding to a site on the GABA receptor channel. The site is different to the site for GABA itself and to the benzodiazepine site, which is also here.
- Does cause some drowsiness at levels needed for seizure control. This is a large drawback and the drug is rarely used except in cases where the seizures are difficult to control.

- Can be used in all forms of epilepsy except absence seizures and is available by injection for status epilepticus.
- **Primidone** (**Mysoline**) is a drug that is converted to phenobarbital by the body. It is occasionally used in epilepsy and may be used in essential tremor.

Phenytoin (Epanutin)

First used in 1935 and stabilizes the cell membrane, preventing excess transmission and decreasing excitability of the neurones.

Used to be the most widely used drug but newer drugs are now preferred due to its side effects and unpredictable metabolism.

- Blocks sodium channels and has some local anaesthetic and antiarrhythmic properties.
- Inhibits calcium entry into the cell and has an effect on the sodium pump.
- It is suitable for partial and generalized convulsions but not absence seizures.
- Causes an increased rate of metabolism of some other drugs (e.g. anticoagulants).
- Metabolism is unpredictable and plasma concentrations vary widely between patients receiving the same dosage. Plasma concentrations are monitored to assist adjustment of dosage.
- Can be affected by the administration of other drugs in an unpredictable manner. It is 80%–90% bound to plasma albumin and there is competition with some other drugs for protein-binding sites. This may increase the level of free drug.

Side effects

Related to plasma concentration.

Mild – vertigo, ataxia, headache, nystagmus. Not sedation.

Larger doses – marked confusion and mental deterioration occur.

- Hyperplasia of the gums, acne and hirsutism occur gradually. Probably due to increased androgen secretion.
- Megaloblastic anaemia associated with folate lack can occur.
- Hypersensitivity reactions, especially skin rashes, are common.
- May cause increased fetal abnormalities and is especially linked to cleft palate.

Sodium valproate

Chemically unrelated to any other epileptic drug.

Discovered quite accidentally in 1963 to have anticonvulsant properties in mice.

It is effective in all kinds of epilepsy and licensed for use in all forms of epilepsy.

Has multiple actions but each contribution to anticonvulsant activity is not understood.

- Sodium channel blockade stabilizes the neuronal membrane. This may be the most important action.
- It also causes a rise in the amount of GABA in the brain. It not only weakly inhibits two enzyme systems that breakdown GABA but also enhances GABA synthesis and release.
- Reduces the excitatory effects of glutamate.
- Inhibits calcium channels.

Well absorbed orally and has a half-life of 15 hours. May take several weeks for the full benefits of treatment to be felt. Can also be used as a mood stabilizer in bipolar depressive illness, in neuropathic pain and in the prophylaxis of migraine.

Side effects

- Compared with many epileptic drugs, it has few side effects. These include nausea, vomiting, abdominal pain and bowel disturbance. The tablets should be taken with food.
- Causes thinning of the hair in about 10% of those taking it.
- Stimulates appetite; therefore it may cause weight gain.
- Tremor, confusion and ataxia.
- Most serious side effect is hepatotoxicity (rare) usually in the first 6 months and more commonly in children. A few cases have been fatal and liver function tests should be done before therapy and for the first 6 months.
- Highly teratogenic with a 30%–40% risk of neural tube defects (BNF, 2019) and a 10% increase in congenital malformations. Not given in pregnancy and not used in women of childbearing age unless with foolproof contraception and under the guidance of a specialist.
- Inhibits liver metabolizing enzymes; therefore it may interact with other antiepileptic drugs.

Tiagabine

Inhibits neuronal uptake of GABA in the brain; therefore it increases the duration of action.

Used in partial seizures.

Topiramate

Mechanism of action is not fully understood.

Licensed as monotherapy in partial and generalized seizures (not absence).

May also be used as migraine prophylaxis.

Side effects include an association with the development of acute glaucoma, usually within 1 month of starting the drug.

Vigabatrin

- Inhibits the breakdown of GABA in the brain by inhibiting the enzyme *GABA transaminase* irreversibly. This means it has a long action and can be administered once daily.
- It is initiated by a specialist when the epilepsy is resistant to other treatments.

Side effects

- Drowsiness, fatigue, gastric upsets, ataxia, tremor.
- Psychoses and depression have occurred.
- Associated with visual field defects.

Zonisamide

- Used as monotherapy for focal seizures and adjunctive treatment for refractory partial seizures.

Benzodiazepines

These drugs act as GABA inducers by binding to the GABA channel.

Diazepam is excellent to use in status epilepticus as it acts very quickly, but causes too much drowsiness to be used as a normal anticonvulsant. *Lorazepam* is also used.

Clonazepam and *clobazam* are occasionally used but cause drowsiness, and their effectiveness may wane after several weeks of continuous treatment.

Convulsive status epilepticus

Most seizures do not last more than 2 minutes. Status epilepticus is when a seizure lasts more than 5 minutes or two or more sequential seizures occur without recovering consciousness between the seizures. Also, it can be when a person has repeated seizures for 30 minutes or longer. It is a medical emergency that needs rapid treatment and early hospitalization. The longer a seizure lasts, the less likely recovery will occur without medication.

Immediate measures include positioning the patient to avoid injury and providing oxygen.

- Intravenous benzodiazepines are used as first line, especially *lorazepam* as it has a longer duration of action than diazepam and carries less risk of thrombophlebitis. *Diazemuls* is an emulsion that reduces the risk of venous thromboembolism associated with intravenous *diazepam*. Absorption from suppositories is too slow in status epilepticus.

- A single dose of *midazolam* (unlicensed use) is sometimes also used by the buccal route or intravenously.
- If seizures fail to respond in 30 minutes, *phenytoin* may be given by slow intravenous injection.
- If these measures fail, anaesthesia with *thiopental* may be used or *propofol* in adults and the patient transferred to the intensive care unit.
- If alcohol abuse is suspected *thiamine* is given and *pyridoxine* also may be administered if there is a deficiency.
- Nonconvulsive status epilepticus is treated depending on the severity of the patient's condition. EEG testing may be needed to confirm this diagnosis. The patient may have complete loss of awareness.

4.4 ANTIPSYCHOTICS

These are drugs used in the treatment of schizophrenia. We have already seen that understanding how drugs work in the CNS is more complex than in any other system because of the complexity of the brain and its functioning. Disorders of brain functioning are usually due to a fault in the neurotransmission process and this is also true in the case of schizophrenia.

The biochemical changes in the brain in schizophrenia are still not understood.

- *Amfetamine* releases dopamine in the brain and produces behaviour indistinguishable from acute schizophrenia.
- All drugs used in the treatment of schizophrenia are dopamine antagonists.
- These facts have led to the *dopamine theory* of schizophrenia.
- Currently glutamate is another neurotransmitter that is being investigated.
- Antagonists of NMDA (glutamate) receptors such as *ketamine* produce psychotic symptoms.

Schizophrenia

Schizophrenia is a psychosis that is characterized by delusions, hallucinations and a lack of insight. It affects about 1% of people during their lifetime and occurs equally in men and women. It usually begins in adolescence or early adulthood and less than 20% of people make a full recovery after the first psychotic episode, which may be triggered by stress. There is some genetic component, involving small contributions from many genes.

The disease may follow a remitting and relapsing course or be chronic and progressive, especially if it has late onset.

Drug treatment, and family or cognitive therapies are the main approaches in preventing a relapse and antipsychotics may need to be taken over a long period or even for life.

Most chronic diseases are managed with drugs rather than cured by them and this is the case in psychiatry. Some psychiatric drugs can compensate for chemical abnormalities in the brain, but they cannot cure them.

The aim is to increase the quality of life for the sufferer and to improve both cognitive and social functioning.

Symptoms of schizophrenia

Symptoms are classified into positive and negative:

1. Positive symptoms include:
   - delusions, often paranoid in nature
   - hallucinations, usually in the form of voices that are heard outside the head and may direct the person's actions
   - thought disorder – wild trains of thought with irrational conclusions, often associated with the feeling that thoughts are inserted or withdrawn by others.
2. Negative symptoms may occur in chronic schizophrenia and include:
   - withdrawal from social contacts
   - a flattening of emotional responses.

The patient with acute schizophrenia usually needs admission to hospital as they are unaware that they are ill and may refuse medication. They can be a danger to themselves or others.

A change in behaviour signifies a change in brain chemistry and a person develops a mental illness when the brain chemistry changes in such a way as to affect his/her ability to function well.

- The goal of drug treatment is to modify the brain's chemical reactions to produce good health and to prevent relapse.
- When drugs reach the brain, they alter the chemical reactions occurring there. The drugs that are used in schizophrenia are all antagonists of the neurotransmitter dopamine.

Drugs used in schizophrenia

The drugs used are antipsychotics, sometimes called *neuroleptics* or *major tranquilizers*. They may also be used short term to alleviate acute anxiety and to control acute behavioural disturbance.

- Before the 1950s no drug treatment was available to treat schizophrenia and most patients remained hospitalized for long periods. ***Chlorpromazine*** in 1956 was the first drug used and it revolutionized psychiatry.

- Acute schizophrenia usually responds better than chronic, and drugs are less effective for negative symptoms in apathetic, withdrawn patients than for positive symptoms such as thought disorders and hallucinations.
- Long-term treatment is often necessary and withdrawal of the drug has to be done with great caution. A patient may appear well while on medication but suffer a disastrous relapse if treatment is withdrawn. This may be delayed for several weeks after stopping the drug.
- Acceptability is the main factor limiting the use of older conventional drugs as they are associated with high rates of side effects affecting movement (extrapyramidal or parkinsonian).
- There is a constant search for new agents with superior efficacy and fewer side effects. These newer drugs are called *atypical antipsychotics*.
- NICE has issued guidance for the treatment of schizophrenia and this is available on its website.

Mechanism of action

All these drugs work by blocking the effects of dopamine in the brain. They are dopamine antagonists but take 2–3 weeks to be maximally effective even though the dopamine receptor is blocked immediately.

- It is mainly the D_2 receptor that is blocked by older antipsychotic drugs and their affinity for these receptors correlates well with their effectiveness.
- This produces a parkinsonian-like syndrome, increased prolactin secretion and reduced drug and fever-induced vomiting. Some may be used as antiemetics.
- They also have antihistamine and sedative effects and block other receptors including serotonergic, alpha-adrenergic and muscarinic receptors. This causes some of their side effects.
- It was thought for a long time that there were only two types of dopamine receptor: D_1 and D_2. Dopamine binds to both. The D_2 receptor is the one that is blocked by typical antipsychotic drugs. Antipsychotic effects require about 80% of these receptors to be blocked.
- It is now known that there are more types of receptor and atypical drugs such as ***clozapine*** are relatively nonselective between D_1 and D_2 but have a high affinity for the D_4 receptor.

Classification of antipsychotic drugs

More than 20 drugs are available (Box 4.1). The differences between them may be minor.

The important division is between older, first-generation typical drugs and the newer, atypical drugs. They are called atypical as they produce fewer extrapyramidal side effects.

BOX 4.1 Drugs used in schizophrenia.

First generation	Second generation (Atypical)
Chlorpromazine	Clozapine
Fluphenazine	Risperidone
Haloperidol	Sertindole
Flupentixol	Quetiapine
Sulpiride	Aripiprazole
Trifluoperazine	Zotepine

Behavioural effects of antipsychotics

- They depress emotional responsiveness and slow response to external stimuli which is useful in thought disorders and delusional beliefs.
- Have a sedative action that helps to control restlessness and confusion. Patients are easily aroused and can respond to questions normally with no loss of intellectual function.
- Aggressive tendencies are strongly inhibited and drugs produce a state of apathy and reduced initiative.

Other clinically useful effects include an antiemetic action and they may be used as antihistamines in allergic reactions.

Side effects of antipsychotic drugs

Extrapyramidal symptoms

These depend partly on the drug and partly on the dose and are much less with atypical drugs. They do not occur with *clozapine*. They are most frequent with older drugs especially *fluphenazine, trifluoperazine* and *haloperidol*.

The extrapyramidal tract is a complex system of motor nerve pathways involving the basal ganglia of the brain. It is the nerve pathway affected in PD where there is a lack of dopamine in the basal ganglia.

Unfortunately, inhibiting the D_2 receptor also blocks dopamine receptors in the basal ganglia and so causes distressing movement disorders including:

- symptoms resembling those of PD
- acute dystonias (abnormal face and body movements)
- akathisia (restlessness)
- tardive dyskinesia (TD) (rhythmic, involuntary movements of the face and jaw).

All these movement disorders are consistent with blocking the dopaminergic nigrostriatal pathway in the brain.

Parkinsonian symptoms

These symptoms occur in more than 50% of those on long-term therapy and include a tremor, a shuffling gait and slow movement with an expressionless face.

Symptoms usually occur gradually and can be helped by the administration of an antimuscarinic drug such as *procyclidine*, but these have their own side effects and should not be given until symptoms occur.

Acute dystonias

Abnormal body and facial movements may occur after only a few doses of the drug and tend to decline with time. They are commoner in young people and include muscle spasms and a protruding tongue. An **oculogyric crisis** may occur where the eyes roll uncontrollably. These are reversible on stopping the drug.

Akathisia

This is a feeling of restlessness and not being able to sit still. It occurs most frequently following a large initial dose of the drug.

Tardive dyskinesia

Unlike the other side effects this does not usually appear until the patient has taken the drug for months or years. It is abnormal movements of the mouth, tongue and trunk, and may become worse if the drug is withdrawn. May be due to an increased sensitivity or over-production of dopamine receptors caused by the drug.

- Begins with jerky tic-like movements of the tongue and face.
- Eventually the whole body may be affected with either tic-like or writhing movements. Patients may flick their tongue in and out of their mouth as often as 20 times in 30 seconds.
- All patients taking these drugs do not develop TD. Advancing age and female sex are the greatest risk factors.
- All antipsychotics can produce TD but there is evidence that clozapine does not.
- Gets worse if the drug is suddenly discontinued or if the patient is given L-dopa.
- There is no satisfactory drug treatment for TD. It is best to discontinue the drug if possible and it may remit, especially in the young. It is also a good idea to reduce the dose to the smallest that will control the schizophrenia.

Other side effects

These vary according to the drug being used and the dose administered.

- Increased prolactin levels leading to milk production in the breasts, gynaecomastia, amenorrhoea and impotence. Less common with atypical drugs.
- Antimuscarinic effects, including dry mouth, constipation and blurred vision.
- Postural hypotension due to blockade of alpha-adrenergic receptors. Greatest in *chlorpromazine, clozapine* and *thioridazine.*
- Hypersensitivity reactions including depression of the bone marrow, jaundice (*chlorpromazine* greatest risk), skin rashes and light sensitivity.
- Agranulocytosis is a particular problem with *clozapine* where there is a 1% −2% risk.
- Hypothermia, especially in the elderly. Great care is needed when these drugs are given to those over 70 due to depressed hypothalamic function.
- Drowsiness and cognitive impairment but *risperidone* causes insomnia and agitation.
- Weight gain with atypical drugs. Risk of insulin resistance and glucose intolerance.
- Some drugs cause QT prolongation on the electrocardiogram (ECG) and this predisposes to torsades de pointes (see Section 5.5).

Neuroleptic malignant syndrome

This is a rare genetic disorder that affects 0.5%−1% of patients taking these drugs. It is due to abnormal D_2 receptors that result in dopamine blockade in the hypothalamus.

Symptoms are high fever, muscular rigidity, hypertension, pallor, urinary incontinence, sweating and fluctuating consciousness.

It occurs at the beginning of the treatment and the drug must be discontinued immediately. It can be fatal, and treatment with *dantrolene*, a muscle relaxant, may be life-saving. A dopamine agonist may be given. Symptoms take about 5−7 days to subside or longer if depot preparations have been used.

Monitoring

- At the start of therapy, a full blood count, urea and electrolytes and liver function test monitoring are required. Then at annual intervals.
- Blood lipids and weight should be monitored every 3 months for the first year, then annually.
- Fasting blood glucose should be measured at the start, at 4−6 months then annually.
- An ECG may be needed if there are cardiovascular risk factors.

Individual drugs

Phenothiazines

The first effective drug used to treat schizophrenia was ***chlorpromazine*** (***Largactil***). It was not designed as a drug to treat schizophrenia, but the parent compound was synthesized in the dye industry. All phenothiazines in use today are chemical modifications of this parent compound. In 1944 it was tested as an antimalarial and found to be of no value in malaria but to have sedative and antihistamine properties.

It was used at first to reduce anxiety preoperatively and to sedate in psychiatry where its ability to suppress psychotic thoughts and behaviours was discovered.

After a week or two the symptoms of schizophrenia begin to improve. Patients stop conversing with their voices and external forces no longer instruct them. Their speech becomes more comprehensive and they become emotionally more responsive.

Chlorpromazine has pronounced sedative effects and produces moderate extrapyramidal and antimuscarinic effects. It is still widely used and is especially useful in violent patients. It can also control agitated states in the elderly without confusion (BNF, 2019). Other drugs in this group include ***promazine*** that is used as an antiemetic mostly.

Prochlorperazine and ***trifluoperazine*** have fewer sedative and antimuscarinic effects but greater extrapyramidal side effects. ***Prochlorperazine*** is mostly used as an antiemetic.

Thioxanthenes

These are similar to the phenothiazines and are antipsychotic and antiemetic in action.

Flupentixol (***Depixol***) is used as a depot preparation and administered every 2—3 weeks. It is less sedating than ***chlorpromazine***.

Butyrophenones

These are less sedative than the phenothiazines.

Haloperidol is especially used in the manic or confused patient. It has a high incidence of extrapyramidal side effects.

Other groups include the diphenylbutylpiperidines (***pimozide***) and the substituted benzamides (***sulpiride***).

See Box 4.2 for information on dosage of antipsychotics.

Atypical (second-generation) antipsychotics

Amisulpride, aripiprazole, cariprazine, clozapine, lurasidone, olanzapine, paliperidone, quetiapine and risperidone

These act on a variety of receptors including dopamine. Others, such as serotonin, alpha-adrenergic, muscarinic and histamine receptors may be

---

BOX 4.2 Dosage of all antipsychotics.

- The minimum effective dose is the threshold dose
- A patient who receives less than the threshold will not benefit from the drug
- Doses much greater than the threshold do not benefit the patient but will increase the side effects and the risk of tardive dyskinesia
- The optimal dose is therefore only just above the threshold dose

---

antagonized too. They have fewer extrapyramidal side effects but do have their own side effects (e.g. glucose intolerance and weight gain). They may be effective in schizophrenia resistant to treatment and for negative symptoms.

Side effects

- Include weight gain (greatest with clozapine and olanzapine), dizziness, postural hypotension and mild extrapyramidal side effects.
- Hyperglycaemia and diabetes can occur, especially with *clozapine* and *olanzapine*.

Clozapine

Clozapine is effective in those who have not benefited from treatment with conventional drugs and are unresponsive or intolerant to other drugs.

The antipsychotic action of conventional drugs and their extrapyramidal side effects are due to a high affinity for the dopamine D_2 receptor. Clozapine has a lower affinity for the D_2 receptor and so produces few, if any, extrapyramidal side effects at clinically effective doses.

- Use is limited because of agranulocytosis and patients have to register with a clozapine patient monitoring service. The white cell count has to be closely monitored throughout treatment.
- Fatal myocarditis and cardiomyopathy have been reported.
- May slow down intestinal peristalsis, which can lead to faecal impaction and intestinal obstruction. If clozapine constipation arises, this should be reported and the next dose withheld until a medical opinion is sought.
- There may be collapse due to hypotension on initiation of treatment so patients need close medical supervision.
- Other adverse reactions include fits, excessive salivation and sedation.

Other second-generation drugs

Olanzapine is used in schizophrenia to treat both positive and negative symptoms and in mania, and to prevent recurrence in bipolar disorder.

Quetiapine is used in schizophrenia and in the treatment of mania, bipolar disorder and depression in bipolar disorder. It is used as an adjunctive treatment in severe depression. The elderly excrete the drug more slowly and need to be prescribed much lower doses to avoid adverse effects.

Risperidone is used for the treatment of those with negative symptoms where other drugs work less well. It is also used to treat mania and can be used for short-term treatment of severe aggression in people with dementia.

Depot injections

Flupentixol, fluphenazine (Modecate), haloperidol, pipotiazine, risperidone, zuclopenthixol (Clopixol)

These are used for long-term therapy when oral treatment is unreliable. They may give rise to a higher incidence of extrapyramidal side effects, but these are less likely with atypical drugs such as *risperidone. Zuclopenthixol* may be used for agitated or aggressive patients. *Flupentixol* can cause overexcitement in such agitated patients. It may worsen the symptoms of mania.

A small test dose is given first with conventional drugs as side effects may be prolonged. Administration is by deep intramuscular injection every 2–4 weeks. Not more than 2–3 mL of oily solution should be administered at the same site and the site must be rotated.

If the dose needs to be reduced to alleviate side effects, the blood levels of the drug will not fall for some time, and it may be a month before there is reduction in the side effects. It must be noted that individual responses differ, and the drug is titrated according to the patient's response.

4.5 ANTIDEPRESSANTS AND MOOD STABILIZERS

Changes in mood include both depression and mania. Depression is a lowering of mood that may range from mild to severe and may be unipolar or bipolar. In bipolar disorder the patient oscillates between depression and mania. Mania is the opposite of depression and there is an elevated mood, extreme confidence and enthusiasm combined with impulsive actions.

Depression has a lifetime incidence of 15%–20% and can occur at any age with an increased tendency in later life. It is often mixed with anxiety and agitation. It may be endogenous where there is no identifiable cause, or reactive when the depression has an identifiable cause such as chronic illness or stressful life events.

Mild depression may not require drug therapy but more severe depression is associated with biological and emotional disturbances that may include:

- appetite or weight disturbance
- sleep disturbance
- apathy and disinterest

- low self-esteem
- poor concentration or indecisiveness
- feelings of guilt or inadequacy
- low mood on waking
- morbid thoughts of suicide or death.

There is an increased risk of suicide in depressed patients.

The biochemical cause of depression is still not understood, but it is thought that there are low levels of certain neurotransmitters at synapses within the brain.

Monoamine theory of depression

This theory arose from the following observations:

- Patients taking *reserpine*, a drug to lower blood pressure, often became depressed and had an increased risk of suicide. This drug reduced the availability of amines such as noradrenaline (norepinephrine) so the theory that depression was due to a reduction of these chemicals in the brain was born.
- Patients taking *iproniazid* for tuberculosis were often very ill but had an elevated mood. It was the first antidepressant but when tried in psychiatry it was too toxic to use in depression. Scientists discovered that this drug interfered with the destruction of amines by blocking the enzyme mono-amine oxidase and went on to develop MAOIs for depression.

The theory is that depression is caused by a deficit of monoamine trans-mitters at certain sites in the brain while mania results from a functional excess. It was originally formulated around noradrenaline (norepinephrine) but it is now realized that serotonin is also important and perhaps other trans-mitters such as dopamine.

Clinical effects of antidepressants take weeks to develop and this may mean it is an adaptive response in the brain that is causing the improvement. This is likely to be a change in receptor numbers.

In drug trials there are usually about 30% of patients who respond to a placebo. This is probably because many cases of depression are self-limiting episodes. Cognitive behaviour therapy (CBT) should be the first line of treatment for depression and CBT should be combined with drug therapy when this is required.

Depression is complex and may respond to different therapies. Some cases are affected by light as in seasonal affective disorder. Research is ongoing to try and understand depression and the response to different forms of treatment. Randomized trials looking at the impact of drugs, CBT and light therapy are in progress.

Antidepressant drugs are effective for treating moderate to severe depression with loss of appetite and sleep disturbance. Improvement in sleeping is often the first benefit of drug therapy. Electroconvulsive therapy is still used in severe depression.

Drug groups used to treat depression

- TCAs (e.g. *amitriptyline*).
- MAOIs (e.g. *moclobemide*).
- SSRIs (e.g. *fluoxetine*).
- Other drugs.

According to the BNF (2019), there is little to choose between different drug groups in terms of their efficacy, and drug choice is tailored to the patient taking account of any previous therapy, medical conditions and suicide risk. SSRIs are better tolerated with fewer side effects and are safer in overdosage, so they should usually be the first line of treatment.

Tricyclic antidepressants

Amitriptyline, clomipramine, dosulepin, doxepin, imipramine, lofepramine, nortriptyline, trimipramine

Other related drugs include *mianserin.*

These drugs block noradrenaline (norepinephrine) and serotonin re-uptake by nerve terminals, thus increasing levels in the brain.

- In addition to their effects on amine uptake, they block other receptors including muscarinic acetylcholine receptors, some histamine receptors and alpha-adrenergic receptors.
- The anticholinergic effects do not contribute to their antidepressant action but are responsible for many of their side effects.
- Some are anxiolytic and produce drowsiness. These may be useful in agitated patients and those with insomnia. *Amitriptyline* is an example. *Imipramine* is less sedative.

Uses

- Moderate to severe depression.
- Panic attacks and some obsessional and phobic states (e.g. *clomipramine*).
- Neuropathic pain where a lower dose than needed in depression is suitable. Probably affect opioid receptors by a serotonin pathway.
- Migraine prophylaxis.

Side effects These are a common reason for discontinuation of the drug.

● Anticholinergic effects are strong with ***amitriptyline*** and weaker with ***desipramine***. They include a dry mouth, blurred vision, constipation and urinary retention.
● Postural hypotension due to alpha-adrenergic blockade.
● Sedation and poor concentration due to blockade of histamine and alpha-adrenergic receptors.
● Ventricular dysrhythmias especially those involving prolongation of the QT interval.
● Cardiotoxicity in overdosage where they may depress myocardial contractility or produce severe arrhythmias. Both the antimuscarinic effects and noradrenergic stimulation contribute to cardiotoxicity.
● Contraindicated in recent myocardial infarction.
● Provoke fits in some people.
● Excessive sweating and tremor.
● Weight gain as they stimulate the appetite.
● Low sodium levels (hyponatraemia) may result, usually in the elderly, due to disordered antidiuretic hormone secretion. This leads to drowsiness, confusion and convulsions.

The drugs should not be stopped abruptly but the dose reduced over a period of about 4 weeks to avoid a withdrawal syndrome with headache, agitation, malaise, sweating and gastrointestinal upset, which could be due to excessive cholinergic activity following prolonged blockade of the muscarinic receptor.

Patients with a recent myocardial infarction or risk of cardiac arrhythmias should not be prescribed TCAs.

Drug interactions
● Strongly potentiate the effects of alcohol, and respiratory depression may follow a bout of drinking.
● Potentiate effects of other centrally acting drugs (e.g. anaesthetics).
● Must not be given with other antidepressants. MAOIs are the most dangerous. The reaction may occur up to 2 weeks after the MAOI is discontinued. Excess stimulation of 5-HT receptors leads to hyperpyrexia, convulsions and coma, which can be lethal. This is called *serotonin syndrome*.
● Increased risk of arrhythmias if taken with other drugs that prolong the QT interval (see Section 5.5).

Danger in overdosage Tricyclics have resulted in many fatalities and their toxicity following an overdose (see Section 9.5) prompted the search for safer drugs.

- Main effects are on the CNS and the heart.
- Excitement and delirium often with convulsions.
- Coma and respiratory depression follow.
- Cardiac dysrhythmias are common with extrasystoles and death may occur from ventricular fibrillation.
- Can deteriorate very rapidly, within an hour after taking the overdose.

Monoamine oxidase inhibitors

Phenelzine (Nardil), isocarboxazid, tranylcypromine

These were the first antidepressants to be used. They increase stores of noradrenaline (norepinephrine) and serotonin by inhibiting breakdown by the enzyme monoamine oxidase.

Response to the drugs is usually delayed for about 3 weeks and is not maximal for a further 1−2 weeks.

Their effects are long lasting as they are irreversible enzyme inhibitors. It takes up to 2 weeks to synthesize a new enzyme, meaning their effects continue after the drug is withdrawn.

They are used only when a patient is unresponsive to other antidepressants because of dangerous dietary and drug interactions.

Drug and food interactions

- Tyramine is an amine that is found in certain foods such as mature cheese, yeast extracts (e.g. Marmite, Bovril and Oxo), fermented soya bean products, broad bean pods, pickled herrings and chianti. It has a pressor effect (raises blood pressure) and this is greatly potentiated when MAOIs are taken as these inhibit the enzyme that destroys tyramine. May give rise to a dangerous rise in noradrenaline and blood pressure with the early warning of a throbbing headache.
- There is danger of this interaction up to 2 weeks after the tablets have been discontinued.
- All those taking MAOIs should be prescribed a warning card with this information.
- Should avoid alcohol while taking the drugs.
- Cough and cold remedies often have sympathomimetics in them, so they should be avoided.
- MAOIs must not be started until 7−14 days after a TCA has been discontinued. The reader is referred to the BNF for further details. Other antidepressants should not be started until at least 2 weeks after MAOIs have been stopped.

- Serotonin syndrome may occur if *pethidine* or *tramadol* is given. Should be avoided for 2 weeks after MAOI is discontinued.
- Opioid analgesics should be avoided as their metabolism in the liver is impaired.
- Many more drug interactions are listed in Appendix 1 of the BNF.

Reversible inhibitors of monoamine oxidase A

Moclobemide

There are two forms of monoamine oxidase enzyme: A and B. For antidepressant action it is MAOA that needs to be inhibited. Both MAOA and MAOB will break down tyramine; therefore if only MAOA is inhibited the interactions with food will be less.

- This drug is also a reversible inhibitor and its effects last less than 24 hours.
- **Large amounts of tyramine-rich food should still be avoided.**
- Risk of drug interactions is claimed to be less.

Selective serotonin re-uptake inhibitors

Citalopram, escitalopram, fluoxetine, fluvoxamine, paroxetine, sertraline

SSRIs are antidepressants lacking many of the adverse effects of the tricyclics. They are less dangerous in overdosage, cause less drowsiness and have fewer anticholinergic side effects. SSRIs are the most frequently prescribed antidepressants and their use has increased year on year since they were first marketed in the 1970s. However, they are not without their own problems and some may increase the risk of self-harm and suicidal behaviour especially in children. For this reason, the MHRA reviewed SSRIs and this report is accessible online at www.mhra.gov.uk.

Mechanism of action

There are at least 15 receptor subtypes for 5-HT so functioning of the 5-HT system is complex (see Section 4.2). TCAs, MAOIs, SSRIs, electroconvulsive shocks and lithium all affect brain 5-HT function in a complex way.

5-HT is synthesized in the neuronal cell body and is stored in vesicles. When an impulse passes down the axon, the 5-HT is released into the synaptic cleft.

There is a high-affinity re-uptake system in the neurone that actively takes up 5-HT and reduces its concentration in the synaptic cleft. SSRIs are targeted at this site.

- *Paroxetine* also has an affinity for M_3 cholinergic receptors found in the brain.
- They have half-lives of 15–24 hours although *fluoxetine* is longer.

- There is a similar delay of 2–4 weeks before they are clinically effective, which is seen with other antidepressants.
- Loss of effect may occur when prescribed over a long period of time.

Uses All drugs are licensed for depression and appear to be equally effective with 50%–70% of patients responding satisfactorily.

Other uses vary from drug to drug and are detailed in the BNF. They include:

- panic disorder
- obsessive-compulsive disorder
- bulimia nervosa
- post-traumatic stress disorder
- social phobia.

Side effects SSRIs are better tolerated than other antidepressants but do have some side effects.

- Gastrointestinal side effects include nausea and vomiting and are dose related, being most severe with *fluvoxamine*. Diarrhoea and abdominal pain are less frequent.
- Anorexia and weight loss.
- Few antimuscarinic side effects, except *paroxetine* that gives a dry mouth and constipation.
- Insomnia, anxiety and agitation may occur.
- Impair platelet aggregation and may provoke upper gastrointestinal tract bleeding if there is previous history.
- Caution is necessary in epilepsy.
- Hyponatraemia (see above) occurs more frequently than with TCAs, especially in the elderly.
- Should be withdrawn slowly to prevent a sudden withdrawal syndrome similar to TCAs (worst in *paroxetine*).
- Some concern regarding increased risk of congenital malformation with some SSRIs in pregnancy. Risk of cardiac abnormality is doubled from 1%–2% with *paroxetine*.
- Does appear to be an increased risk of suicide and self-harm in the first few weeks of use compared to other drugs. Most frequent in the young but can occur at any age. *Fluoxetine* is the only SSRI that the MHRA says has a favourable risk/benefit balance in the young.

SSRIs are much safer than TCAs if an overdose is taken.

Drug interactions Metabolized by cytochrome P450 enzymes and interact with drugs also metabolized by this pathway or that inhibit these enzymes (e.g. erythromycin).

Interact with dopaminergic and serotonergic drugs resulting in serotonin syndrome.

Other antidepressants

Serotonin and noradrenaline re-uptake inhibitors

Venlafaxine

- Has a greater effect on serotonin re-uptake at lower doses.
- Low affinity for muscarinic, histaminergic and adrenergic receptors.
- May be more effective than SSRIs for major depression.
- Not used in heart disease, and ECG done prior to treatment.
- NICE recommends not to be prescribed in uncontrolled hypertension, and blood pressure should be monitored, discontinuing the drug if it increases.
- More dangerous than SSRIs in overdose.
- Improvement may begin earlier than other antidepressants.

Selective noradrenaline re-uptake inhibitors

Reboxetine

- Increases serotoninergic transmission by increased noradrenergic activity.
- May cause insomnia, sweating, postural hypotension and dizziness.

Presynaptic α_2-adrenergic antagonist

Mirtazapine

- Reduces negative feedback control on 5-HT release in areas of the brain.
- Does block histamine receptors but has low affinity for muscarinic and α_1 receptors.
- Causes drowsiness and sedation.
- Increased appetite and weight gain may occur.

St John's wort

- Popular herbal remedy for treating mild depression. Does induce metabolizing enzymes in the liver and so interacts with some other drugs (see Section 9.1).
- Antidepressants should not be prescribed alongside St John's wort due to possible interactions.

Electroconvulsive therapy

This is stimulation of the brain through electrodes placed on either side of the head. The patient has to sign consent and is lightly anaesthetized and paralysed with a muscle relaxant to avoid injury from induced seizures.

- May cause confusion and memory loss, sometimes for a few weeks.
- Used in major depression with response rates of 60%–80% and appears the most effective treatment for suicidal depression.

Although this book concentrates on the drugs used to treat depression, it must be remembered that simple measures, such as introducing an **exercise regime**, are sometimes very effective. **Psychological support** must be given alongside any treatment, and **CBT** is available for recurrent depression. Box 4.3 summarizes some key points of antidepressants.

Bipolar disorder and mania

Bipolar disorder is present when both manic and depressive episodes occur. In mania the patient feels elated and cheerful. He may have grandiose ideas of wealth and fame and spend a lot of money, often dressing flamboyantly. He does not sleep much and does several things at once. There may be outbursts of aggression. Hypomania is a milder form of mania and sometimes is present at the same time as depression so that the patient may be laughing one minute and crying the next. This is known as a mixed affective state. The patient is unwilling to go to hospital with mania and feels nothing is wrong and that they have never felt better. Drugs are used for acute states and long-term control.

BOX 4.3 Some key priorities according to the NICE quick reference guide: depression.

- Antidepressants are not routinely recommended for the initial treatment of mild depression
- Selective serotonin re-uptake inhibitors are the drugs recommended for moderate and severe depression; these are safer than tricyclic antidepressants and less likely to be discontinued due to side effects
- Warn patients of delay in onset of antidepressant effect and possible side effects
- See after 2 weeks to review; take extra care and monitor if there is a high risk of suicide
- Continue for at least 6 months after remission and then review
- Withdraw drugs gradually over a period of 4 weeks, sometimes longer, and warn patients that there may be withdrawal symptoms, although these are usually mild
- Consider changing to another drug if no response only after a month or, if some response, wait 6 weeks

---

Antimanic drugs

Benzodiazepines (e.g. *lorazepam*) may be used at first but should not be used long term because of the risk of dependence. Antipsychotics (see Section 4.4) are usually needed and *olanzapine, quetiapine* or *risperidone* are used with either *lithium* or *valproate* added if response to antipsychotic drugs is poor. Valproate must not be used if there is a chance of pregnancy as it is highly teratogenic and can produce neural tube defects and congenital malformations.

Some anticonvulsants are mood stabilizers and *carbamazepine* may be used for prophylaxis if lithium does not work. Sometimes patients need an antidepressant drug while also taking a mood stabilizer. NICE has produced guidance for the management of bipolar disorder and this is available on its website.

Lithium

Increases 5-HT function and 5-HT and noradrenaline (norepinephrine) turn-over in the brain. Not a complex molecule like other antidepressants but a simple metallic ion.

- It controls the manic phase of bipolar illness; it is also effective in unipolar illness and is used as prophylaxis for mania or depression.
- It is able to control the mood swings and thus reduce both manic and depressive phases.
- Given in an acute attack it is only effective in controlling mania, and since other agents work just as well and are safer for this, its main use is in long-term prophylactic control of manic-depressive illness.
- Produces no enduring sedative effects and does not slow down thoughts or subdue feelings.
- Mania is prevented but happiness is not. Depression is lifted but the ability to feel sadness is not.
- The anticonvulsant *carbamazepine* has a similar prophylactic effect against mood swings. It is used in patients unresponsive to lithium.

Pharmacokinetics Lithium is clinically effective at a plasma concentration of 0.5−1 mmol/L, and above 1.5 mmol/L it is toxic and so the therapeutic window is very narrow. Serum lithium concentrations have to be monitored.

Excreted by the kidney in two phases. About half the oral dose is excreted in the first 12 hours but the remainder is taken up by the cells and takes 1−2 weeks to eliminate. This means that lithium accumulates slowly over 2 weeks until a steady state is reached. Renal disease or sodium depletion reduces the excretion rate. Diuretics also have this effect.

Main toxic effects of lithium
- Nausea, vomiting and diarrhoea.
- Tremor and hyper-reflexia.

- Renal effects: polyuria.
- Serious renal tubule damage with prolonged treatment in some cases, so need to monitor renal function.
- Long-term use may result in hypothyroidism and mild cognitive and memory problems.

It is dangerous in overdosage and may be fatal. Acute lithium toxicity results in neurological deficits that range from confusion and motor impairment to coma, convulsions and death if the plasma concentration reaches 3−5 mmol/L.

4.6 ANXIOLYTICS AND HYPNOTICS

Anxiolytics are literally drugs to 'break up anxiety' and hypnotics are agents that induce sleep. Sedatory and hypnotic drugs are depressants of the CNS. They cause loss of consciousness in large doses and eventually respiratory depression. There are some newer drugs used in anxiety that do not cause drowsiness but act on 5-HT receptors in the brain.

Anxiety

Anxiety is a normal response to something we are frightened of. An anxiety state arises when this fear is inappropriate and not associated with real events. The fear may be more anticipatory and interferes with daily living. Anxiety is often associated with depression although there are many types of anxiety disorder.

Symptoms include worry, nervousness, apprehension and fear. Usually there is difficulty in getting off to sleep at night. Physiological symptoms include sweating, tachycardia and epigastric discomfort. These are due to stimulation of the sympathetic nervous system.

Anxiety states are not totally understood but there is involvement of specific areas of the brain and certain neurotransmitters. There may be excess serotonergic and adrenergic activity. Inhibitory transmission via GABA may be decreased and excitatory glutamate may be increased. Both genetic predisposition and environmental triggers contribute.

Insomnia

Sleeping tablets used to be given as an aid to sleep to practically all inpatients in the 1960s! They are no longer prescribed except in exceptional circumstances or for very occasional use.

It is recognized that sleep patterns are variable and people require different amounts of sleep that may also vary during an individual's lifespan. If there is an inability to get to sleep or maintain sleep then insomnia is present.

Usually simple measures such as avoiding caffeine, regular exercise in the daytime, noise reduction and not having a daytime nap will help. However, sometimes it is still necessary to use hypnotics but for very short periods.

Drugs should not be prescribed for anxiety without also offering psychological support.

Anxiolytic and hypnotic drugs

Drugs that are used for anxiety will usually induce sleep if taken at night and, likewise, most hypnotics are also anxiolytic.

Benzodiazepines

An important class of drug discovered by accident in the early 1960s. Their hypnotic and anxiolytic actions were unexpected and they became widely prescribed before it was realized that both tolerance and dependence occur with long-term use. They are now used in anxiety only for short periods in extreme cases.

Mechanism of action

They act on the GABA$_A$ receptor and enhance the response to GABA by facilitating the opening of GABA-activated chloride channels. The GABA receptor mediates inhibitory neurotransmission in the brain.

Benzodiazepines only act in the presence of GABA and do not open the channel themselves.

There are also binding sites on the GABA$_A$ receptor for alcohol, volatile anaesthetics, barbiturates, *propofol* and *etomidate*.

Clinical effects and uses

- Reduction of anxiety and aggression.
- Sedation and sleep induction.
- Anterograde amnesia.
- Anticonvulsant.
- Reduction of muscle tone.

Different doses of the same drug may be used to achieve the above effects. *Diazepam* is used in small doses to reduce muscle spasm; in higher doses as an anxiolytic and hypnotic; and intravenously in status epilepticus. Commonly used drugs are listed in Table 4.3.

- Benzodiazepines are only used short term in anxiety because of withdrawal effects. The shorter-acting drugs produce withdrawal symptoms more readily. Longer-acting drugs allow the use of smaller doses and so have less sedatory effects.

TABLE 4.3 Duration of action and uses of some benzodiazepines.

Duration of action	Drug	Uses
Ultrashort	Midazolam	Intravenous sedation and light anaesthesia
Short (12–18 h)	Lorazepam	Anxiety, insomnia, status epilepticus, perioperatively
	Oxazepam	Anxiety
	Temazepam	Insomnia, perioperatively
	Lormetazepam	Insomnia
Medium (24 h)	Alprazolam	Anxiety
	Nitrazepam	Insomnia
Long (24–48 h)	Diazepam	Anxiety, insomnia, alcohol withdrawal, status epilepticus, febrile convulsions, muscle spasm, perioperatively
	Chlordiazepoxide	Anxiety, alcohol withdrawal
	Flurazepam	Insomnia
	Clonazepam	Anticonvulsant, status epilepticus

- When used for sleeping a shorter-acting drug gives fewer 'hangover effects' the next day. Regular use is discouraged because tolerance and dependence occur but occasional use (e.g. by shift workers) may be effective.
- Reduce muscle tone by a different action and do this in smaller doses than those needed for sedation. May be used in back pain to reduce muscle spasm. Also used in cerebral spasticity or postoperative muscle spasm.
- All are anticonvulsant in action but *clonazepam* is effective without causing sedation.
- They are not antidepressants or analgesics.
- *Diazepam, lorazepam* and *midazolam* are available by injection and may be given intravenously.
- *Midazolam* is used while conducting unpleasant procedures such as a colonoscopy or minor surgery. It sedates but the patient remains conscious and cooperative. There are no unpleasant memories of the procedure due to anterograde amnesia.
- Intravenous *midazolam* or *lorazepam* are used to control status epilepticus. Diazepam is also available rectally to control fitting.

Unwanted effects

- Drowsiness, impaired coordination and increased reaction times. This affects driving or the operation of dangerous machinery.

- Some benzodiazepines are metabolized in the liver to a metabolite with further activity. Repeated dosing can lead to a build-up in the body. This can be especially dangerous in the elderly prescribed sleeping tablets as these may increase confusion and falls.
- Light-headedness and impaired memory.
- Depressant action of other drugs and alcohol is increased.
- Tolerance (the requirement of increasing doses to produce the same effects) may occur.

Withdrawal syndrome

- With long-term use dependence can occur.
- Stopping the drug produces rebound insomnia and increased anxiety that is rather like an increase of the original symptoms and may encourage further prescribing. There may be tremor and dizziness.
- If the drug is long acting, the withdrawal syndrome may occur up to 3 weeks after stopping the drug. It can occur within hours in short-acting drugs.
- Sudden withdrawal of short-acting drugs can produce confusion and occasionally convulsions.
- Benzodiazepine dose should be slowly reduced in small steps.
- These drugs should not be used to treat short-term mild anxiety or insomnia unless it is causing extreme distress. In severe anxiety their use should be limited to 2—4 weeks.

Effects in overdosage

Benzodiazepines are less dangerous than many other drugs. Usually they just cause prolonged sleep but can occasionally cause severe, life-threatening respiratory depression, especially if taken with other drugs or alcohol (see Section 9.5).

Flumazenil is a benzodiazepine antagonist that can be used to reverse the effects of midazolam after minor procedures, thus allowing the patient to wake up and go home sooner. It has a rapid onset of action but its effects only last about 2 hours so there may be some re-sedation. It is occasionally used in overdosage but only by experts as it can be dangerous if the patient has taken a mixed overdose, especially TCAs, or in those dependent on benzodiazepines when it can produce convulsions.

Other sedatory drugs acting on the gamma-aminobutyric acid receptor

Zopiclone and *zolpidem* bind to sites on the $GABA_A$ receptor that are close to but different from the benzodiazepine site. They are licensed for short-term use (up to 4 weeks) in insomnia.

Barbiturates

These were the largest group of drugs used for insomnia and anxiety until the 1960s. CNS depressants and their effects range from reduction of anxiety to unconsciousness and death from respiratory depression.

- Bind to a different site on the $GABA_A$ receptor.
- They were widely abused in the 1950s and produce tolerance and dependence. Withdrawal can produce convulsions.
- Induce drug-metabolizing enzymes (P450 system); therefore they are involved in drug interactions.
- Rarely used today but *phenobarbital*, a long-acting barbiturate, is occasionally used as an anticonvulsant.
- *Thiopental* is a barbiturate anaesthetic agent.

Other anxiolytic drugs

Buspirone

This is an anxiolytic drug that is a partial antagonist at the $5\text{-}HT_{1A}$ receptor. It may also have some antidepressant action but has no sedative action.

- Takes up to 2 weeks to relieve symptoms and initially may produce an increase in anxiety symptoms.
- Has no effect on GABA receptors and does not stop withdrawal symptoms from benzodiazepines.
- Probably decreases 5-HT input into the hippocampus and lessens the degree of unpleasantness caused by incoming stimuli, thereby reducing anxiety.
- It does not control panic attacks or severe anxiety states.
- No reports of tolerance or dependence.
- Side effects include dizziness, headache and nausea.

Selective serotonin re-uptake inhibitors

- Recommended by NICE as the first drugs to be used in generalized anxiety disorder. Only some SSRIs are licensed for generalized anxiety (e.g. *paroxetine*).
- Some SSRIs are licensed for post-traumatic stress (e.g. *sertraline*), bulimia nervosa (e.g. *fluoxetine*) and obsessive–compulsive disorder (e.g. *sertraline*).

Beta blockers

Sometimes used in anxiety to control the tremor and palpitations but do not reduce fear and worry (e.g. *propranolol*).

NICE guidance is available for the management of anxiety and panic disorder. This is available on their website at **www.nice.org.uk**.
Benzodiazepines should not be used beyond 2–4 weeks.
CBT has the longest duration of action.
First-line drugs are SSRIs.

Panic disorder

NICE guidance does not recommend the use of benzodiazepines.

CBT has evidence for the longest duration of effect.

Some SSRIs are licensed for panic disorder (e.g. *citalopram*) and these are the drugs of choice. Other antidepressants are used if SSRIs are ineffective including *imipramine, clomipramine* and *moclobemide*.

4.7 ATTENTION DEFICIT HYPERACTIVITY DISORDER

- This is a behavioural disorder that is characterized by hyperactivity and inattention as well as some impulsivity. It can lead to social and educational problems.
- The symptoms usually exist together, but in some the hyperactivity may dominate while in others it could be the inattention.
- The symptoms usually occur in children between 3 and 7 years of age but may not be recognized until later.
- The problems tend to continue into adulthood and may make employment difficult.

In children with moderate attention-deficit/hyperactivity disorder (ADHD) psychological treatments should be tried first and drug treatment is only started under specialist care. The aim of drug treatment is to control the symptoms and improve quality of life. Drugs used are **CNS stimulants** and are sympathomimetics (e.g. *methylphenidate, atomoxetine* and *amfetamines*).

Methylphenidate

- This is a first-line drug and is used as part of a treatment programme.
- It may also be used in narcolepsy.
- It shares similar stimulant properties to *amfetamine.*
- It may produce growth retardation in children and growth should be monitored. Growth usually returns to normal once the drug is stopped.

Guanfacine is an alpha-2 adrenoreceptor agonist that is used when stimulants are not tolerated or are ineffective.

4.8 NEURODEGENERATIVE DISORDERS

In the adult, neurones cannot be replaced if they are damaged and treatment of disorders where there is degeneration of nerve cells is limited. The two most common disorders are Parkinson's disease (PD) and Alzheimer's disease (AD), which are both forms of chronic neurological disorder that become increasingly common with age and are increasing in incidence as we live longer.

Parkinson's disease

PD was first described by James Parkinson in 1817. It is progressive but does not usually shorten the lifespan.

- It is due to a loss of dopaminergic cells in the basal ganglia, an area of the brain that has a role in regulating motor function. There is a reduced ability of the cells in the substantia nigra to manufacture dopamine.
- In the basal ganglia two transmitters, dopamine and acetylcholine, are usually in balance. When there is a reduction in dopamine the acetylcholine has excess activity.
- The symptoms of PD are due to a decline in dopamine and a relative excess of acetylcholine.
- The dopamine produced by the brain is reduced by 60%—80% before any symptoms appear.
- There is deposition of protein aggregates called Lewy bodies in the cytoplasm and these may be associated with dementia in about 20% of cases.
- In two-thirds of cases the first symptoms occur between the ages of 50 and 60 years.
- The cause in most cases is not known. There is a genetic component in some cases and others may be due to atherosclerotic changes. Neurotoxins in the environment may be implicated but research continues to identify these.

Signs and symptoms

The loss of cells from the substantia nigra and the progress of the disease occur at variable rates and to a variable extent. Some patients may become rapidly disabled in a few years and others may have a mild, slowly progressive disorder that does not need treatment for several years. The majority of cases fall in between these two extremes and the condition slowly becomes more incapacitating over a period of about 10 years.

Major features

- Resting tremor.
- Muscle rigidity.
- Difficulty in initiating motor movements.

The tremor is present only at rest at first and is reduced or eliminated by movement. It usually starts in one hand or arm and takes 2–3 years to spread to the other hand and arm. It is rhythmic and may be described as a 'pill-rolling movement'. Eventually the tremor spreads to include the lips, face, tongue and lower limbs. It is increased by stress, fatigue and cold.

Rigidity is cogwheel in quality and occurs throughout the full range of movement of the joints. It is present in the limbs, trunk and neck and may lead to a stooped posture with the body and head flexed forward. This may lead to falls. There is a slowness or poverty of movement (bradykinesia) and a lack of spontaneous movement (akinesia).

- At first this leads to a difficulty with fine movements, such as fastening buttons, and writing becomes smaller.
- When the legs are affected this leads to a 'shuffling gait'. The person starts walking slowly but then speed builds up, often culminating in a fall.
- There is hesitation at doorways and difficulty in entering.
- There is a need to make a deliberate effort to initiate all movement.
- As spontaneous movement declines there is a mask-like expression.
- The hands no longer swing on walking.
- The eyes do not blink and there is a staring expression.
- The speech becomes monotone and dysarthria occurs as speech is weak and slurred.
- There is difficulty in eating and increased salivation that is embarrassing and tends to lead to a desire to eat alone.
- Difficulty in performing two movements at once (e.g. rising from a chair and shaking hands).
- Nonmotor symptoms include depression, dementia, sleep disturbances, bladder and bowel changes, swallowing problems and weight loss.

Drug therapy

Drugs used either enhance dopaminergic activity or decrease cholinergic activity. None of the drugs delay progression of the disease. The aim is to control the symptoms and increase quality of life. Physiotherapy and occupational therapy may be useful alongside referral to a dietician.

Dopaminergic drugs

Drugs may:

- be a precursor of dopamine (***levodopa***)
- prevent destruction of dopamine (***selegiline, rasagiline***)

- be a dopamine agonist (e.g. *pramipexole, ropinirole, rotigotine, bromocriptine*)
- cause the release of dopamine (e.g. *amantadine*).

Levodopa

Co-beneldopa (Madopar) is levodopa and benserazide.
Co-careldopa (Sinemet) is levodopa and carbidopa.
This is the drug of choice for the motor symptoms of PD.
Levodopa is the precursor of dopamine. Dopamine cannot itself be used as it does not cross the BBB. Levodopa can cross the BBB and is converted to dopamine by the enzyme dopa decarboxylase within the brain.
Pharmacokinetics. Absorbed from the small intestine and transferred across the BBB by active transport.
Converted to dopamine in the peripheries, reducing the amount available for the brain but also producing unwanted effects.

- To reduce unwanted conversion the levodopa is combined with a dopa-decarboxylase inhibitor (carbidopa or benserazide) that cannot cross the BBB; therefore it only prevents conversion to dopamine in the peripheries.
- This inhibits about 80% of the conversion outside the brain and leaves 5% −10% of the oral dose available to cross the BBB. Only about 1% of the dose would be available without this inhibition and 10 times the dose would be needed to have the same effects in the brain.
- Levodopa has a short half-life but the dopamine produced is able to be stored in the neurones when the disease is in its early stages. This produces a stable response.
- Therapeutic effects of levodopa decrease as the disease progresses leading to motor fluctuations with 'on' periods after medication and 'off' periods when there is weakness and restricted mobility. The duration during which each dose of medication is beneficial is reduced.
- Modified release preparations are available to allow a continuous supply of the drug to the neurones.

Side effects

- Conversion to dopamine in the peripheries causes nausea and vomiting due to stimulation of the CTZ of the vomiting centre (see Section 6.3). *Domperidone* may be needed for this. It is a dopamine antagonist that works on the CTZ but cannot enter the basal ganglia.
- Postural hypotension due to peripheral vasodilation.
- Excessive dopamine in the CNS leads to involuntary writhing movements especially of the face and neck (dyskinesia), and akathisia (restlessness).
- Impulse control disorders can occur including pathological gambling, binge eating and hypersexuality. Patients and relatives should be informed of this risk. If an impulse control disorder occurs the medication will be withdrawn or the dose reduced.

- A schizophrenia-like syndrome with hallucinations and confusion can occur. There may be insomnia and nightmares.
- Sudden onset of daytime sleeping can occur. Must refrain from driving until these effects have stopped.
- Gastrointestinal bleeding may occur.

Selective monoamine oxidase B inhibitors

Selegiline is a specific enzyme inhibitor that delays the destruction of dopamine in the neurones. Interactions that occur with MAOI antidepressants and certain foods do not occur as this drug is selective for the neuronal enzyme.

Selegiline can be used as the sole medication early in the disease, in an attempt to delay the destruction of neuronal dopamine. Later in the disease it prolongs the action of levodopa and reduces the dose needed by about one-third.

Catechol-O-methyltransferase inhibitors

Entacapone, tolcapone, opicapone Used to reduce 'end of dose' motor fluctuations later in the disease. Inhibit the enzyme that breaks down about 30% of the levodopa.

- Do not cross the BBB but double the half-life of levodopa and increase the motor response to each dose. When *entacapone* is started, the dose of levodopa may need to be reduced.
- *Tolcapone* is only used if *entacapone* fails.
- *Entacapone* is available as a triple combination with *levodopa* and *carbidopa*.

Dopamine receptor agonists

Apomorphine, bromocriptine, cabergoline, pergolide, pramipexole, ropinirole Direct agonists at the dopamine receptors in the CNS. They have a longer duration of action than levodopa and tend to cause less 'on–off' effects but do not appear to be effective in those where the effects of levodopa have decreased with time.

Main side effects are nausea and vomiting, confusion, delusions and sleep disturbances.

Pramipexole may be neuroprotective but this needs further investigation.

Apomorphine is given by subcutaneous injection or continuous infusion. It has a rapid action of short duration. It is used by expert units for severe motor problems late in the disease. High doses cause respiratory depression. This is antagonized by naloxone as *apomorphine* is an opioid derivative.

Bromocriptine, cabergoline and *pergolide* have been associated with pulmonary, peritoneal and pericardial fibrotic reactions and echocardiography should be done before treatment is started and at regular intervals of 6–12 months. The patient should be monitored for dyspnea, persistent cough and chest pain.

Amantadine

First used as an antiviral drug. Appears to stimulate the release of dopamine stored in the nerve terminals. Tolerance develops so its use is limited but it may be used late in the disease to reduce dyskinesia.

Muscarinic antagonists

Orphenadrine, procyclidine, trihexyphenidyl These were the only drugs available at one time but are rarely used nowadays due to antimuscarinic side effects (see Section 2.3). They restore the balance between dopaminergic and cholinergic activity but have little effect on the bradykinesia and are less effective than levodopa for treating the tremor.

They are used occasionally in young people with early PD and a severe tremor but are not first choice. There is a risk of aggravating dementia in the elderly.

Beta-adrenergic antagonists

May be used for symptomatic treatment of postural tremor in some patients but are not drugs of first choice.

Care in the community

Although this is a pharmacology book it must be emphasized that PD is a chronic degenerative condition where patients need an individual plan of care that they are involved in making. Communication is vitally important and knowledgeable professionals are needed to support and provide reliable information to both the patient and their carers. Many areas now have a PD nurse specialist and this is a big step forward.

Physiotherapy, occupational therapy and speech therapy should be available to those with PD, and palliative care requirements should be considered. Those with PD are very prone to falls and will need aids to reduce these.

It is extremely important that medication is given regularly and at the same time of day so that blood levels are maintained and the patient's symptom control is optimized.

Medication for PD should not be suddenly withdrawn as there is a risk of neuroleptic malignant syndrome (see Section 4.4).

Lewy body dementia in PD may sometimes respond to anticholinesterase inhibitors (see Section 2.3).

Depression may be present and is usually treated with an SSRI (see Section 4.5).

National Institute for Health and Care Excellence guidance

NICE guidance on PD was reviewed in 2017 and is available on the website www.nice.org.uk. It emphasizes the aspects of care in the preceding section, and for those with early PD it gives them the option to select their first-choice drug therapy:

- Levodopa should be used in as low a dose as possible to maintain good function.
- A dopamine agonist may be used but not an ergot derived drug.
- MAO-B inhibitors such as *selegiline* may be used.

The guidance states that, eventually, levodopa will be required with adjuvant drugs as the condition progresses.

Dementia

Dementia is a chronic disorder of behaviour and intellectual function due to organic brain disease. It usually starts with short-term memory loss and forgetfulness progressively leading to disorientation in surroundings that are unfamiliar together with mood and personality changes, restlessness and sleep disorders. As the disease progresses, social behaviour deteriorates and there may be self-neglect. The person may also become aggressive but there is no impairment of consciousness.

- **Alzheimer's disease (AD)** is the commonest cause of dementia, mostly occurring in the elderly but sometimes having an earlier onset. Genetic factors play a part in some forms of early-onset disease.
- Brain size decreases with enlarged ventricles and shrunken gyri. This can be seen on a computed tomography or magnetic resonance imaging scan.
- Under the microscope the brain tissue is changed and there are senile plaques of amyloid deposited together with an abnormal form of protein that forms neurofibrillary tangles. Clinical symptoms appear in parallel with the neurofibrillary tangles. The areas of the brain most affected are those of memory and language.
- There appears to be a loss of nicotinic and certain muscarinic acetylcholine receptors in parts of the brain.
- Recent research implicates changes in other neurotransmitters such as noradrenaline and serotonin.
- Other forms of dementia include vascular dementia (due to cerebrovascular disease), dementia with Lewy bodies, frontotemporal dementia and mixed dementia.

Drugs used in Alzheimer's disease

Acetylcholinesterases

Donepezil, galantamine, rivastigmine Increase the activity of acetylcholine by inhibiting the enzyme that destroys it.

- ***Donepezil*** is a reversible inhibitor of acetylcholinesterase with a high degree of selectivity for the CNS.
- ***Galantamine*** is a reversible competitive inhibitor that has some agonist action at nicotinic receptors as well.
- ***Rivastigmine*** has a prolonged action as it is a slowly reversible inhibitor.
- These three drugs are recommended as monotherapy for managing mild to moderate AD.

All are absorbed from the gastrointestinal tract and can be given orally. They may cause nausea and vomiting, diarrhoea and abdominal pain. In some patients they may cause insomnia and confusion.

N-methyl-D-aspartate receptor antagonists

Memantine is a noncompetitive antagonist of the excitatory transmitter glutamate at its NMDA receptor (see Section 4.2). It seems to prevent glutamate-induced toxicity to neurones without interfering with memory and learning. ***Memantine*** is recommended for monotherapy if patients are intolerant of the three above; it is also recommended in severe AD.

It can be given with an acetylcholinesterase (AChE) in AD in moderately severe or severe disease. Side effects include diarrhoea, insomnia, dizziness, hallucinations and headaches.

National Institute for Health and Care Excellence guidance

This was revised in 2018 and includes guidance on the support of carers and those working with patients with AD. This includes individually tailored care plans and recorded notes of the care and interventions given. Dementia-care training should be given to all care staff.

Tests of cognitive ability are used to help diagnosis but dementia should not be ruled out because the patient has a normal score. Sometimes other drugs, such as antidepressants and antipsychotics, may be prescribed under specialist supervision.

Vascular dementia

This may occur in those with cerebrovascular disease and is common over the age of 85 or following a stroke. Deterioration is due to multiple small infarcts within the brain. The presentation is usually more acute than in AD and may occur in steps as more infarcts occur. Treatment is targeted towards control of blood pressure and aspirin to prevent thrombus formation. The drugs used above may be of some use.

Lewy body dementia

This may occur in PD (see above) and is due to the deposition of abnormal proteins called Lewy bodies in the brain. It can develop without PD too. The disease is similar to AD and there may be a good response to anticholinesterases in some instances.

Motor neurone disease

This is a neurodegenerative condition that affects the brain and spinal cord. Progressive muscle weakness follows the degeneration of motor neurons.

Symptoms may include muscle cramps, muscle wasting and stiffness, loss of dexterity and eventually loss of respiratory function. There may be some cognitive dysfunction. The disease may present as isolated and unexplained symptoms; for example, trips and falls, speech problems, fatigue.

There are several forms of the disease and the commonest is amyotrophic lateral sclerosis.

The consultant neurologist will be involved in care alongside the multidisciplinary team.

There is no cure but drugs may help to maintain body functions and manage symptoms. Alongside drugs physiotherapy, nutrition advice, exercise programmes and social support will be needed.

NICE guidelines have been revised in 2016 and updated in 2018. They are very comprehensive and available on the website www.nice.org.uk/guidance/ng42

- For muscle cramps *quinine* (unlicensed use) is recommended as first line treatment. If this fails, *baclofen* may be given or sometimes *dantrolene* or *gabapentin*.
- An antimuscarinic drug may be prescribed for drooling of saliva and *glycopyrronium* is recommended in the BNF as this has fewer CNS side effects. Specialist use of botulinum toxin is sometimes used.
- *Riluzole* is licensed for use in amyotrophic lateral sclerosis to extend the time until mechanical ventilation is needed.

Section 5

Cardiovascular system

Section Outline

5.1 CARDIOVASCULAR SYSTEM – OVERVIEW

Heart and circulatory disease is the biggest killer in the UK and cardiovascular disease (CVD) was the cause of 168,472 deaths in the UK in 2017 (British Heart Foundation, 2019). Approximately 460 people a day die from CVD and approximately 110 of those dying from CVD will be under 75. The laying down of fatty plaques in the large arteries of the body produces **atherosclerotic CVD**, which may lead to angina, myocardial infarction (MI) and strokes.

The death rate from CVD varies over the UK with the highest death rates being in the north of England, central Scotland and the south of Wales. The south east of England has the lowest mortality from coronary heart disease (CHD).

CHD is the leading cause of death in the UK and is responsible for 66,000 deaths a year (an average of 180 deaths per day). The incidence of MI is higher in men than women and rises with age but it is also the commonest cause of premature death, causing 22,000 deaths in those under 75 each year. Someone dies from CHD in the UK about every 8 minutes and 1 in 7 men and 1 in 12 women die from CHD. CHD kills twice as many women as breast cancer.

In the 1960s, 7 out of 10 heart attacks were fatal in the UK, whereas today 7 out of 10 people will survive a heart attack. The British Heart Foundation (BHF) releases many statistics about heart disease. These can be found in full on their website (www.bhf.org.uk).

Many of the risk factors for CVD have been identified and some of these are not modifiable such as age, sex and heredity, including race. Premature death from CHD is higher in men and women of Asian origin. The disease is familial and children whose parents have heart disease are more likely to develop it themselves.

A Nurse's Survival Guide to Drugs in Practice. https://doi.org/10.1016/B978-0-7020-7658-9.00005-6

Risk factors that can be modified include:

- hypertension
- abnormal blood lipid levels
- obesity
- diabetes
- physical inactivity
- smoking
- excessive alcohol intake.

It is by reducing these risk factors further that the incidence of CVD can be decreased. Other contributory factors include an individual's response to stress.

Deaths from CHD have been declining in the UK since the 1970s. In 1969, the age-standardized death rate from CVD in the UK was 1045 per 100,000 of the population. In 2017 it was 246 per 100,000, and deaths in adults in the UK have fallen by a massive 50% in the last 15 years (BHF, 2019). This is partly due to better diet and better education but is also due to the increased availability of new drugs both in treatment and prevention of CVD.

Even though deaths have declined we can still do much more to prevent CVD. Around 60% of the British population still do less than the recommended 30 minutes of physical activity five times a week. It is estimated that around 28% of adults in the UK are obese (BMI over 30) and one-third are overweight. Obesity has increased by 50% in adult men and women, and since 1991 the incidence of type 2 diabetes has doubled in men and increased by about 80% in women. It must be remembered that 'prevention is better than cure' and those working in healthcare must take every opportunity to provide health education and support to patients in the battle against CVD.

The emphasis in this book is on the drugs used both in prevention and treatment of CVD but it must be remembered that changing our diet to a healthier one by reducing salt and animal fats, eating at least five (or better still, seven) portions of fruit and vegetables a day, losing weight and doing some physical activity are all just as important in both the prevention and the management of CVD.

Clinical assessment of cardiovascular risk

To prevent CVD, not only those already presenting with atherosclerotic CVD or diabetes but also apparently healthy individuals at high risk (CVD risk of >10% over 10 years) of developing atherosclerotic disease need to be identified and targeted. People in all these three groups need lifestyle and risk factor management, including drug therapy if necessary.

- Ideally, all people over 40 years of age with no history of CVD or diabetes and not already on treatment for hypertension need to be screened in primary care every 5 years for their CVD risk. Younger patients with a family history of CVD should also be screened for risk.

- Presenting features are used alongside risk calculators such as QRISK2 (www.qrisk.org) and JBS3 (www.jbs3risk.com/pages/risk_calculator.htm) are used. The risk calculators base their calculation of lipid profile, systolic blood pressure (SBP), gender, age, ethnicity, smoking status, body mass index (BMI), chronic kidney disease, diabetes mellitus, atrial fibrillation (AF), treated hypertension, rheumatoid arthritis, social deprivation and a family history of premature CVD. Calculators may underemphasize the risk in some, for example, those already taking medication for hypertension.
- The risk calculators are used to estimate the risk of developing CVD over the next 10 years.

Lifestyle targets

The aim is to work with patients and their families so that they:

- discontinue smoking
- make healthier food choices (e.g. increasing fruit and vegetable content of the diet)
- increase physical exercise
- achieve optimal weight
- reduce alcohol consumption.

Alongside these targets, blood pressure (BP) and blood cholesterol should be rigorously controlled.

Primary prevention of CVD includes the use of drugs to control BP and reduce blood lipids. Aspirin as an antiplatelet is not used for primary prevention due to the limited benefit gained versus the risk of bleeding associated with the drug.

5.2 HYPERTENSION

Hypertension is often called 'the silent killer'. The person with raised BP may feel physically fit and be unaware of the damage that is occurring to their cardiovascular system. The World Health Organization (WHO) has identified hypertension as one of the most important prevalent and preventable causes of early death and illness.

Optimal blood pressure and hypertension

The optimal BP for an adult is 120/80 mmHg and the upper limit of normal is 140/90 mmHg (Table 5.1).

TABLE 5.1 Definitions of hypertension, as documented in the National Institute for Health and Care Excellence guidelines (2019).

Optimal blood pressure	<120/80 mmHg
Normal blood pressure	<130/85 mmHg
High normal blood pressure	130/85 mmHg–139/89 mmHg
Hypertension Stage 1 hypertension	Clinic measurements of 140/90–159/99 mmHg or average home measurements of 135/85 mmHg to 149/94 mmHg
Stage 2 hypertension	Clinic measurements of 160/100–179/119 or average home measurements above 150/95 mmHg
Stage 3 or severe hypertension	Clinic systolic BP >180 mmHg or higher or clinic diastolic of 120 mmHg or higher.
White coat effect	A discrepancy of more than 20/10 mmHg between clinic and average HBPM (home blood pressure monitoring) measurements

Information taken from NICE, 2019b.

- Antihypertensive treatment was shown to reduce the risk of heart attack by approximately 40% and stroke by about 30% in those aged 65–74 years as far back as 1992 (MRC Working Party, 1992) and prevent premature death.
- Stroke is the third most common cause of death in the UK. It causes approximately 36,000 deaths each year in the UK and there are more than 100,000 strokes each year in the UK which is a stroke every 5 minutes (BHF, 2019).
- Stage 1 hypertension is asymptomatic but needs to be controlled by lifestyle modifications and drugs if necessary.
- Drugs may be needed for life.
- True hypertension has to be identified by taking several readings over a period of weeks or by using 24-hour ambulatory BP monitoring (ABPM).
- The hypertensive patient should also be screened for possible secondary causes of the raised BP such as renal artery stenosis, Cushing's syndrome or Conn's syndrome.
- Guidelines for the management of hypertension are provided by the National Institute for Health and Care Excellence (NICE) in association with the British Hypertension Society (BHS) and the Royal College of Physicians.
- In 2015, one in four men and one in five women worldwide had hypertension with fewer than one in five of these having the problem under control (WHO, 2019). One of the global targets of the WHO is to reduce the prevalence of hypertension by 25% by 2025.
- In England, at least one in four adults have high BP with around 40% of these undiagnosed. At least half of all heart attacks and strokes are associated with high BP (PHE, 2019).

The latest NICE guidelines came out in 2019 and are available in full from www.nice.org.uk.

NICE guidance states the following:

- Advice on lifestyle modification should be given to all people with high, borderline or high-normal BP.
- Antihypertensive drug therapy should be started in those of any age with sustained SBP >160 mmHg or sustained diastolic BP (DBP) >100 mmHg.
- Treatment decisions are made in those with sustained SBP between 140 and 159 mmHg and/or sustained DBP between 90 and 99 mmHg according to the presence or absence of CVD, other target organ damage or an estimated CVD risk of >20% over 10 years.
- A target clinic BP of less than 140/90 mmHg should be the aim.
- In people with diabetes mellitus drug treatment should start if BP is raised above 140/85 mmHg. This is because diabetes increases the risk of CVD.
- Risk charts are used as an aid but should not replace clinical judgement and are not appropriate in those with established disease in whom treatment should be started if BP is more than 140/90 mmHg.
- The charts should not be used when BP is persistently above 160/100 mmHg or when there is already damage to other organs from the raised BP. In these cases, antihypertensive drugs should be used.

Hypertensive crisis

Malignant hypertension is a term that was used to describe a condition when the DBP was >140 mmHg with evidence of small vessel damage such as retinal haemorrhages or proteinuria. It carried a poor prognosis. The patient:

- may have headaches
- may have visual disturbances − blurring of vision
- may be confused.

Needs urgent treatment as the untreated mortality is 80%.

BP is not usually reduced rapidly as this may lead to stroke, blindness or a MI.

The aim is to gradually reduce BP over several hours.

Parenteral drugs are only used in hospital to reduce very high BP in:

- gross ventricular failure due to hypertension
- hypertensive encephalopathy with fits
- eclampsia with fits.

Today, the term **hypertensive crisis** is used to describe the patient whose SBP is over 180 mmHg or DBP is over 120 mmHg.

A hypertensive crisis may be divided into a **hypertensive emergency** when the severe hypertension is associated with end organ damage or **hypertensive urgency** when there is no end organ damage with the severe hypertension.

Target blood pressure

A target BP to be obtained should be set. The BHS suggests <140/85 mmHg for those without diabetes. A target BP of 130/80 mmHg should be the aim in already established CVD or diabetes.

This may not be possible in some patients even with the appropriate drug treatment.

Normal regulation of blood pressure

To understand how drugs used for the treatment of hypertension work, it is necessary to understand how BP is controlled within the healthy body.

Two factors determine BP. These are cardiac output (CO) and systemic vascular resistance (SVR):

$$BP = CO \times SVR$$

CO is dependent on stroke volume (the amount of blood leaving one ventricle in one contraction) and heart rate. SVR is dependent upon the diameter of the arterioles. In vasoconstriction the BP is higher. Vasodilation causes a fall in BP.

The nervous system and the endocrine system are involved in the normal regulation of BP. Two main systems maintain BP within fairly narrow limits:

- autonomic nervous system (ANS) − neural and chemical
- renin-angiotensin-aldosterone system (RAAS).

Short-term blood pressure control

There are sensory receptors (baroreceptors) found in the arch of the aorta and the carotid arteries that detect changes in pressure within these arteries and send impulses to the vasomotor centre (VMC) in the medulla of the brain. The baroreceptors detect any sudden change in systemic BP. This is shown in Figures 5.1 and 5.2.

A rise in BP leads to

- Increased impulses from the baroreceptors to the VMC.
- This results in inhibition of the VMC and a decreased stimulation of the sympathetic nervous system (SNS) leading to peripheral vasodilation of both arterioles and veins and a fall in BP.
- Reduction in venous return and CO contribute to this.
- Impulses also go to the cardiac centres where the parasympathetic nervous system (PNS) is stimulated and heart rate and contractile force are reduced.

A fall in BP leads to

- Stimulation of the VMC.
- Increased sympathetic vasoconstriction.
- Impulses from the cardiac centre that lead to increased CO.

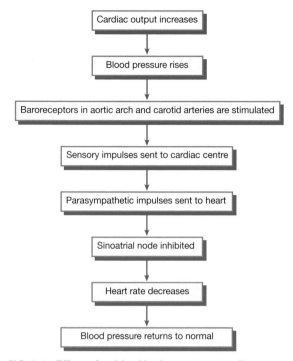

FIG. 5.1   Effects of a rising blood pressure on cardiac output.

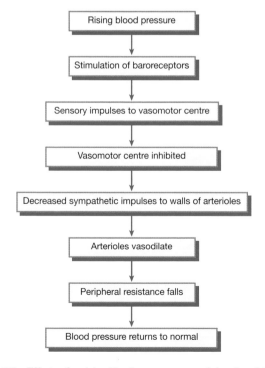

FIG. 5.2   Effects of a rising blood pressure on peripheral resistance.

The baroreceptors protect against sudden changes in BP such as those occurring when changing position (e.g. standing from reclining).

Hormones carried in the bloodstream also influence BP. They may act directly on the smooth muscle of the arterioles or may act on the VMC.

- *Adrenaline* (epinephrine) and *noradrenaline* (norepinephrine) are released by the adrenal gland in stress and they enhance the action of the SNS, increasing BP.
- **Nitric oxide** (NO) is secreted by the endothelial cells lining the blood vessels and is a vasodilator released on stimulation of the PNS. The action of NO underlies the effects of nitrates (see Section 5.4).
- *Antidiuretic hormone* (ADH) increases reabsorption of water and by increasing blood volume increases BP.
- *Atrial natriuretic peptide* (ANP) and **B-type natriuretic peptide (BNP)** secretion result in increased sodium and water loss. These are secreted when the atria (ANP) or ventricles (BNP) of the heart are stretched due to water retention or raised BP.
- *Inflammatory chemicals* such as histamine are potent vasodilators — there is a fall in BP in anaphylaxis. They also increase capillary permeability leading to fluid loss from the bloodstream.
- *Alcohol* causes BP to fall. It inhibits ADH, depresses the VMC and promotes vasodilation, especially in the skin.

The renin-angiotensin-aldosterone system

This system regulates renal blood flow. If renal BP drops (as it will when systemic BP falls) the release of renin by the renal arterioles is increased. Stimuli for renin release also include sodium depletion and direct stimulation by the SNS.

Renin is an enzyme that acts on circulating angiotensinogen and converts it to angiotensin I. This is split by angiotensin converting enzyme (ACE) to give angiotensin II (Fig. 5.3).

Angiotensin II raises BP because it:

- is a potent vasoconstrictor
- increases salt and water retention by stimulating the release of *aldosterone* from the adrenal cortex. *Aldosterone* acts on the distal convoluted tubule of the nephron to preserve sodium. Water follows sodium passively into the blood. Increased potassium is lost in the urine. The increased blood volume increases BP.

Reducing blood pressure

The drugs used to treat high BP work by interfering with the systems described above. Remember the equation BP = CO × SVR. We could reduce BP by lowering vascular resistance or reducing CO.

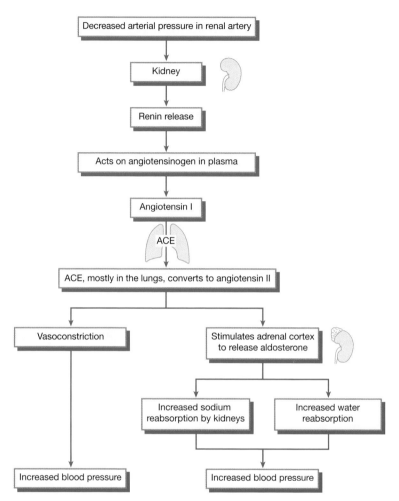

FIG. 5.3   Effects of the renin–angiotensin–aldosterone system. *ACE*, Angiotensin converting enzyme.

- Vasodilation will reduce SVR. Many antihypertensive drugs are vasodilators.
- May act by modulating the mechanisms responsible for BP control; for example, the SNS and its neurotransmitter noradrenaline (norepinephrine) or the RAAS.
- May have a direct effect on the blood vessel wall and relax smooth muscle.
- Hypertension may also be treated by reducing CO, although this is less common.

Blood pressure measurement

Large variations in BP throughout the 24-hour cycle are normal. The systolic pressure will rise following exercise so patients should sit quietly for 10 minutes before their BP is taken. Ideally the BP should be taken at least twice at a 5-minute interval and the lowest reading recorded.

All adults should have their BP measured at least every 5 years and those with high-normal BP or who have had high BP readings at any time should be checked annually.

To identify hypertension (persistently raised BP above 140/90 mmHg) the patient should return at monthly intervals (re-evaluation sooner if severe hypertension), at least twice, and the BP should be taken under the best conditions available. Ambulatory BP recording over a 24-hour period may be offered or if unsuitable, home BP monitoring should be done and readings recorded in a diary.

Measurement should involve:

- a properly maintained and calibrated measuring device
- BP taken in both arms
- relaxed and comfortable setting
- removal of tight clothing
- the patient quiet and seated with his/her arm outstretched and supported, ensuring that the hand is relaxed
- standing BP recorded in the elderly or those with diabetes to identify postural hypertension (fall in BP when standing of 20 mmHg or more)
- the mean of at least two readings.

Do not treat on the basis of an isolated reading.

'White coat hypertension'

In many people the anticipation of measurement causes the BP to rise due to an alerting reaction. This may be by 10/20 mmHg and may be sufficient in about 10% of patients to lead to misdiagnosis so ABPM or home measurement is used to gain correct readings. White coat hypertension may be a CVD risk itself but not all studies support this.

There is still substantial underdiagnosis, undertreatment and poor rates of BP control in the UK, although the situation is improving.

Management of hypertension

As the cause of essential hypertension is not known it cannot be treated, although the risk factors can be targeted by changing lifestyle.

Lifestyle modification

Extremely important in all those with high BP and also recommended for those with high–normal BP as this may often evolve to hypertension with ageing (Table 5.2).

Lifestyle modifications that help to reduce risk of CVD include stopping smoking and hypertensive patients should be encouraged to give up smoking. This may not reduce BP but will reduce CVD risk by up to 50% in 1 year in a heavy smoker.

Relaxation therapies such as yoga and biofeedback may reduce BP, but the research results are varied and conflicting. The patient may wish to pursue these but they are not routinely provided on the National Health Service (NHS).

The implementation of lifestyle changes is always difficult and patients will need enthusiasm and determination, especially to sustain these measures over time. The support of the healthcare team and the family will be needed.

Drug treatment of hypertension

On average one drug may reduce BP by 7%–8% but the individual response to a drug varies greatly. One drug may produce a large drop in BP in one person

TABLE 5.2 Lifestyle interventions for blood pressure reduction.

Intervention	Recommendation	Expected SBP reduction
Weight reduction	Body mass index 20–25 kg/m^2	5–10 mmHg per 10 kg weight loss
Dietary Approaches to Stop Hypertension (DASH) eating plan	Diet rich in fruit and vegetables – at least 5 portions daily	8–14 mmHg
	Reduce saturated fat and total fat content	2–8 mmHg
Restrict salt in diet	<2.4 g sodium or <6 g sodium chloride (salt) daily (5 g = 1 tsp)	4–9 mmHg
Physical activity	Regular aerobic activity, e.g. brisk walking 30 min most days	2–4 mmHg
Alcohol only in moderation Excessive consumption associated with raised BP	Men <21 units/week Women <14 units/week	Up to 10 mmHg
Reduce excessive coffee consumption	Less than 5 cups daily	1–2 mmHg

BP, Blood pressure; *SBP,* systolic blood pressure.

and little or no response in another. This is probably due to the variety of factors involved in the pathogenesis of high BP.

Classes of drug commonly used to treat hypertension include:

- thiazide diuretics (e.g. *Bendroflumethiazide*)
- calcium channel blockers (CCBs; e.g. *amlodipine*)
- ACE inhibitors (ACEIs; e.g. *ramipril*)
- angiotensin II receptor blockers (ARBs; e.g. *losartan*)
- alpha-adrenergic receptor antagonists (e.g. *doxazosin*)
- beta-receptor blocking drugs (e.g. *atenolol*)
- older agents; very little used now — interfere with activation of SNS (e.g. *methyldopa*).

Diuretics

Diuretics are described in greater detail in Section 6.2.

Thiazide diuretics

Bendroflumethiazide, hydrochlorothiazide. These are the commonest diuretics prescribed in hypertension. They are cheap, easy to use and can be given once daily. They are well absorbed through the gut and excreted through the kidney.

Mechanism of action

- BP is lowered through a combination of increased renal excretion of sodium and water, thus reducing blood volume and CO, and a reduction in peripheral resistance, the mechanism of which is not entirely understood.
- Reflex increase in renin production due to the decreased fluid volume may attenuate the BP lowering.
- Have antihypertensive action when used alone and also potentiate the action of other antihypertensive drugs.
- Excretion of sodium, magnesium and potassium is increased.
- Excretion of calcium is decreased and there is evidence that they may reduce bone loss in postmenopausal women.
- There is no dose—response curve and a small dose is just as effective in hypertension as a large dose. This is good as most side effects occur at larger doses.

Dose

Bendroflumethiazide. The usual treatment is 2.5 mg daily. A higher dose than 2.5 mg should not be used in hypertension as there is no benefit and the metabolic side effects increase.

- Maximum effect in 4—6 hours. Duration of action 8—12 hours.

Other clinical uses of thiazides include mild heart failure (HF) and oedema where the dose given may be larger.

Side effects

- Hypokalaemia − this is unusual with the small dose recommended in hypertension as it is dose dependent.
- Hyperglycaemia due to increased insulin resistance. This means other drugs may be better in patients with diabetes. Impaired glucose tolerance is worse if a beta blocker is prescribed as well.
- Altered lipid profile − small increase in low-density lipoprotein (LDL) cholesterol and triglycerides.
- Hyperuricaemia (raised uric acid levels) may result in gout.
- Erectile dysfunction in some patients.
- Efficacy is reduced in those taking nonsteroidal anti-inflammatory drugs (NSAIDs).
- Rashes.
- Blood dyscrasias.

Other thiazide-like diuretics with a similar action include *chlortalidone* and *indapamide*.

Cautions

- Contraindicated in those with gout. Compete with uric acid for excretion in the kidney.
- Avoid in those receiving lithium as there is a high risk of lithium toxicity.
- Monitor effect on blood glucose in diabetes.

Loop diuretics such as *furosemide* have a stronger diuretic action but are less effective in hypertension than thiazides. They may be used if there is advanced renal impairment or if fluid retention is involved.

Potassium-sparing diuretics such as *amiloride* and *spironolactone* may be used, if necessary, to limit potassium loss with thiazides (not usual). They should not be used as first-line management of hypertension but may be useful in resistant hypertension where aldosterone may be involved.

Angiotensin converting enzyme inhibitors

By blocking the formation of angiotensin II, these drugs vasodilate and lower BP as well as reducing cardiac preload and afterload. They also have some diuretic action. They are used for the treatment of hypertension, HF and to reduce further renal damage in diabetic nephropathy. They are also given following a MI where they reduce mortality.

The evidence base for their use in diabetes is very strong. When used to control BP, they appear to reduce the progression of nephropathy. They reduce proteinuria and stabilize renal function. They are always first-choice antihypertensives in those with diabetes unless contraindicated.

Early evidence from the ASCOT study (McDougall et al. 2005) showed a greater reduction in MI and stroke following treatment of hypertension with ACEIs or CCBs than with treatment with a beta blocker.

They are first-line treatment for hypertension in those under 55 years of age, unless of African or Caribbean descent when a CCB or a diuretic should be used initially. This is because ACEIs are less effective in these patients. Younger people and Caucasians tend to have higher renin levels relative to older people or the black population of African descent. In those over 55 years, a diuretic may be used first.

Captopril was the first drug. Now there are many (Box 5.1).

Mechanism of action

- All inhibit ACE that converts angiotensin I to angiotensin II. They thus reduce the formation of angiotensin II. This causes vasodilation and a reduction in BP.
- The same enzyme, known this time as *plasma kininase*, inactivates bradykinin, a powerful vasodilator. The effect of this is further vasodilation.
- They affect the venous system, and by vasodilation reduce cardiac load, making them useful in HF (see Section 5.6).
- They do not decrease cardiac contractility.
- They prevent renal absorption of sodium by lowering production of aldosterone and so have a diuretic effect, causing sodium loss and potassium retention.
- Acute fall in BP can occur with the first dose of these drugs especially in dehydration, HF or accelerated hypertension. They should be used with care in the elderly and those on diuretics. This acute fall is rarely seen when they are used to treat uncomplicated hypertension.
- Some are prodrugs and are converted to the active agents in the liver.

BOX 5.1 Angiotensin converting enzyme inhibitors.

Captopril
Co-zidocapt
Enalapril
Fosinopril
Imidapril
Lisinopril
Perindopril
Quinapril
Ramipril
Trandolapril

Renal function and electrolytes should be checked before starting ACEIs and monitored during treatment.

Cautions Chronic renal disease and peripheral vascular disease (PVD), where there may also be renal artery stenosis that is undiagnosed.

Contraindications

- They should be avoided in pregnancy as they are teratogens (see Section 7.5).
- Not given to patients with known hypersensitivity to them — danger of anaphylaxis.
- Avoid in bilateral renal artery stenosis — may precipitate renal failure as they reduce glomerular filtration rate (GFR). Renal blood flow is affected by angiotensin II, which vasoconstricts the efferent arterioles of the glomeruli of the kidney, thereby increasing GFR. By reducing angiotensin II levels, ACEIs reduce GFR. ACEIs can induce or exacerbate renal impairment in patients with renal artery stenosis. This is especially a problem if the patient is also taking an NSAID and a diuretic.

ACEIs should be avoided in severe bilateral renal artery stenosis as they reduce GFR and may cause progressive renal failure.

Side effects

- Persistent dry cough in 10%–20% of users — more common in women and can still develop many months into treatment. ACE is involved in the breakdown of bradykinin and this is also inhibited. Accumulation of kinins may cause the cough.
- Dizziness and hypotension, especially in volume-depleted patients.
- Disturbances of taste (especially with captopril).
- Rashes.
- Angioedema in 1% but commoner in the black population — 4%.
- Should be avoided in women of child-bearing age — maldevelopment of the renal tract in the fetus.

Angiotensin receptor blockers

Introduced in 1995. These drugs do not lessen the formation of angiotensin II but block the cell receptors for type 1 angiotensin II (AT_1). This leads to vasodilation and a fall in BP.

They have the potential to inhibit angiotensin II action more than ACEIs because there are other enzymes in the body that can make angiotensin II as well as ACE.

Losartan was the first drug to be introduced. Now there are many (Box 5.2).

● As they do not inhibit ACE formation, they do not inhibit the breakdown of bradykinin and other kinins. They thus do not cause a cough and are less likely to cause angioedema.
● Would appear to have the advantages of ACEIs without the disadvantages.
● Often well tolerated in patients who are intolerant of other drugs.
● Used if intolerant to ACEIs in hypertension and HF. They are sometimes prescribed in addition to ACEIs in HF (see Section 5.6).
● The maximum effect on BP usually occurs within 3—6 weeks.

Cautions As in ACEIs — renal artery stenosis.

Contraindications See ACEIs. Avoid in pregnancy and breastfeeding.

Side effects
● Usually mild and are better tolerated than ACEIs.
● Hypotension and dizziness may occur.
● Hyperkalaemia occasionally.
● Angioedema but less frequent than with ACEIs.

BOX 5.2 Angiotensin II receptor antagonists (ARBs).

Azilsartan
Candesartan
Eprosartan
Irbesartan
Losartan
Olmesartan
Telmisartan
Valsartan

Calcium channel blockers

These drugs are used in both angina and hypertension. They dilate peripheral arterioles and so reduce BP. They are also effective in large vessel stiffness, one of the common causes of an elevated SBP in the elderly.

Mechanism of action Act through the inhibition of the transfer of calcium ions across cell membranes and into the smooth arterial muscle cells. Some also affect myocardial muscle.

- Calcium is needed for muscle contraction.
- Reduce BP by **vasodilation** following relaxation of smooth muscle in arterioles.
- There are two groups of CCBs based on their chemical structure.
- The groups differ in their affinity for cardiac conducting tissues, cardiac muscle and vascular smooth muscle:
  - dihydropyridines − *amlodipine*, *felodipine*, *nifedipine* and most others
  - non-dihydropyridines, also known as rate limiting − *verapamil*, *diltiazem.*
- Non-dihydropyridines also influence myocardial muscle cells and reduce myocardial contractility.
- They affect the cells within the specialized conducting system of the heart and the propagation of electrical impulses may be depressed.
- *Verapamil* and *diltiazem* should be avoided in HF as they may depress cardiac contraction.
- *Verapamil* and *diltiazem* reduce CO whereas the dihydropyridines have little effect on cardiac muscle but are potent vasodilators and have some mild diuretic effects.
- *Diltiazem* is less likely to reduce cardiac contractility than *verapamil* and is sometimes used for the control of hypertension.
- Longer-acting dihydropyridines are better than short-acting ones as they lower BP very effectively and do not activate a reflex sympathetic response (which would cause tachycardia).
- All are well absorbed from the gastrointestinal tract.
- CCBs are suitable for those with angina, asthma and PVD.

Side effects
- Headache.
- Flushing.
- Dose-dependent ankle oedema due to an effect on capillary permeability.
- Gum hypertrophy may occur.
- Non-dihydropyridines (*verapamil* and *diltiazem*) cause less oedema but are negative inotropes and are dangerous in HF or when given with beta blockers (also negative inotropes).
- CCBs are dangerous in overdosage (see Section 9.5).

Alpha-adrenoceptor blocking drugs (alpha blockers)

Block the α_1 adrenoceptor in the smooth muscle of the blood vessels (see Section 2.2). Stimulation of the alpha receptor brings about vasoconstriction and so blocking it causes vasodilation and a fall in BP.

- Short-acting drugs had the side effect of postural hypotension but in those administered once-daily (*doxazosin* and *terazosin*) this is less of a problem.
- Caution should still be taken with the first dose as postural hypotension may occur within 30—90 minutes. The first dose should be taken when going to bed.
- Alleviate some symptoms of **benign prostatic hypertrophy** so may have dual use in this group of patients.
- Used in the short-term management of **phaeochromocytoma** (benign tumour of the adrenal medulla that releases adrenaline [epinephrine]). Tachycardia is then controlled by the use of a cardioselective beta blocker.

Side effects
- Postural hypotension.
- Drowsiness, dizziness, lack of energy.
- May exacerbate stress incontinence in women.

Beta-adrenoceptor blocking drugs (beta blockers)

Beta blockers are antagonists at the beta adrenoceptor for noradrenaline (norepinephrine) (see Section 2.2). They were developed for their antianginal properties in the 1960s but were then found to lower BP.

Atenolol is one of the most frequently prescribed beta blockers for hypertension. It is water soluble and cardioselective.

BP-lowering mechanism is complex and not fully understood but includes the following:

- Reduction in CO by reducing force and rate of cardiac contraction. At first this may be offset by reflex vasoconstriction and this may limit the initial effect on BP. A longer-term effect occurs over days as the vascular resistance is restored to pre-treatment levels.
- Reduction in renin secretion by the kidney.
- Some also have a central effect on the VMC.

They are effective, safe and well absorbed from the gastrointestinal tract.

Drugs differ in their selectivity for β_1 receptors, their lipid solubility, their duration of action and their partial agonist activity.

- Some (e.g. *propranolol*) block both β_1 receptors (heart rate and force) and β_2 receptors (vascular and bronchial smooth muscle) whereas others (e.g. *atenolol* and *bisoprolol*) are cardioselective and work mostly on the β_1 receptor.
- Partial agonists (e.g. *oxprenolol*) give less bradycardia and less cold peripheries.
- Lipid-soluble drugs are able to enter the brain and may give nightmares. *Atenolol* is water soluble and does not.
- Some are metabolized by the liver. Others are water soluble and excreted by the kidney. Care is needed in renal impairment as they may accumulate and dose reduction may be needed.
- Cardioselective drugs are less likely to affect airway resistance or raise serum cholesterol levels. *Atenolol, bisoprolol, metoprolol, nebivolol* and *acebutolol* are cardioselective. They are not cardio specific and do have limited action on the β_2 receptor.
- Useful to control hypertension in those with angina or who have had an MI.

Beta blockers should be avoided in asthma, heart block and PVD.

Side effects

- Bronchospasm – contraindicated in asthma.
- Bradycardia.
- Cold hands and feet.
- Fatigue – aching limbs on exercise.
- Vivid dreams.
- Impaired concentration and memory.
- Erectile dysfunction.
- Impaired response to hypoglycaemia and impaired blood glucose control.
- Increasing evidence that they increase the likelihood of diabetes, especially if combined with a thiazide diuretic.
- Worsening dyslipidaemia – reduce high-density lipoprotein (HDL) cholesterol and increase triglycerides.

Vasodilator drugs

These drugs are not usually given to control hypertension. Reducing BP too quickly can be dangerous and even in accelerated hypertension an oral agent such as *labetalol* is preferred. They may be seen in theatre, critical care and other exceptional situations.

Minoxidil

- Opens adenosine triphosphate (ATP)-sensitive potassium channels in vascular smooth muscle cells, causing hyperpolarization and relaxation of the smooth muscle in the blood vessels. This leads to vasodilation.
- The potassium channels are normally kept closed by intracellular ATP, which is apparently antagonized by *minoxidil*.
- It is a potent vasodilator which causes severe fluid retention and oedema.
- Vasodilation is accompanied by increased CO and tachycardia. For these reasons a loop diuretic and a beta blocker must be used alongside this drug.
- It is given in severe hypertension resistant to other drug combinations.

Hydralazine

- A potent vasodilator that acts mainly on arteries and arterioles, causing a fall in BP.
- This is accompanied by reflex tachycardia and increased CO.
- Not used alone as it causes fluid retention.
- Occasionally given by mouth with other drugs if hypertension is resistant to treatment.
- May also be used in HF combined with a nitrate.

Side effects include flushing, tachycardia, palpitations, headache and dizziness.

Diazoxide

- A vasodilator that may be used occasionally in severe hypertension associated with renal disease and is given by intravenous injection or infusion.
- The drug results in a rapid fall in BP.
- Probably works by opening potassium channels.

Side effects include tachycardia, hyperglycaemia and salt and water retention.

Sodium nitroprusside

- May be used for controlled hypotension in anaesthesia where it is given by intravenous infusion. Very rarely used in hypertensive crisis.
- May also be used occasionally in HF.
- It releases NO, which causes an increase in cyclic guanosine monophosphate (GMP) in vascular smooth muscle cells. This causes vasodilation.
- **Side effects** are associated with the rapid reduction of BP and include headache, dizziness, nausea, abdominal pain, perspiration, palpitations, apprehension and retrosternal discomfort.

Other vasodilators Vasodilators are used in some types of **pulmonary hypertension** under specialist supervision. These drugs include bosentan, epoprostenol, iloprost and sildenafil.

Centrally acting antihypertensive drugs

Methyldopa Converted in the adrenergic nerve endings to a false transmitter that stimulates α_2 receptors in the medulla and reduces sympathetic outflow.

- It is a prodrug that is metabolized in the brain to the active form.
- Oral administration leads to active absorption by an amino acid transporter.
- Safe in pregnancy and so still seen sometimes to control hypertension.
- Not given if depression present — can make this worse.

Clonidine
- This drug has a central effect probably by action at the imidazoline receptor, but also works on the postsynaptic α_2 receptors to inhibit the activity of adrenergic neurones.
- Withdrawal of this drug has to be accomplished slowly to avoid a hypertensive crisis.
- Also used in the treatment of menopausal hot flushes and migraine.

Moxonidine
- This is an agonist at the imidazoline receptor which is important in the regulation of sympathetic drive. The receptors are situated in the VMC and stimulation leads to decreased sympathetic activity and increased vagal tone.
- Has a role if the more commonly used drugs are contraindicated or fail to control the hypertension. Given orally and has to be withdrawn slowly.
- Abrupt withdrawal has to be avoided.

Choices of antihypertensive drug — guidelines, combination therapy and evidence

Guidelines for the management of hypertension are provided by NICE (2019b) working with the BHS. The first NICE guidelines were published in 2004 and updated in 2006 following publication of the ASCOT study. This was a large, randomized, controlled trial that showed reduction in stroke, coronary events and cardiovascular death, and all-cause mortality was greater in patients taking CCBs and ACEIs for BP control than in those patients taking beta blockers and diuretics. Risk of stroke was 23% less and risk of cardiovascular events was 16% less. The risk of developing diabetes was 30% less (Table 5.3).

Beta blockers are not used as first-line therapy for hypertension unless there is history of angina or MI.
If a beta blocker is withdrawn, the dose should be stepped down slowly.

TABLE 5.3 NICE recommendations for choosing antihypertensive drug treatment (2019b).

Step 1	Younger than 55 years but not of black African or African-Caribbean family origin or those with type 2 diabetes of any age or family origin	55 years or older and do not have type 2 diabetes, or black African or African-Caribbean family origin patients of any age who do not have type 2 diabetes
	Angiotensin converting enzyme (ACE) inhibitor or if not tolerated, an angiotensin receptor blocker (ARB)	Calcium channel blocker (CCB) or, if not tolerated, a thiazide-like diuretic
Step 2	Discuss with the person whether they are taking their medication correctly. ACE inhibitor or ARB + CCB **or** ACE inhibitor or ARB + thiazide-like diuretic In those of black African or African-Caribbean family origin who do not have type 2 diabetes, consider an ARB in addition to Step 1 treatment	
Step 3	Review medication and ensure the patient is taking the optimum tolerated doses Discuss adherence ACE inhibitor or ARB + CCB + thiazide-like diuretic	
Step 4	This is now regarded as resistant hypertension Confirm clinic BP with ambulatory BP measurements and discuss adherence Consider fourth antihypertensive drug or seek specialist advice Further diuretic therapy, e.g. spironolactone if potassium is below 4.5 mmol/L Or an alpha blocker or beta blocker if potassium more than 4.5 mmol/L If blood pressure remains uncontrolled, seek specialist advice	

Information taken from NICE, 2019b.

Hypertension control in the UK is not optimal and some patients may need to take several drugs to control their BP.

Fixed-dose combinations of drugs in one tablet may sometimes be used. By putting more than one medication in each tablet, compliance is increased as the patient only has one tablet to take. The drugs should be prescribed individually first, to ensure that the patient can tolerate them and to establish the right dose. If a combined tablet is used, it is more difficult to identify individual side effects.

Dosage (Table 5.4)

- Ideally the drug should only need to be taken once daily.
- An interval of at least 4 weeks is necessary sometimes for the full response to be observed.

TABLE 5.4 Compelling and possible indications and contraindications, and cautions for the major classes of antihypertensive drugs.

Class of drug	Compelling indications	Possible indications	Cautions	Compelling contraindications
Alpha blockers	Benign prostatic hypertrophy		Postural hypotension, HF*	Urinary incontinence
ACE inhibitors	HF, LV dysfunction, post-MI, established CHD, type 1 diabetic nephropathy, secondary stroke prevention¶	Chronic renal disease, type 2 diabetic nephropathy, proteinuric renal disease	Renal impairment‡	Pregnancy Renovascular disease
ARBs	ACE inhibitor intolerance, type 2 diabetic nephropathy, hypertension with LVH, heart failure in ACE-intolerant people, post-MI	LV dysfunction post-MI, intolerance of other antihypertensive drugs, proteinuric renal disease, HF†	Renal impairment‡	Pregnancy Renovascular disease§
Beta blockers	MI, angina	HF¶	HF¶, PVD, diabetes (except with CHD)	Asthma/COPD, heart block
CCBs (dihydropyridine)	Elderly, ISH, angina, CHD	Elderly, angina, MI		
Other CCBs (rate limiting)			Combination with beta blockade**	Heart block, HF, gout**
Thiazides/thiazide-like diuretics	Elderly, ISH, HF, secondary stroke prevention			

ACE, Angiotensin converting enzyme; ARBs, angiotensin II receptor blockers; BP, blood pressure; CCBs, calcium channel blockers; CHD, coronary heart disease; COPD, chronic obstructive pulmonary disease; HF, heart failure; ISH, isolated hypertension; LVH, left ventricular hypertrophy; MI, myocardial infarction; PVD, peripheral vascular disease.

* HF when used as monotherapy;

†ACE inhibitors or ARBs may be beneficial in chronic renal failure but should only be used with caution, close supervision and specialist advice;

‡caution with ACE inhibitors and ARBs in peripheral vascular disease because of the association with renovascular disease;

§ACE inhibitors and ARBs are sometimes used in people with renovascular disease under specialist supervision;

¶in combination with a thiazide/thiazide-like diuretic;

¶beta blockers are increasingly used to treat stable heart failure; however, beta blockers may worsen heart failure;

** thiazide/thiazide-like diuretics may sometimes be necessary to control BP in people with a history of gout, ideally used in combination with allopurinol.

Reproduced from The Joint British Societies' Guidelines on Prevention of Cardiovascular Disease in Clinical Practice (2005), BMJ Publishing Group and British Cardiac Society with permission.

- When the first drug is tolerated well by the patient but is insufficient to control the BP then either substitution or addition of a drug may be tried.
- If the hypertension is mild and the response to the first drug was very small then substitution may be used effectively.
- In other cases, it is better to add drugs stepwise and in small doses until BP is controlled.
- The treatment can be stepped down later if BP falls below target levels.

Other measures to reduce cardiovascular risk

Patients are often prescribed aspirin and/or a statin to further prevent their risk of CVD but only when their BP is under control due to the risk of haemorrhage.

Hypertension in the elderly

Trial data show older people benefit as much, if not more, than younger ones if they are treated. The Hypertension in the Very Elderly Trial (HYVET) (Beckett et al. 2008) began in 2001 and randomized 3845 patients over 80 years of age with hypertension into groups taking a low-dose diuretic and an ACEI or a placebo. The trial was stopped early (2007) due to significant reduction in strokes and cardiovascular mortality in the treated group.

- BP in the elderly is more variable and so measurements should be taken on several occasions at different times of the day before diagnosis is confirmed.
- It is necessary to take the BP both sitting and standing as postural hypotension is common.
- May need to treat to the standing levels to prevent episodes of hypotension.
- In those aged 60−80 diuretics have been shown to be effective in four large trials.
- The new NICE guidelines (2019b) recommend treating stage 1 hypertension in all, including those over 80 years of age. This is a new directive.

Hypertension and stroke

Although stroke mortality has fallen by approximately 45% in the last 30 years in the UK, there are over 100,000 strokes annually. The incidence of stroke doubles every decade over 55 years of age.

- Hypertension is the most important treatable factor for the prevention of stroke. After a stroke it is usual to initiate antihypertensive therapy within 2 weeks.
- Other drugs, such as antiplatelet agents, should also be used in thrombotic stroke. Aspirin 75 mg daily has been found to reduce the incidence of further cardiovascular events by about 20% if the history is of ischaemic stroke.

- If AF is present, anticoagulation may reduce the incidence of a further stroke by over 60%
- Statins should also be considered if total cholesterol (TC) is above 3.5 mmol/L.

Hypertension and diabetes mellitus

- Hypertension is twice as common in those with diabetes and should be treated aggressively.
- Reduction of BP in those with diabetes has been shown to reduce both mortality and morbidity by very large margins.
- Progression of such complications as retinopathy and nephropathy have been reduced.
- The target clinic BP should be below 140/80 mmHg and further cardio-vascular benefit is likely if BP is lowered to >130/80 mmHg. The latter should be the target if kidney, eye or CVD are present.
- In patients with hypertension and diabetes in the Hypertension Optimum Treatment (HOT) trial (Hansson et al. 1998), if a DBP of <80 mmHg was aimed for instead of 90 mmHg, the incidence of major cardiovascular events was halved.
- Trials in diabetes that used ACEIs for BP lowering have shown the incidence of nephropathy to be vastly reduced with these drugs.

Ethnic minority groups

Black men and women in America do have higher BPs and rates of hypertension than white counterparts. According to Thomas et al. (2018), approximately 75% of black men and women in America develop hypertension by the age of 55 years. The figure for white men is 55% and for white women is 40% at the same age. Within the black population there is a higher incidence of strokes, renal failure and left ventricular hypertrophy (LVH), although CHD morbidity and mortality remain lower than in whites.

The hypertension is usually sensitive to salt restriction. The black population have lower renin levels usually and BP responds better to diuretics or CCBs.

In British South Asians there is a high rate of type II diabetes and an increased risk of stroke as well as CHD. There is no evidence that response is any different to antihypertensives, but the high prevalence of diabetes may influence drug choices.

The importance of communication

- Patients may not understand the need for long-term treatment in the absence of symptoms.

- Taking time to explain to patients and relatives is worthwhile.
- Simplifying the drug regimen helps and drugs that only need to be given once daily should be used where possible.
- NICE has developed tools to help organizations implement their guidance. These are available from their website (www.nice.org.uk).

- SBP is more important than DBP as a determinant of CVD risk and adverse outcome, especially in those over 55 years.
- Aim is now to reduce BP to below 130/80 mmHg.
- Many people will require at least two drugs for effective control of BP.
- Hypertension should not be treated in isolation – drugs may be needed to reduce other CVD risk factors (e.g. aspirin and statins).

5.3 ATHEROSCLEROSIS AND LIPID-LOWERING DRUGS

Lipids within the body are essential both as energy providers (triglycerides) and as constituents of cell membranes and building blocks for other molecules (cholesterol). Although very necessary, raised levels of lipids within the bloodstream are the predominant cause of CVD where they become deposited within the arterial walls as atheroma (derived from the Greek word for gruel or porridge).

Lipid transport and atheroma formation

Both cholesterol and triglycerides are lipids. Atheroma is derived mostly from cholesterol but high triglyceride levels in the blood are also linked to heart disease.

- The process of atheroma deposition can start in childhood with the laying down of fatty streaks in the artery walls.
- The streaks continue to develop slowly, increasing in size to become collagen-covered plaques that cause narrowing of affected arteries.
- Eventually the artery may be narrowed to such an extent that oxygenated blood to the area supplied by the artery is insufficient to meet the metabolic demand and ischaemia results.
- This may present as angina if a coronary artery is affected or as poor circulation in the legs if the femoral arteries are affected (PVD). In cerebrovascular disease it is the blood supply to the brain that is affected.
- Plaques may become unstable and leak. When this occurs, platelets are attracted to the area and a thrombus may result. This could completely block the artery and result in a heart attack or stroke.

Raised cholesterol levels are an important risk factor for CVD.

Cholesterol is a lipid that is not used as a fuel for energy but is essential for life. It was first isolated from gall stones in 1784 and is used in the body for:

- the manufacture of cell membranes
- the synthesis of vitamin D
- the synthesis of steroid hormones (e.g. cortisol, oestrogen, progesterone, testosterone)
- the production of bile salts.

Sources of cholesterol

Approximately 15% of cholesterol is in the diet. The remaining 85% is made by the liver from acetyl CoA, a product of fat metabolism. Saturated fatty acids (mostly obtained from eating animal fats) increase production of cholesterol. To reduce cholesterol levels, a diet low in saturated fat should be eaten.

Sitostanol ester (from plants) reduces the reabsorption of cholesterol into the bloodstream and is incorporated into **Benecol** products, such as margarine, which lower cholesterol levels.

Raised levels of lipids in the bloodstream are called **hyperlipidaemia**. A high cholesterol level is **hypercholesterolaemia**. Some people have a hereditary high level of cholesterol, and diet alone is unlikely to lower the blood levels sufficiently.

Hyperlipidaemia results from a familial tendency interacting with a diet high in animal fats.

Elimination of cholesterol

- Cholesterol is broken down by the liver and converted into bile salts to be eliminated from the body. This is the only exit route for cholesterol.
- Some cholesterol is reabsorbed from the large bowel and transported back to the liver to be reused. A high-fibre diet binds to the bile acids and promotes the excretion of cholesterol by preventing reabsorption.
- Sometimes cholesterol is present in bile at virtually the limit of its solubility. It can then crystallize out to form gall stones.

Lipid transport in the bloodstream

- Lipids are insoluble and have to be transported around the body using carriers called **lipoproteins** that are lipid-containing protein complexes.
- Lipoproteins are mixtures of triglycerides, phospholipids and cholesterol. They include:
  - LDL
  - IDL (intermediate density lipoprotein)
  - VLDL (very low-density lipoprotein)
  - Lipoprotein (a)
  - HDL.
- The most important lipoproteins in the development of atherosclerosis were considered for many years to be LDL and HDL but now IDL, VLDL and lipoprotein(a) are also considered important.
- Cholesterol is now split (for ease of management) into HDL cholesterol and non-HDL cholesterol. HDL cholesterol is 'good' and non-HDL cholesterol is 'bad'.
- LDL carries about 70% of the TC. It delivers cholesterol to the peripheral tissues and is one of the 'baddies' of CHD, alongside other 'non-HDL' forms of cholesterol.

Elevated levels of non-HDL cholesterol are associated with an increased risk of atherosclerosis and CHD.

- Body cells have receptors for LDL on their surface that they can autoregulate. When the cell has enough cholesterol for its needs it will reduce the number of receptors on its surface. Excess LDL thus remains in the bloodstream and may be deposited in the arteries.
- HDL is made in the liver and small intestine. It picks up excess cholesterol from the cells and takes it to the liver for breakdown and transport into bile. It is the 'goody' of CHD as it scavenges and eliminates cholesterol. About 20%–30% of cholesterol is transported as HDL.

High levels of HDL are associated with a reduced risk of atherosclerosis.

- When a TC level in the blood is measured, this includes HDL and non-HDL cholesterol.
- The TC to HDL cholesterol ratio is used as a measure for risk assessment for CVD, and to obtain this, fasting blood lipid levels have to be measured.
- CVD risk is determined by the levels of LDL and HDL cholesterol. The higher the LDL, the higher the risk. Risk is inversely related to HDL cholesterol levels.
- Lowering the level of LDL and raising the level of HDL cholesterol slows the progression of atherosclerosis and may even induce regression.
- Acceptable levels are:
  - TC   <5 mmol/L
  - Cholesterol/HDL ratio   <4
  - LDL cholesterol   <3 mmol/L
  - Non-HDL cholesterol   <4 mmol/L
  - Triglycerides   <1.7 mmol/L

(https://www.nhs.uk/conditions/high-cholesterol/)

Role of low-density lipoprotein in atherosclerosis

- LDL is the main carrier of cholesterol to the liver and the body cells.
- Damage to the endothelial lining of the blood vessels, especially in areas of turbulence, such as the bifurcation of an artery, allows LDL to penetrate the blood vessel wall. Smoking or hypertension could be involved in causing damage.
- LDL is deposited below the inner lining (intima) of the blood vessel.
- Oxidation of the LDL occurs with time and this attracts white blood cells (WBCs, macrophages) to the area. These scavenge the LDL, accumulating cholesterol, and become foam cells.
- When the WBCs die, their contents become deposited as atheroma.
- A collagen cap is formed over the atheroma and as this grows the vessel is narrowed.
- With time, the plaque may become unstable and rupture may occur. This leads to the aggregation of platelets and blood clot formation as in an MI.

It is estimated that around half the adult population in the UK are living with a raised cholesterol level above 5 mmol/L (BHF, 2019) (Table 5.5). This not only reflects the high intake of dietary fat eaten, but also is dependent on genetic factors. Cholesterol levels are incorporated into risk factor tables for CVD.

TABLE 5.5 Values for serum lipid levels in the bloodstream.

	TC (mmol/L)	LDL (mmol/L)	HDL (mmol/L)	TGs (mmol/L)
Desirable	<4.0	<2	>1.2	<1.7
Less desirable	4.0–4.7	2–3		
Borderline	4.8–6.0	3.0–4.0	1.0–2.0	1.7–2.2
High risk	>6.0	>4.0	<1.0	>2.2

LDL, Low-density lipoprotein; *HDL,* high-density lipoprotein; *TC,* total cholesterol; TGs, triglycerides.

Cardiovascular mortality rises with:
- increasing TC levels
- increasing LDL levels
- low HDL levels
- high triglyceride levels.

Familial hypercholesterolaemia

- An inherited condition that is an autosomal dominant trait.
- Prevalence in the UK of about 1 in 500.
- Cholesterol is raised to twice normal levels (usually >9 mmol/L).
- 50% of men have CHD by the age of 55 years with women about 20 years later.
- CHD mortality rate at least 10 times that of the general population.
- Need early identification and treatment to lower blood lipids.

Secondary causes of hyperlipidaemia include hypothyroidism, diabetes, obesity, nephrotic syndrome, alcohol abuse and liver disease. Some drugs (e.g. thiazide diuretics) can also raise blood lipids.

Lifestyle and cholesterol levels

- Raised cholesterol levels need to be treated alongside other risk factors for CVD. Drugs should be used alongside, and not instead of, lifestyle changes.
- A healthier diet typically reduces cholesterol by 5%–10%. If fat is restricted to <30% of calories with <7% as saturated fat and fibre increased, there can be a fall of about 8%–15% in LDL.

- Other important factors include weight loss, BP reduction, reduced insulin resistance and increased intake of fruit and vegetables.
- Weight loss itself can lower cholesterol — a 10 kg loss can lower LDL by about 7% and raise HDL by 13%. A BMI of 20–25 should be aimed for.
- Regular exercise is beneficial and appears to increase HDL.
- Alcohol should be restricted to less than 14 units a week with several alcohol-free days each week. Binge drinking should be avoided.

Lipid-lowering drugs

These act by reducing the formation of lipids or hastening their removal from the body (Table 5.6).

There is evidence that therapy that lowers LDL and raises HDL will lower the incidence of atheroma and related disorders. It may reduce the progression of coronary artery disease (CAD).

Drug therapy must be combined with adherence to diet, weight loss (if needed) and reduction in BP if appropriate, as well as stopping smoking.

Lipid-lowering drugs include statins, fibrates, anion-exchange resins, nicotinic acid and ezetimibe. No drugs yet independently raise HDL levels.

Benefits of lipid lowering

- One systemic study (Gao et al. 2014) indicated that intensive therapy that lowers LDL by about 30% probably does reduce atheromatous progression and even leads to some regression of the plaque.
- A 10% reduction in TC lowers the risk of death from CHD by 10% and of non-fatal MI by 21%.

TABLE 5.6 Effects of some lipid-lowering drugs.

Drug	LDL	HDL	TGs
Statins	Lower	Raise	Modest effect
Fibrates	Modest effect	Raise	Lower
Anion-exchange resins	Lower		May aggravate
Nicotinic acid		Raise	Lower
Fish oils		Raise	Lower

LDL, Low-density lipoprotein; *HDL,* high-density lipoprotein.

Statins

Atorvastatin, fluvastatin, pravastatin, rosuvastatin and simvastatin

These are the most potent lipid-lowering drugs and first choice to lower cholesterol levels.

They are compounds developed from fungi that inhibit an enzyme needed by the body to produce cholesterol. The first one was *lovastatin* and was approved in America in 1987.

They are used as primary prevention if the 10-year total CVD risk, using risk assessment, is greater than 10%. This used to be 20% but has been halved in the latest NICE guidelines and means that an extra 4.5 million people could be eligible for statins, helping to prevent up to 28,000 heart attacks and 16,000 strokes a year (NICE, 2018e). *Atorvastatin* is the drug of choice, and for primary prevention NICE recommends atorvastatin 20 mg daily. The guidelines include the use for all ages including those over 85 years old. However careful assessment of factors that could make treatment inappropriate should be carried out.

Their use in secondary prevention is discussed below.

Mechanism of action

- An important enzyme needed by the liver in the synthesis of cholesterol is **HMG CoA reductase** (hydroxymethylglutaryl coenzyme A reductase).
- If this enzyme is inhibited, the cells will reduce their manufacture of cholesterol.
- Statins competitively and potently inhibit this enzyme, thus limiting the rate of synthesis of cholesterol and reducing levels in the blood.
- This leads to an increase in LDL receptors on cell surfaces as there is less cholesterol available for them. This is good because the additional receptors further increase removal of LDL from the bloodstream.
- There is also a small fall in plasma triglycerides and a small rise in HDL (about 3%−10%).

Cholesterol lowering potency varies. They are grouped by NICE into three different intensity categories:

- low intensity if the reduction is 20%−30%
- medium intensity if the reduction is 31%−40%
- high intensity if the reduction is above 40%.

In 2004, simvastatin became available as an over-the-counter medicine at a dosage of 10 mg/day.

It has to be dispensed by a pharmacist and is licensed for primary prevention in people with a moderate (10%) 10-year risk of CHD.

As part of the NHS Long-Term Plan to reduce heart disease and stroke, high-dose statins could soon be available over the counter in High Street pharmacies (2019).

Evidence for clinical effectiveness

- Initial evidence showed that statins reduced the incidence of coronary events and reduced total mortality in patients up to the age of 75 years with a serum cholesterol of 5 mmol/L or greater. Newer evidence shows that there are benefits at any age and at lower levels of cholesterol. They can reduce the incidence of CHD by 50%−60%.
- Benefits are seen not only in those with a history of CVD (secondary prevention) but also in those with no history (primary prevention), even when cholesterol levels are within the 'normal' range.
- Statins also reduce the incidence of nonhaemorrhagic stroke when used for secondary prevention in CHD.
- May lower blood cholesterol by one-third in familial hyperlipidaemia.
- They are generally more effective than any other drugs in lowering LDL.
- Need to adopt diet and lifestyle changes alongside their use.

Pharmacokinetics

- All of these drugs are well absorbed from the gut.
- All have short half-lives of about 2 hours except *atorvastatin* (14 hours).
- All effective if given once daily.
- All work slightly better if given at night when the liver synthesizes more cholesterol.
- Results can be seen after a week and are maximal after 4−6 weeks of treatment.
- Metabolized by cytochrome P450 enzymes in the liver, and this is the source of many important interactions. Grapefruit juice inhibits metabolism of statins and may produce more side effects.

Side effects

- Uncommon but include gastrointestinal disturbances (abdominal pain, flatulence, diarrhoea, nausea and vomiting), headache, rash, muscle cramps and elevation of liver enzymes.
- Statins may increase the anticoagulant effects of warfarin. *Atorvastatin* appears least likely to increase the anticoagulant effects.
- Reversible **myositis** (inflammation and degeneration of muscle) is a rare but significant side effect. Myalgia, myositis and myopathy have all been reported. Can occur in approximately 1 in 1000 cases.
- **Creatine kinase** (**CK**) is an enzyme that is elevated in muscle breakdown. The level should be taken if the patient complains of aching or painful muscles, and if elevated to more than five times the upper limit of normal, the statin should be discontinued.
- **Rhabdomyolysis** (pathological breakdown of skeletal muscle) is rare (approximately 1 case in every 100,000 treatment years) and appears to be dose dependent. This can lead to renal failure if the products of muscle

breakdown damage the kidneys. The risk is increased if the drugs are combined with fibrates, which are also used to lower blood lipids. The risk appears greatest with **gemfibrozil** and statins should **not** be prescribed with this drug.

- Risk of myopathy is less with **pravastatin** and **fluvastatin** – perhaps because they have less muscle penetration (hydrophilic).

Monitoring requirements

- Before starting treatment, a full lipid profile should be done including TC, HDL-cholesterol, non-HDL cholesterol and triglycerides.
- Thyroid function and renal function should be assessed.
- Liver enzymes should be measured before treatment, after 3 months and at 12 months, according to NICE guidelines (2018e).
- CK should be measured before statin therapy is started if there is a history of muscle pain. It should be repeated if over five times the upper normal limit and if it remains at this level, the statin should not be started.

Cautions

- Patients should be advised to report unexplained muscle pain promptly.
- Muscle toxicity can occur with all statins but is more likely when higher doses are used.
- Caution is needed with any history of muscular disorders, a high alcohol intake, renal impairment or hypothyroidism.
- Any abnormalities in blood results seen above in the monitoring section.

Contraindications

- Liver disease.
- Pregnancy and breastfeeding.

Current thoughts

- The benefits of statins appear to be greater than those that would occur just due to a decrease in LDL cholesterol. Atherosclerosis can be thought of as an inflammatory process and it is possible that they are having an anti-inflammatory action.
- C-reactive protein (CRP) is a protein produced by the liver that is raised in inflammation. It has been used as a marker for inflammation (e.g. in rheumatoid arthritis) for many years. Statins can reduce CRP by up to 60%.
- Lower CRP levels may be important in the prevention of CVD, and research into these areas continues.
- Statins also reduce platelet adhesion, may stabilize the atheromatous plaque and be antithrombotic.

- Eighteen years ago, a long-term follow-up in the West of Scotland Coronary Prevention Study (WOSCOPS) showed that 5 years of statin therapy still benefited patients in terms of reduced mortality 10 years later (Freeman et al. 2001).

Primary prevention
- In those asymptomatic patients at increased risk of CHD due to raised serum cholesterol but with no existing disease.
- The risk of CVD is greater in men, in people over the age of 50 years, in those with a family history of CVD and in some ethnic backgrounds such as South Asians.
- Those at risk should be identified by their presenting risk factors as well as the use of risk calculators and clinical judgement.

Secondary prevention
- All patients with symptomatic CVD − previous MI, angina, non-haemorrhagic stroke, coronary bypass surgery.
- Heart UK recommends that all those with acute atherosclerotic CVD should commence statin therapy in hospital. Even when TC is <4.0 mmol/L statin therapy should not be delayed. Research shows risk is reduced whatever the cholesterol level.
- In diabetes mellitus, given to all patients over 40 years of age with type 1 or type 2 diabetes. Also considered in younger patients if poor glycaemic control, low HDL cholesterol and raised triglyceride, hypertension or family history of premature CVD.

Cholesterol-absorption inhibitors
Ezetimibe

- A newer drug that inhibits intestinal absorption of cholesterol.
- Can lower LDL cholesterol by about 15%−20% when added to diet (Pandor et al. 2009).
- Well tolerated but no randomized, controlled trial evidence yet available for long-term safety.
- Can be used in combination with a statin or alone if statin not tolerated.
- Recommended in conjunction with a statin for the treatment of hypercholesterolaemia
- Increased risk of rhabdomyolysis if used with a statin.

Fibrates
Bezafibrate, ciprofibrate, fenofibrate and gemfibrozil

- Reduce triglycerides mostly − have variable effects on LDL and raise HDL.

- A statin is always used first unless serum triglycerides are above 10 mmol/L or the patient cannot tolerate a statin.
- May be added to statin therapy on specialist advice if triglycerides remain high even when LDL has been reduced. Added in type 2 diabetes if triglycerides over 2.3 mmol/L. Greater risk of myositis if combined with a statin.
- Appear to stimulate the formation of lipoprotein lipase, which reduces triglyceride levels. It stimulates clearance of LDL from the liver.
- Increase cholesterol excretion in bile and so may increase risk of gall stones.

Side effects Gastrointestinal disturbances; for example, nausea and vomiting, headache and itching.

Can cause myositis especially if renal function is poor.

Anion-exchange resins

For example, colestyramine, colestipol, colesevelam

- Bind bile acids in the intestine and prevent their reabsorption.
- This promotes the conversion of cholesterol into bile acids in the liver and increases LDL receptor activity, increasing clearance of LDL from blood.
- They reduce LDL but can aggravate hypertriglyceridaemia.

Side effects Interfere with absorption of fat-soluble vitamins and bleeding has been reported due to vitamin K deficiency.

Nicotinic acid

- This is a vitamin that raises HDL cholesterol and reduces triglycerides.
- Inhibits triglyceride synthesis in the liver.

Side effects

- Causes flushing that is less if taken in the evening.
- Palpitations.
- Gastrointestinal disturbances.
- May impair glucose tolerance and increase the risk of gout.

Fish oils (omega-3 [ω-3] fatty acids)

- Present in fish oil supplements (e.g. **Maxepa**).
- Can lower triglyceride levels but do not have a reliable effect on cholesterol levels.
- Can be used with statins or other lipid-lowering drugs.

Benecol (and other similar margarines)

- **Benecol** contains plant stanol ester, which helps block the uptake of cholesterol in the gut. Therefore, with **Benecol** less cholesterol enters the bloodstream.
- Normally 50% of cholesterol is absorbed into the bloodstream. **Benecol** reduces this amount to about 30%. The rest simply passes out of the body.
- **Benecol** can reduce levels of LDL by up to 14%. The amount of HDL cholesterol is unchanged. Results are usually seen within as little as 2−3 weeks.
- Average daily portion reduces LDL by about 0.5 mmol/L in 50- to 59-year-old age group − reduction in risk of CVD of about 25% (Law, 2000).

Combinations of drug therapies

Potential for side effects is greater when statins are combined with other drugs. This is especially true of myositis. Fibrates and statins may be needed when triglycerides are high but specialist advice is needed, and *gemfibrozil* should not be combined with a statin.

5.4 ISCHAEMIC HEART DISEASE

Angina describes the pain that occurs in ischaemic heart disease (IHD) when the blood flow through the coronary arteries that supply the heart muscle with oxygenated blood is insufficient to meet the heart's metabolic requirements.

Types of angina

- **Stable angina** (angina of effort) where there is a constant narrowing of a coronary artery. Blood supply to the heart muscle is sufficient at rest, but when metabolic demand increases, pain due to lack of oxygen supply to the ischaemic cardiac muscle occurs. The commonest precipitating factor is exercise but other forms of stress such as emotion, cold or even a heavy meal can bring on the pain.
- **Variant angina** (Prinzmetal's) due to spasm of the coronary artery. There may be atheroma present but not necessarily. The vessel goes into spasm and narrows. This can occur at any time and is not related to exercise.
- **Unstable angina** (acute coronary syndrome) is a more severe pain that may come on at rest and has a worse prognosis. There is usually some rupturing of an atheromatous plaque and it is difficult to differentiate this pain from that of an MI.

Management of angina

Lifestyle modification (see Section 5.1) is always the starting point of treatment. Drug therapy not only aims to relieve symptoms and reduce the frequency and severity of attacks, but also attempts to prevent a MI.

The pain of angina is usually treated with nitrates which are vasodilators. Nitrates together with some other drugs, such as channel blockers and beta blockers, are used to prevent or reduce attacks of angina. Antiplatelet drugs and statins are prescribed to prevent further progression to a MI. Many of these drugs are discussed in detail elsewhere in this book (Table 5.7).

Nitrates

Glyceryl trinitrate, isosorbide mononitrate, isosorbide dinitrate

Nitrates are extremely effective in relieving the pain of angina but are also used to prevent attacks occurring. They are vasodilators and are commonly given as glyceryl trinitrate (GTN) sublingually in the form of a spray or a tablet.

The action of amyl nitrate was discovered in 1867. The drug produced flushing and tachycardia with a fall in BP when inhaled and was first used to relieve angina the same year. GTN replaced amyl nitrate. It was actually developed to be an explosive and is the major ingredient of dynamite.

TABLE 5.7 Summary of antianginal drugs.

Drug group	Examples	Contraindications
Beta blocker	Atenolol Bisoprolol	Asthma, severe bradycardia, heart block, severe peripheral vascular disease, heart failure (specialist)
Dihydropyridine calcium channel blocker	Amlodipine Felodipine Modified release nifedipine	Unstable angina, heart failure, aortic stenosis
Rate-limiting calcium channel blocker	Diltiazem Verapamil	Heart failure, bradycardia, heart block
Nitrate	Glyceryl trinitrate Isosorbide mononitrate Isosorbide dinitrate	Mitral or aortic stenosis
Potassium channel activator	Nicorandil	Hypotension, left ventricular failure
Sinus node inhibitor	Ivabradine	Heart failure, heart block, bradycardia

Mechanism of action Nitrates relax smooth muscle and so dilate blood vessels. They are prodrugs that are changed by the body into NO, which then stimulates the secondary messenger cyclic guanosine monophosphate (GMP). The cyclic GMP activates a protein kinase and this leads to a cascade of effects in smooth muscle culminating in relaxation.

Nitrates relieve the pain of angina by several mechanisms.

- Nitrates have their main effects on the cardiovascular system.
- There is a reduction in cardiac oxygen consumption, secondary to venous and arterial vasodilation, which has reduced the workload of the heart.
- Veins are dilated more than arteries, reducing venous return and thus the work of the left ventricle.
- Systemic arteries are dilated and this also reduces the workload of the heart.
- In angina the diseased coronary vessel cannot respond by vasodilation but nitrates can divert the blood to the ischaemic area by dilating the collateral circulation (Fig. 5.4). These are other smaller blood vessels that have developed to supply the ischaemic area of heart muscle.
- Relaxation of the blood vessel wall relieves coronary spasm in variant angina.

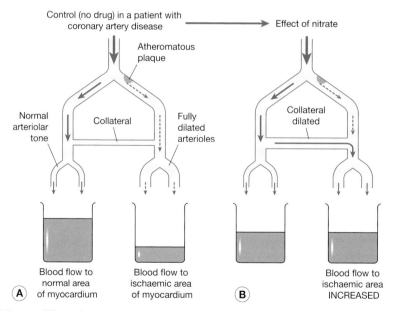

FIG. 5.4   Effect of organic nitrates on the coronary circulation. (A) Control. (B) Nitrates dilate the collateral vessel, thus allowing more blood through to the underperfused region (mostly by diversion from the adequately perfused area).

Nitrates may cause a reduction in BP and a reflex tachycardia, but even so, oxygen demand is reduced.

Pharmacokinetics

- GTN is rapidly inactivated by hepatic metabolism and suffers a very large first-pass effect when given orally. It is given sublingually, transdermally or intravenously to avoid this.
- GTN has a rapid onset of action and given sublingually starts to work within 2 minutes. Duration of action is only up to 30 minutes.
- If given intravenously the onset of action is immediate and the duration is 3−5 minutes.

Routes of administration   GTN is extremely effective given sublingually for the relief of angina. This may be in the form of a 300-microgram tablet which is placed under the tongue and allowed to dissolve.

The patient should be warned that if the pain is not relieved in 2−3 minutes with sublingual GTN they should consult a doctor.

GTN tablets must be kept in glass bottles with foil, a foil-lined cap and no cotton wool. They should be discarded after 8 weeks.

- An aerosol spray is an alternative and popular method of sublingual administration with a longer shelf life than the tablets. It may be administered prior to an activity likely to cause angina.
- GTN also may be given transdermally in the form of patches that are applied to the skin surface and provide a slow release throughout the day. The patches should be replaced every 24 hours and may be removed for an 8-hour period (usually overnight) in each 24 hours to prevent tolerance developing.
- Longer-acting nitrates are used in the form of ***isosorbide mononitrate*** (ISMN) and ***isosorbide dinitrate*** (ISDN). ISDN comes in sublingual or intravenous forms and as modified-release tablets that are taken orally twice daily.
- In MI and left ventricular failure (LVF), GTN may be administered intravenously by *Tolerance.*
- If high levels of nitrates are maintained throughout 24 hours, for 1 week or more, partial tolerance develops. This means the antianginal effect is lost, although not totally.
- Tolerance is avoided by 'eccentric' prescribing and allowing the level of nitrate to fall for a period in every 24 hours. This is achieved by a nitrate-free period of at least 6 hours in each 24 hours. If ISMN is prescribed twice daily it could be given at 10 a.m. and 4 p.m., giving a nitrate-free period of 18 hours overnight when there is less risk of angina.

Adverse effects
- Throbbing headache due to vasodilation of arteries supplying the head. Tolerance usually develops to this side effect while the antianginal property remains.
- Postural hypotension and dizziness. May occasionally cause fainting.
- Palpitations.
- Flushing due to vasodilation.

Nitrates and sildenafil

- Nitrates should not be used concurrently with *sildenafil* (*Viagra*) — a large and sudden drop in BP occurs in the majority of patients. Both drugs cause vasodilation.
- *Sildenafil* blocks the enzyme that normally destroys NO.
- Could range from no symptoms to mild symptoms of dizziness and lightheadedness to syncope to lowering of the supply of blood to the heart muscle, which could lead to the conversion of an area of myocardial ischaemia to infarction.

Nitrate use
- Angina treatment and prophylaxis.
- Intravenous GTN is used to treat MI.
- Acute LVF following MI.

Beta-adrenergic antagonists

These are first-line drugs for prevention of angina attacks. This is because they slow the heart rate and force of contraction thus reducing the oxygen demands of the heart. The heart no longer responds to noradrenaline released on stimulation of the SNS so heart rate will greatly increase with exercise or emotion.

The slower heart rate also gives more time for coronary perfusion which occurs in cardiac diastole. Thus, myocardial blood supply is improved.

Atenolol is most frequently used as it is cardioselective (see Section 2.2). Acute heart failure (AHF) is a contraindication but in stable HF *bisoprolol* may be prescribed by a specialist (see Section 5.6).

Side effects Bronchospasm may occur so the drugs are usually not given to patients with asthma.

May potentiate PVD and the patient may experience cold hands and feet. Other side effects are as described in Section 2.2.

Calcium channel blockers
Amlodipine, diltiazem, felodipine, nicardipine, verapamil (Box 5.3)

These act by blocking calcium channels in smooth muscle and cardiac muscle (see Section 5.2).

BOX 5.3 Dihydropyridine calcium channel blockers.

Amlodipine
Clevidipine
Felodipine
Lacidipine
Lercanidipine
Nicardipine
Nifedipine
Nimodipine

- Vascular effects — vasodilation. Mainly affects the small arteries and arterioles. Peripheral resistance and arterial pressure usually fall. Reduce arterial spasm as they relax the smooth muscle.
- Cardiac effects — they slow the heart rate and decrease the force of cardiac contraction. This is seen in rate-limiting drugs such as *verapamil* and *diltiazem.*
- Lower the oxygen requirements of the ischaemic myocardium. Due to reduction in contractility of the myocardium and reduction in BP.
- Dihydropyridines such as *amlodipine* act chiefly on the smooth muscle in the blood vessels and produce arterial vasodilation and so reduce the symptoms of angina. They can sometimes be added to beta blockers and also have useful antihypertensive action.

Long-acting or modified-release forms are chosen as short-acting drugs such as *nifedipine* may produce a reflex tachycardia and was shown in one study to give increased mortality in IHD. Nifedipine is not recommended for angina prophylaxis.

Rate-limiting CCBs such as *verapamil* and *diltiazem* affect the cardiac calcium channels, slowing the heart rate and reducing contractility. This means they are not prescribed alongside a beta blocker but may be useful first-line drugs if the patient cannot take a beta blocker.

Diltiazem or verapamil should not be combined with beta blockers. This is extremely dangerous and may result in profound bradycardia or HF.

- Do not increase bronchospasm so may be safely prescribed in asthma.
- Do not exacerbate PVD so cold peripheries that may be a side effect of beta blockade are not a problem.
- Do not blunt cardiovascular response to exercise.

Side effects. Flushing, headache, peripheral oedema and constipation.

Nicorandil

- A drug that dilates both arteries and veins because of nitrate generating properties and potassium channel opening properties.
- Controls the symptoms of angina as well as other drugs described.
- Side effects include headache and flushing, dizziness and nausea.

Ivabradine

Licensed for treatment of angina in patients in normal sinus rhythm.

Selectively inhibits the cardiac pacemaker current and so reduces the rate of depolarization within the sinoatrial (SA) node of the heart. This reduces heart rate without reducing the force of cardiac contraction.

- Should not be prescribed in patients with bradycardia or some other cardiac conditions.
- Can be used in combination with dihydropyridine CCBs, *nicorandil* or nitrates but should not be given with rate-limiting CCBs as it may induce a severe bradycardia.
- Side effects include bradycardia, first-degree heart block, headaches, dizziness and blurred vision.

Acute coronary syndromes

Acute coronary syndrome (ACS) includes unstable angina and non-ST elevation MI (NSTEMI) as well as ST elevation MI (STEMI).

Unstable angina and non-ST elevation myocardial infarction

Initial treatment includes oxygen, nitrates, aspirin (before arrival at hospital) and clopidogrel in addition to heparin. Diamorphine is used, if necessary, for the pain.

In unstable angina there may be pain at rest or the pain is sometimes that of crescendo angina where it rapidly worsens in frequency or severity. This is an emergency as it usually means there is some rupture of an atheromatous plaque and the patient may progress to have a MI. These patients are admitted to hospital. The drugs used in their care are all described elsewhere but will be briefly summarized here.

- Aspirin may halve the risk of death and so should always be given unless contraindicated. *Clopidogrel*, another antiplatelet drug, may also be prescribed.
- *Heparin* will be started (see Section 5.7).
- Cardioselective beta blockers are started.
- GTN may be needed by infusion.
- Coronary angiography is indicated.

ST-segment elevation myocardial infarction

Occurs when there is complete blockage of a coronary artery by a thrombus. Blood supply to the affected area of cardiac muscle is compromised, and irreversible damage to the heart muscle will occur unless the blood supply is rapidly re-established. The patient will usually have severe chest pain, may be hypotensive, sweating and nauseous or vomiting. He/she is also likely to be frightened.

The aims here are to provide pain relief and emotional support, to re-establish the blood flow to the myocardium and to reduce mortality.

About half those who die following an MI die within the first few hours, usually from arrhythmias, especially ventricular fibrillation (VF), and access to defibrillation is essential.

- Oxygen, nitrates and an opioid analgesic such as *diamorphine* provide initial support and relieve the pain but will also reduce anxiety and dilate peripheral blood vessels.
- An antiemetic such as *metoclopramide* may be needed as the patient is often nauseated. The opioid may add to this.
- *Aspirin* is given for its antiplatelet effect and may be chewed or dissolved in water. It may have been administered by the paramedic before the patient arrives in hospital.
- *Clopidogrel* should also be given. *Prasugrel* is an alternative in patients having percutaneous coronary intervention (PCI). *Ticagrelor* is also an alternative.
- Re-establishment of the coronary blood flow and limitation of the infarct size are achieved either by percutaneous coronary angioplasty (the preferred method) or by the use of 'clot-busting' thrombolytic drugs that break down the thrombus (e.g. *alteplase, tenecteplase*). These drugs are discussed in Section 5.7.
- *Glycoprotein IIb/IIIa inhibitor* can be used to reduce the risk of immediate vascular occlusion in intermediate and high-risk patients.
- If patients cannot be offered PCI within 90 minutes of diagnosis, a thrombolytic drug alongside either unfractionated heparin (UFH), a low molecular weight heparin (LMWH) or *fondaparinux sodium* should be given.
- *Heparin* is used with alteplase, reteplase and tenecteplase. This is to prevent re-thrombosis.
- Nitrates may be used to relieve the ischaemic pain and may be given by infusion if the sublingual route is not effective.
- Beta blockers (e.g. *atenolol, metoprolol, bisoprolol*) may be given (unless contraindicated). They reduce rate and contractility of the heart so reducing oxygen demand. It is hoped that this may allow the cardiac muscle to

survive the period of ischaemia. Beta blockers also reduce the risk of rupture of the heart.

- ACEIs have been shown to reduce mortality in acute MI and are started within 24 hours unless there are contraindications.
- If there is diabetes or raised blood glucose, insulin is given.

Long-term management

To protect the myocardium, several drugs should be started while the patient is still in hospital and continued on discharge.

- Aspirin 75 mg daily.
- Beta blockers if not contraindicated.
- An ACEI, especially if there is decreased function of the left ventricle.
- CCBs (e.g. *verapamil*) are only used if the patient cannot have a beta blocker.
- Statins are given to try and prevent further coronary events.

Rehabilitation is important following an MI and lifestyle advice as well as emotional support are given. Both physical and psychological wellbeing need to be optimized. Instruction should be given as to how much exercise should be done and lifestyle advice given. This will include stopping smoking and eating healthily. The patient needs to know when they can drive, return to work and when sexual activity may be recommenced.

5.5 CARDIAC ARRHYTHMIAS

An arrhythmia is any deviation from the normal rhythm of the heart.

The heart beat

- Heart rate and rhythm are controlled by the SA node situated in the wall of the right atrium.
- The SA node is under the influence of the ANS.
- The natural rate of electrical impulse generation from the SA node is about 80 times a minute.
- The PNS slows this rate to around 60−70, acting via the vagus nerve (the so-called 'vagal brake').
- The impulses spread throughout the atria and then via the atrioventricular (AV) node (where transmission is delayed allowing time for the atria to empty) through the AV bundle (bundle of His) and then dividing into the right and left bundle branches that give rise to the Purkinje fibres conducting the impulse throughout the ventricles (Fig. 5.5).

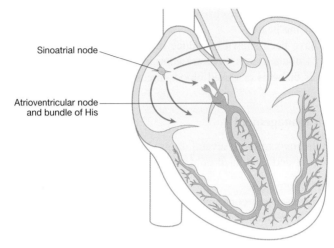

Sinoatrial node

Atrioventricular node and bundle of His

FIG. 5.5 **The conduction system of the heart.**

Cardiac arrhythmias

Arrhythmias result from a disturbance in the generation or transmission of these impulses.

- Arrhythmias may be due to over-excitability of the heart or to defects in the conduction system.
- They may be classified according to the site of origin of the abnormal rhythm — atrial, junctional or ventricular — and on whether the rate is fast (tachycardia) or slow (bradycardia).
- Arrhythmias may be intermittent or continuous.

The conduction system of the heart is very susceptible to damage, especially by ischaemia, and the commonest cause of cardiac arrhythmia is IHD. The majority of deaths following a MI result from VF and not direct failure of contraction of the muscle.

Clinical features

The patient with an arrhythmia may present with:

- palpitations: these are an awareness of one's own heartbeat
- dizziness, feeling faint or losing consciousness: these are due to reduced blood supply to the brain.

Types of arrhythmia

The arrhythmia is diagnosed by taking an electrocardiogram (ECG). Sometimes it may be difficult to do this as the abnormal beat may not be present for a sufficient length of time.

- The commonest arrhythmia is AF where the pulse is irregularly irregular. It occurs in approximately 10% of those over 65 years of age. Over a million people in the UK have AF and it contributes to one in five strokes (Stroke Association, 2019). The atria are fibrillating and the ventricles are contracting independently of the atria.
- Supraventricular tachycardia is also quite common. Here the pulse is extremely rapid, but regular.
- Ventricular tachycardia is much rarer but much more dangerous as it can lead to VF where the electrical activity in the ventricles is completely chaotic and there is no CO. This type of arrhythmia is responsible for most deaths immediately following a MI. The treatment for VF is defibrillation.
- Bradyarrhythmias include the various types of heart block.
- When electrical activity completely stops, this is asystolic arrest.

Heart block

- Heart block results from damage to the conducting system.
- In complete heart block the atria and ventricles beat completely independently.
- The rate is determined by whichever pacemaker in the ventricles takes over (escape rhythm).
- If the AV conduction completely fails there are periods of unconsciousness known as Stokes−Adams attacks. An artificial pacemaker is needed in these cases.

Sick sinus syndrome

- Also known as SA disease or sinus node dysfunction.
- There is usually some fibrosis of the SA node.
- Episodes of sinus bradycardia or sinus arrest occur.
- Bradycardia−tachycardia syndrome may occur where patients experience paroxysmal atrial tachyarrhythmias followed by periods of asystole.

Wolff−Parkinson−White syndrome

- A congenital condition due to the presence of an accessory conducting system between the atria and the ventricles.
- It is associated with supraventricular tachycardia due to re-entry.
- In some cases, episodes may be infrequent and settle on their own without treatment.
- When treated with antiarrhythmic drugs the accessory tissue may respond differently to normal conducting tissue.

- *Digoxin* and *verapamil* enhance conduction and so are **contraindicated in Wolff–Parkinson–White (WPW).**
- *Adenosine, amiodarone, flecainide* or *disopyramide* may be used.
- Long term, catheter ablation is often used and is 95% successful (NHS, 2019).
- For others, daily medication, such as amiodarone, may be prescribed.

Long QT syndrome

- May be congenital or acquired and may lead to torsade de pointes which is a dangerous and atypical form of ventricular tachycardia that may cause palpitations and syncope but may end spontaneously.
- In congenital long QT, torsade can be provoked by increased adrenaline as in exercise or emotion.
- Acquired long QT syndrome may be caused by some drugs (e.g. *sotalol, erythromycin, terfenadine*) or by electrolyte disturbances such as low potassium levels in the blood (hypokalaemia), low magnesium (hypomagnesaemia) and low calcium levels (hypocalcaemia).

It is not always clear what is the cause of an arrhythmia and treatment may be difficult (Box 5.4).

Mechanisms underlying arrhythmias

There are four basic mechanisms that underlie pathological cardiac arrhythmias.

1 Delayed after-depolarization, which triggers ectopic beats

This is a repetitive discharge that does not rely on the arrival of an impulse from elsewhere. The after-depolarization occurs immediately after the action potential if an abnormally high calcium is present, and is encouraged by agents such as *noradrenaline* and *digoxin* that increase intracellular levels and reduced by drugs that block calcium entry. Raised calcium can also delay repolarization, shown as a longer QT interval on the ECG. Many drugs increase the QT interval by binding to ion channels. This carries a risk of dangerous ventricular arrhythmias.

BOX 5.4 Some causes of cardiac arrhythmias.

Ischaemic heart disease
Congenital abnormalities of conduction pathway (e.g. Wolff–Parkinson–White syndrome)
Arrhythmogenic drugs (e.g. digoxin, some antiarrhythmic drugs)
Metabolic disturbances (e.g. hypokalaemia)
Endocrine disturbances (e.g. hyperthyroidism)
Long QT syndrome and torsade de pointes

2 Re-entry – resulting from partial conduction block

In the normal heart rhythm, the impulse dies away after it has activated the ventricles because it is surrounded by refractory tissue. Re-entry occurs when the impulse succeeds in exciting regions of the myocardium when the refractory period has subsided. A simple ring of tissue can result in this if there is a transient or unidirectional block present. This is known as a 'circus rhythm'. The re-entrant rhythm will persist only if the time taken for propagation around the ring is greater than the refractory period. It may be halted by drugs that prolong the refractory period.

Re-entry may also occur if there is slowing of action potential propagation which often occurs following an MI. This is due to inactivation of fast sodium channels leaving only slow sodium channels to support propagation of the action potential.

Re-entry is thought to be the mechanism behind many types of arrhythmia.

3 Abnormal pacemaker activity

Pacemaker activity is usually confined to the SA node and the conducting tissue but can occur in other parts of the heart under pathological conditions.

Increased sympathetic activity encourages this. Myocardial ischaemia causes an increase in sympathetic activity and also an increase in the release of *adrenaline* from the adrenal gland, both of which encourage the appearance of abnormal pacemakers.

4 Heart block

Heart block results from ischaemic damage to, or fibrosis of, the AV node or other areas of the conducting system.

It is not always clear which of the above mechanisms are responsible for an arrhythmia.

Treatment options:

- Sometimes, if asymptomatic, there is no treatment required although the patient should receive follow-up appointments.
- Simple clinical intervention such as vagal manoeuvres.
- Drug treatment
- Electrical such as cardioversion for tachyarrhythmia or pacing for bradyarrhythmia.
- In unstable patients with adverse features, drugs act more slowly and less reliably so electrical treatment is usually preferred (Resuscitation Council, 2015).

Drugs used in the treatment of arrhythmias

Drugs that modify the rhythm and conduction of the heart are used to treat arrhythmias. Most drugs that are used in treatment may actually precipitate arrhythmias themselves (pro-arrhythmogenic) or depress ventricular contractility and so need to be used with caution. This is a field for the specialist and only a brief description of drugs will be given here.

Aims of antiarrhythmic therapy are:

- to reduce ectopic pacemaker activity
- to prevent circus movement in re-entrant circuits.

Currently available drugs achieve this role by:

- blocking sodium or calcium channels
- prolonging the effective refractory period
- antagonizing the effects of catecholamines at the β_1 receptor.

Drugs decrease the automaticity of ectopic pacemakers more than nodal tissue but many antiarrhythmic drugs will depress normal conducting tissue when dosages are increased and produce a drug-induced dysrhythmia. Some are proarrhythmic even at 'therapeutic' concentrations if acidosis, sinus tachycardia or electrolyte imbalance are present.

When to treat arrhythmias

Only when they are producing symptoms or are in danger of becoming life-threatening. If ectopic beats are spontaneous with a normal heart, they rarely require pharmacological treatment.

- The benefit of treatment must outweigh the potential risk. In serious arrhythmias such as ventricular tachycardia that may progress to VF this is always the case, whereas multiple supraventricular ectopic beats are harmless and do not require treatment.
- Research in the form of the Cardiac Arrhythmia Suppression Trial (CAST) showed that prophylactic treatment of ectopic beats with *flecainide* (class I antiarrhythmic drug) following a MI actually increased mortality.
- There may be factors precipitating the arrhythmia that can themselves be removed, for example, hypokalaemia, drugs such as *digoxin*, acidosis, hypoxia.
- Sometimes a nondrug treatment may be preferred; for example, cardiac pacing or ablation of accessory conduction pathways.

The British Resuscitation Council has produced algorithms for the treatment of life-threatening arrhythmias. These are available on its website at www.resus.org.uk.

Adrenaline is used in cardiac arrest. Activation of the β_1 adrenoreceptors repolarizes the damaged or hypoxic myocardium by stimulating the Na^+/K^+ pump. This may restore function.

Atropine is an antimuscarinic drugs that blocks vagal activity and is used to treat bradycardia. Its use can sometimes allow sympathetic activity that was hidden to become overt and result in sinus tachycardia or, extremely rarely, ventricular tachycardia or VF.

Vaughan Williams classification of antiarrhythmic drugs

Antiarrhythmic drugs are classified according to their electrophysiological actions into four classes. This allows several drugs with similar properties to be classed together. The classification was first proposed by Vaughan Williams (1918−2016) in 1970 and has been constantly updated (Table 5.8). The latest update was in the journal *Circulation* for the centenary of Vaughan Williams' birthdate (Ming et al. 2018). This revision does make it much clearer which drugs are useful for which arrhythmias. Table 5.9 lists the trials that are linked to information in this chapter.

Another classification method is to divide the drugs into those used only in supraventricular arrhythmias, those used only in ventricular arrhythmias and those that may be used in either (Table 5.10).

Class I drugs

- Block sodium channels. Have been referred to as membrane stabilizers because they inhibit action potential propagation in excitable cells. Make the cells less responsive to excitation.
- This is also the mode of action of local anaesthetics and some anticonvulsants (e.g. *phenytoin*). This drug may be used to reduce *digoxin*-induced arrhythmias.
- They reduce the rate of depolarization in phase 0 of the action potential.
- Show the property of use-dependence. The more the sodium channels are opened, the more they will block.
- Class I drugs are less used now than in the past. This is due to the better safety profile of some other drugs.

TABLE 5.8 Vaughan Williams classification of antiarrhythmic drugs.

Class	Mechanism of action	Repolarization time	Examples
Ia	Membrane stabilization	Prolongs	Quinidine
Ib	Sodium blockade	Shortens	Lidocaine
Ic		Unchanged	Flecainide
II	Beta-adrenergic blockade	Unchanged	Esmolol
III	Increase refractory period by repolarizing K^+ currents	Prolongs	Amiodarone Sotalol
IV	Calcium channel blockade	Unchanged	Verapamil Diltiazem
IV-like (not classified)	K^+ channel opener	Unchanged	Adenosine

TABLE 5.9 Clinical trials mentioned in this chapter.

Trial	Date	Full title	Reference
AIRE	1993	Acute Infarction Ramipril Efficacy Study	Lancet 1993; 342:821–828
CAPRICORN	2001	Carvedilol Post-Infarct Survival Control in Left Ventricular Dysfunction	Lancet 2001; 357:1385–1390
CHARM	2003	Candesartan in HF Assessment of Reduction in Mortality and Morbidity	Lancet 2003; 362:772–776
CIBIS-II	1999	The Cardiac Insufficiency Bisoprolol Study II	Lancet 1999; 353:9–13
CONSENUS	1987	Effects of enalapril on mortality in severe CHF Cooperative North Scandinavian Enalapril Survival Trial	N Engl J Med 1987; 316:1429 –1435
COPERNICUS	2003	Carvedilol Prospective Randomized Cumulative Survival	JAMA, 2003; 289(6):712–718
MERIT-HF	1999	Metoprolol Randomized Trial in Congestive Heart Failure	Lancet 1999; 353:2001–2007
OPTIME-CHF	2002	Outcomes of a Prospective Trial of Intravenous Milrinone for Exacerbations of Chronic Heart Failure	JAMA 2002; 287:1541–1547
RALES	1999	Randomized Aldactone Evaluation Study	N Engl J Med 1999; 341(10):709 –717
SOLVD	1991	The Studies of Left Ventricular Dysfunction. Enalapril	N Engl J Med 1992; 327:685 –691
TRACE	1999	Trandolapril Cardiac Evaluation Study	Lancet 1999; 354:9–12

- **Amiodarone** has similar effects on the sodium channel but is not included in class I because of other important properties.
- Class I drugs are further divided according to their effects on repolarization time:
  - class 1a – prolong repolarization time (e.g. **quinidine**)
  - class 1b – shorten repolarization time (e.g. **lidocaine**)
  - class 1c – repolarization time is unchanged (e.g. **flecainide**).

TABLE 5.10 Drugs used for specific cardiac arrhythmias.

Arrhythmia	Drug	Class	Uses
Drugs only used in supraventricular arrhythmias	Adenosine* Verapamil Esmolol	IV II	Paroxysmal supraventricular tachycardia (PSVT) + in WPW SVT − not WPW
	Digoxin		Control of ventricular rate Slows ventricular response in atrial fibrillation
Drugs used in ventricular arrhythmias	Procainamide Disopyramide Lidocaine* Mexiletine Flecainide Propafenone Sotalol Amiodarone*	Ia Ia Ib Ib Ib Ic III III	Ventricular arrhythmias including ventricular tachycardia, especially after myocardial infarction Nodal and ventricular tachycardias, ventricular fibrillation
Drugs used in supraventricular and ventricular arrhythmias	Amiodarone* Beta blockers Disopyramide Flecainide Propafenone	III II Ia Ib Ic	As above + SVT, atrial fibrillation and flutter

SVT, Supraventricular tachycardia; *WPW,* Wolff−Parkinson−hite.
*Most frequently used.

Class 1a Lengthen the action potential duration and refractory period (e.g. disopyramide)

Used to be used much more frequently than today. Effective for both supraventricular and ventricular arrhythmias.

Class 1b Inhibit fast sodium current. Shorten action potential duration (e.g. lidocaine)

- Abortion of premature beats.
- Act selectively on diseased or ischaemic tissue.
- They are useful in the control of ventricular arrhythmias after a MI.

Lidocaine

- Acts exclusively on sodium channels.
- Also used as a local anaesthetic. Has a short half-life of 2 hours.
- Cannot be given orally due to its large first-pass metabolism.

- Its antiarrhythmic action is confined to the ventricular muscle and conducting system.
- May be used in an intravenous infusion to suppress ventricular dysrhythmias.
- It has no effect on atrial dysrhythmias.
- Adverse effects are mainly on the central nervous system. Include drowsiness, disorientation and convulsions (especially in the elderly).
- Used mostly to suppress ventricular tachycardia and VF after cardioversion, cardiac surgery and anaesthesia.
- Lowest proarrhythmic action of all class I drugs.

Contraindications Sinoatrial disorders, all grades of AV block, severe myocardial depression, porphyria.

Class 1c Minimal effect on refractoriness. Inhibit fast sodium channel. Delay conduction in His−Purkinje system (e.g. flecainide, propafenone)

Flecainide

- Potent sodium channel blocker but also blocks some potassium channels, which may explain its ability to treat atrial arrhythmias.
- Negative inotropic effect (reduces cardiac contractility).
- Slows conduction in all cardiac cells including WPW syndrome.
- Half-life of 14 hours.
- Does have proarrhythmic effects.
- In trials many years ago to see if *flecainide* suppressed the incidence of dysrhythmias following MI when there were asymptomatic premature beats, the drug had to be discontinued when mortality in the treated group was 7.7% compared with 3.0% in controls. There was induction of lethal ventricular dysrhythmias in some patients (Teo et al. 1993).

Class II drugs

Beta-adrenoreceptor antagonists (e.g. *atenolol, esmolol*). Counteract the dysrhythmic effects of catecholamines and prolong the refractory period of the AV node.

- Especially useful if arrhythmias precipitated by stimulation of SNS in exercise or emotion.
- Beta blockers are effective for a range of supraventricular dysrhythmias.
- They may be used in WPW syndrome and in *digoxin*-induced dysrhythmias.
- Used in sinus tachycardia, paroxysmal atrial tachycardia, exercise-induced ventricular arrhythmias, hereditary long QT syndrome and phaeochromocytoma (with an alpha antagonist).

- Benefits following an MI are probably due to antiarrhythmic activity. Excellent record in reducing mortality post MI.
- HF may be precipitated if a patient is dependent on sympathetic drive to maintain output. Negative inotropic effects may produce problems in overt congestive cardiac failure but some beta-adrenergic antagonists are used in stable HF (see Section 5.6).

Interactions

Concomitant administration of *verapamil* or *diltiazem* increases the risk of bradycardia and AV block. These drugs also reduce cardiac contractility and can induce HF if given with a beta blocker.

Stable HF is no longer a contraindication for beta blockade.

Class III drugs (e.g. amiodarone, sotalol)

All class III agents act by lengthening the action potential and increasing the refractory period. This means they must prolong the QT interval and, if there is hypokalaemia or bradycardia, may predispose torsade de pointes. *Amiodarone* has shown itself to be the least likely to do so.

Amiodarone

Effective in both ventricular and supraventricular arrhythmias and increasingly used for life-threatening arrhythmias.

- Prolongs the refractory period of myocardial cells and the AV node.
- Unlike many antiarrhythmic drugs, it causes little cardiac depression.
- Powerful inhibitor of abnormal automaticity. Suppresses ectopic activity.
- It prevents atrial and ventricular re-entrant rhythms.
- Lengthens cardiac action potential, probably due to blocking potassium channels.
- Slows the sinus rate and AV conduction.
- It does have some alpha- and beta-blocking properties and some weak class IV effects.
- Weak coronary and peripheral vasodilator actions.
- In low doses it is also effective for recurrent AF.
- Does have many serious side effects in long-term administration.

Pharmacokinetics

- Extremely lipid soluble and effective orally with variable and slow absorption.
- Widely distributed in the body with little remaining in the blood.
- It is stored in fat and many other tissues and has a very long estimated half-life of approximately 54 days (range 25−110 days) after repeated dosing due to slow release from the stored sites. A loading dose is necessary because of this.

- It may take weeks or months to achieve a steady-state plasma concentration. This is important when drug interactions are likely.
- Eliminated mostly in bile and some in sweat and tears.
- Hypokalaemia can render the drug ineffective and predisposes ventricular arrhythmias.

Uses
- It is an effective agent against most cardiac arrhythmias. May be used for paroxysmal supraventricular, nodal and ventricular tachycardias, AF and flutter and VF. It is effective in chronic ventricular dysrhythmias.
- Often the drug of choice in life-threatening arrhythmias. The risk of sudden death is not increased by its use.
- Reported to be effective in 60% who have not responded to other drugs.
- In AF it slows the ventricular response and may restore sinus rhythm.
- It may be used to maintain sinus rhythm following direct current (DC) conversion for atrial flutter or fibrillation.
- It is effective in supraventricular tachycardia associated with WPW syndrome.
- Antianginal action probably due to beta blocking and calcium channel blocking effects. Used in unstable angina with severe ventricular arrhythmias.

Administration Orally, 200 mg, three times daily for 1 week; reduced to 200 mg twice daily for a further week and then 200 mg daily or the minimum dose required to control the arrhythmia.

When given intravenously, it is administered by infusion via a central venous catheter over 20–120 minutes with ECG monitoring. May receive further infusion with maximum of 1.2 g in 24 hours. Amiodarone causes phlebitis if given into a peripheral vein.

For VF or pulseless ventricular tachycardia it is given by intravenous injection of 300 mg over at least 3 minutes.

Adverse effects
- Has less proarrhythmic effects than most other antiarrhythmic drugs. Adverse cardiac effects – bradycardia, heart block, induction of ventricular dysrhythmias. Torsade de pointes is more likely if hypokalaemia is present and electrolytes should be closely monitored.
- May cause hypotension when given intravenously at high doses or if given too quickly.

Extracardiac adverse effects are frequent and serious. They often limit the long-term use of amiodarone. Approximately 26% of patients discontinue the drug due to intolerance. A long half-life means that the effects of the drug continue for a period of time after it has been discontinued.

- Microdeposits accumulate in the cornea and may give visual haloes and photophobia. They rarely interfere with vision but may affect night driving. The deposits are dose related and reversible when the drug is discontinued.

- Photosensitivity is common and a bluish discoloration of the skin may occur. Total sun block should be worn to prevent this.
- Structurally related to thyroxine and has complex effects on thyroid hormones. Contains a high concentration of iodine. Rise in T_4 and small decrease in T_3. Five per cent develop hyperthyroidism or hypothyroidism. Thyroid function should be monitored by laboratory testing every 6 months in long-term treatment.
- Nausea and vomiting in almost half those with congestive cardiac failure; constipation.
- The most serious complication is pulmonary fibrosis. This is slow in onset but may be irreversible. Regular chest x-rays are needed to monitor.
- Rarely, liver damage can occur. Liver function tests should be monitored every 6 months and the drug discontinued if severe liver function abnormalities occur.
- Neurological symptoms may be due to peripheral neuropathy, an infrequent side effect.
- Teratogenic and also to be avoided in lactation.

Interactions
- Beta blockers and CCBs augment the depressant effect on the AV node.
- Should not be used with other drugs that lengthen QT interval including class Ia and III antiarrhythmics, tricyclic antidepressants and thiazide diuretics.
- Effects of *digoxin* and *warfarin* are enhanced. Plasma digoxin may rise 100%.

Sotalol

- Nonselective beta-adrenoreceptor antagonist that also has class III antiarrhythmic properties. Unlike other beta blockers, it also prolongs the cardiac action potential and the QT interval by delaying the slow outward K^+ current.
- Prolongation of the action potential can lead to life-threatening torsade de pointes in about 5% of those treated. This has led to a decline in its use.
- Torsade is more likely if hypokalaemia is present and so electrolytes need to be closely monitored.
- Prolongs cardiac refractoriness but has also has class I effects.

Class IV drugs
CCBs (e.g. *verapamil*, *diltiazem*).
   Inhibit slow calcium channel-dependent conduction through the AV node. Shorten the plateau of the action potential and reduce the force of cardiac contraction. They suppress premature ectopic beats but decrease cardiac contractility.

Verapamil

- Controls supraventricular tachycardias such as AF and is effective in paroxysmal supraventricular tachycardia.
- It should not be used in WPW syndrome.
- It is not effective for ventricular dysrhythmias and can be fatal, by myocardial depression, if given in wide complex ventricular tachycardia.
- Intravenous administration is now rarely used as the safer, short-acting and extremely effective drug, *adenosine* (see below), is now available to terminate supraventricular tachycardia.
- Must not be given to a patient recently taking beta blockers due to the risk of hypotension and asystole.
- Adverse effects are mainly due to the depression of cardiac contractility and may cause bradycardia.
- Displaces *digoxin* from its plasma binding sites and also reduces its renal elimination. This means the dose of digoxin will need to be reduced and the plasma concentration checked.

Drugs not classified in the Vaughan Williams system

Adenosine

Adenosine plays an important role in the body where it combines with phosphate groups to form the high-energy molecule ATP. It also has important effects on breathing, heart muscle, nervous conduction and platelets as well as its effect on the cardiac conduction system that forms the base for it use in arrhythmias.

Adenosine increases potassium conductance and inhibits calcium influx. It slows AV conduction as well as dilating coronary and peripheral arteries. It has less effect on the SA node.

The adenosine receptor, A_1, is responsible for its effect on the AV node. The receptor is linked to cardiac potassium channels. Adenosine hyperpolarizes cardiac conducting tissue and thus slows the rate of rise of the pacemaker potential.

Pharmacokinetics

- It is rapidly metabolized and its half-life in plasma is only about 10 seconds. It must be given intravenously. Peak action 10 seconds.
- Given as a rapid intravenous bolus of 3 mg (some doctors may use 6 mg) over 2 seconds (with cardiac monitoring) followed by a saline flush to obtain high concentrations in the heart. If it does not work within 1–2 minutes, a further 6 mg bolus is given and then 12 mg after 1–2 minutes if necessary.
- At the correct dose, the effect occurs as soon as the drug reaches the AV node, within about 15–30 seconds.

Indications
- Adenosine is used as the first-line drug to rapidly terminate paroxysmal supraventricular tachycardia including that seen in WPW syndrome.
- Also useful in differentiating between broad-complex tachycardias of ventricular or supraventricular origin. If supraventricular then AV block with adenosine allows the P waves to be seen and the diagnosis can be made.
- Ventricular tachycardias do not usually respond to adenosine unless exercise induced.
- Not used to treat AF or flutter.

Contraindications Heart block, sick sinus syndrome.
Asthma — bronchoconstriction may be precipitated in asthma patients and can last for 30 minutes. It is not known why this occurs.

Adverse effects
- Adverse effects are not serious due to the brevity of action, but headache, facial flushing, chest pain and transient dysrhythmias e.g. bradycardia may occur in 10%—20% of patients.
- Bronchoconstriction in asthma.
- Transient new arrhythmias including torsade de pointes may occur in about 65% of patients.

Drug interactions Less effective if caffeine or theophylline have been used. These compete for the adenosine receptor.
Dipyridamole inhibits breakdown so dose must be reduced.
Unlike *verapamil*, may be used after a beta blocker.
Dronedarone
- A multi-channel blocking antiarrhythmic drug
- Used to maintain sinus rhythm after cardioversion in stable patients with paroxysmal or persistent AF when other treatments are unsuitable.

Magnesium
Magnesium is regarded as the body's own calcium antagonist. It weakly blocks calcium channels and inhibits sodium and potassium channels. Magnesium deficiency predisposes to arrhythmias.

- Used intravenously to treat torsade de pointes and arrhythmias after *digoxin* overdose.
- Given intravenously after an MI it may help to prevent the occurrence of dysrhythmias and perhaps prevent ischaemic damage.
- The drug of choice in the prevention of recurrent seizures in eclampsia.

Potassium

Hypokalaemia predisposes to serious ventricular arrhythmias, especially after MI. It also makes the arrhythmia more difficult to terminate. The risk is further increased if digoxin is also being administered.

Hyperkalaemia is also arrhythmogenic so potassium has no place in the management of arrhythmias in those with normal potassium levels but the aim should be to maintain a normal serum potassium concentration.

Atrial fibrillation

This is the most common cardiac arrhythmia seen in practice which affects about 1.3% of the population in England and Wales (NICE, 2018b). Men are affected more than women and the incidence increases with age.

- The patient may present with a variety of symptoms such as dizziness, palpitations or exercise intolerance but may be asymptomatic and so early diagnosis can be difficult. This is likely to mean that the prevalence of AF is underestimated.
- The atria are fibrillating and the ECG shows a typical undulating baseline without discrete P waves.
- Therapy aims to control the ventricular rate, to restore and maintain sinus rhythm and to prevent thromboembolism.
- The risk of stroke in those with AF is five times higher than in those with a normal heart rhythm (NICE, 2018b).
- Clots form more easily within the fibrillating atria and measures should be taken (i.e. anticoagulation) to prevent this. Clots formed in the atria may escape into the circulation and are a common cause of stroke.
- There is an increased risk of mortality in those with AF. The mortality rate is double that of those without AF, independent of other risk factors.
- Conditions that increase the risk of developing AF include hypertension, valvular heart disease, diabetes mellitus, HF and chronic or acute alcohol use.
- Alleviation of symptoms and prevention of complications are the aims of treatment.

Treatment of AF

- Antiarrhythmics may be used either to restore the normal heart rhythm and to maintain this ('rhythm control') or to control the ventricular rate ('rate control') in those patients who remain in AF.
- Anticoagulation therapy is very important to reduce the incidence of stroke. This used to be with older therapies such as heparin and warfarin but newer antithrombotic agents that are direct acting oral anticoagulants (DOAC) are being used more frequently as alternatives to warfarin.

- Non-pharmacological management includes electrical cardioversion which 'shocks' the heart back into a normal rhythm and catheter or surgical ablation to create lesions which stop the abnormal impulses that cause AF.
- In a life-threatening acute presentation of new-onset AF, emergency electrical cardioversion is used.
- If not life-threatening, pharmacological cardioversion using intravenous amiodarone or flecainide can be used.
- For urgent rate control a beta-blocker or verapamil may be given intravenously.
- Beta blockers or rate-limiting CCBs (e.g. diltiazem) are the drugs recommended as first-line management for rate control in persistent AF.
- *Digoxin* is usually only effective for controlling the ventricular rate at rest and so should only be used as monotherapy in sedentary patients with non-paroxysmal AF. Digoxin is also use when AF is combined with congestive HF.
- If a single drug does not control the AF then a combination of two drugs may be prescribed.
- Some patients under specialist care may sometimes administer single doses of flecainide orally when an episode begins.
- To maintain sinus rhythm, a beta-blocker may be used and if ineffective, *flecainide* or *propafenone* may be used or *amiodarone*.

The NICE has produced guidelines for the management of AF that can be found on the website www.nice.org.uk.

In AF, stroke prevention is of vital importance in all patients. All patients with AF are assessed for risk of stroke and this is balanced with their risk for bleeding before anti-coagulation. Full details are found in the BNF (2019), Chapter 2.

Paroxysmal supraventricular tachycardia

The patients may learn to terminate the arrhythmia themselves by using vagal manoeuvres such as a Valsalva manoeuvre, immersing the face in ice cold water or carotid sinus massage. These should be performed with ECG monitoring.

If required, *adenosine* is the drug of choice, producing transient AV block within 15−30 seconds.

Verapamil is sometimes used but not when a beta-blocker has been recently administered and not for WPW syndrome.

For recurrent episodes, catheter ablation may be used with an aim to produce a lifelong 'cure'.

Alternatives for chronic therapy are CCBs, beta blockers, flecainide or propafenone.

It can be seen that therapy in cardiac arrhythmias is complex but it is hoped that this section has enabled the reader to understand the action of some of the drugs that may be used in these situations.

5.6 CARDIAC FAILURE

Chronic heart failure (CHF) is a clinical syndrome where any cardiac abnormality (in contraction and/or relaxation) impairs the heart's ability to function as a pump. This results in the common symptoms of breathlessness and fatigue together with signs such as fluid retention. There are many different causes and HF itself is not a diagnosis. If the patient presents with HF we need to establish the cause.

The prevalence of CHF is increasing as the population lives longer and there are about 920,000 people in the UK today with CHF (BHF, 2018). There are probably as many again with damaged hearts who have not yet developed symptoms of heart disease.

The most common cause of CHF in the UK is CAD and many patients will have had an MI in the past. Other causes include hypertension and LVH, arrhythmias such as AF, congenital heart disease, cardiomyopathies, valve disease, chronic obstructive pulmonary disease and extracardiac causes such as hyperthyroidism and anaemia.

Investigations involved in diagnosis include the measurement of N-terminal pro-B type natriuretic peptide (NT-proBNP) in those with suspected HF. Those with very high levels above 2000 ng/L are referred urgently for specialist assessment and echocardiography.

Lifestyle advice is important in both the prevention and treatment of HF. Education, weight control, dietary modification, smoking cessation and physical activity are all areas where advice should be given.

Cardiac function

This depends on preload, afterload, contractility, heart rate and rhythm.

- *Preload* is the volume of blood left in the left ventricle at the end of diastole (i.e. immediately before ejection). Increased preload is due to salt and water retention.
- *Afterload* is the force the heart muscle must generate to overcome the resistance in the aorta and the peripheral arteries (i.e. the total peripheral resistance).
- *Contractility* is the force of ventricular contraction independent of loading. Calcium is essential for cardiac contraction.

HF occurs when CO is insufficient to maintain adequate perfusion of the tissues. The fall in CO leads to adaptations by the body. Initially these adaptations help and maintain the circulation but eventually they have deleterious effects.

Adaptive changes in chronic heart failure

- Activation of the SNS and the RAAS occurs.
- This causes elevation of heart rate and increases peripheral resistance. The workload of the heart is increased, increasing the need for oxygen and energy.
- Stimulation of RAAS contributes to sodium and water retention in HF.
- HF may be:
  - acute or chronic
  - systolic (large heart, reduced ejection fraction) or diastolic (near normal heart size and normal ejection fraction).
- The treatment and management can be complex and differs according to the type of HF present.
- NICE updated their guidance for all types of HF in 2018 and the reader is referred to these guidelines (available at www.nice.org.uk) for greater detail than is given in this text.

Acute heart failure

There is rapid onset of signs and symptoms secondary to abnormal cardiac function. Commonly this is acute LVF with pulmonary oedema and severe shortness of breath. It could be hypertensive AHF or secondary to an MI and may occur without previous heart disease being present. It may be new in onset or the patient may already have CHF.

- There is reduced CO, reduced perfusion of the tissues, increased pressure in the pulmonary circulation and tissue congestion.
- The patient presents with acute pulmonary oedema and breathlessness.
- The dyspnoea is directly related to high left atrial pressure which raises the pressure in the pulmonary circulation and leads to the development of pulmonary oedema.
- The patient is literally 'drowning in their own secretions'.
- Need immediate symptomatic relief. Dyspnoea is the dominant symptom.
- There is a possibility of imminent cardiorespiratory death and so this is an emergency where the emphasis is on drugs given intravenously.
- Oxygen is administered.

Drugs used in the treatment of acute heart failure

The main aim is to reduce preload by the use of diuretics (e.g. *furosemide*).
Nitrates and opiates are no longer routinely used in the treatment of AHF (NICE, 2018b).
Loop diuretics (e.g. *furosemide*) are used in AHF because they are strong and have a rapid effect.

- The dose is titrated according to response and symptom relief.
- If already taking diuretics, a higher dose may be required.

- May be combined with thiazides or spironolactone if necessary.
- May be used with other drugs such as nitrates (if myocardial ischaemia present) or inotropes (if cardiogenic shock [CS] is present).

Cardiogenic shock

This is tissue hypoperfusion occurring because of HF. It may lead to progressive multi-organ failure. There is peripheral vasoconstriction and the patient is cold and sweating with a low SBP (systolic <90 mmHg). The patient may be confused and oliguria may be present. It develops gradually in patients at risk of CS through mild shock, then severe shock followed by refractory CS when advanced mechanical circulatory support is required. Early intervention is essential as the reversibility of CS is time-dependent and usually only possible before the advanced stage (Dwornik, 2016).

Aetiology may be:

- cardiomyopathic — due to ischaemia, myocarditis or cardiac myopathy
- mechanical — related to valvular or structural pathology
- arrhythmic.

Most frequently secondary to LV failure due to MI (Dwornik, 2016).

Mortality is high and ranges between 50% and 70%. Survival can be improved with early recognition and circulatory support (Aissaoui, 2012).

The aim is to reduce the load on the heart, preserve cardiac function and to maintain an optimal BP so that the kidneys receive an adequate blood supply.

In this case inotropic agents (e.g. *dobutamine*) increase the force of cardiac contraction and may be needed. Dobutamine has a pulmonary vasodilatory effect and improves peripheral perfusion. It does have a systemic vasodilatory action and a positive chronotropic effect and so may exacerbate hypotension and arrhythmias. *Milrinone* is an alternative inotrope that has less arrhythmogenicity compared to catecholamines.

Sometimes if perfusion does not occur with inotropes it may be necessary to use vasopressors (drugs that constrict the blood vessels). These drugs are only used briefly and in specialist units as they increase afterload of the failing heart. An example is *noradrenaline* (see Section 2.2).

Mechanical circulatory support to provide sufficient organ and tissue perfusion may be required if the above fail.

Chronic heart failure

The number of people living with HF in the UK increased by 23% between 2002 and 2014 from 750,125 to 920,616. This is 1.6% of the population. The rise is partly due to improved survival from IHD, partly due to an ageing population and partly due to a rise in cardiovascular risk factors (Taylor et al. 2019).

The survival rate at 1 year after diagnosis has increased by 6.6% from 74.2% in 2000 to 80.8% in 2016. Survival at 5 years increased by 7.2% from 41.0% in 2000 to 48.2% in 2012 (Taylor et al. 2019).

Chronic HF is dominated by salt and water retention. The prognosis is improving but is still poor and is dependent on severity at presentation. Increased sympathetic activity leads to increased cardiac contraction but at the expense of increased preload, afterload and oxygen demand. The more severe the failure, the higher the level of catecholamines released. The already weakened heart is forced to work harder — a vicious circle that has to be broken.

Drugs used in chronic heart failure

Updated recommendations for the pharmacological management of HF have been produced by NICE (2018b). They are available at www.nice.org.uk and are shown in Fig. 5.6.

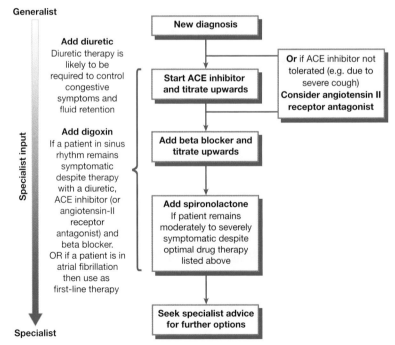

FIG. 5.6 **Recommendations for the pharmacological management of heart failure.** *ACE,* Angiotensin converting enzyme. *Reproduced from National Collaborating Centre for Chronic Conditions, 2003. Chronic Heart Failure, National Clinical Guideline for Diagnosis and Management in Primary and Secondary Care. Royal College of Physicians, London. Copyright © Royal College of Physicians. Reproduced by permission.*

The aim is to relieve symptoms (fatigue, breathlessness and oedema), decrease acute exacerbations, improve exercise tolerance and prolong life. We want to increase quality of life with drugs that do not have too many side effects. In practice this means using ACEIs as soon as possible.

The emphasis is on prevention of progressive damage to the myocardium. Drugs used to achieve improvement in symptoms are:

- diuretics
- digoxin
- ACEIs.

Drugs used to achieve improvement in survival work by:

- angiotensin blockade – ACEIs, angiotensin receptor blockers
- beta receptor blockade
- aldosterone blockade.

Failure of the heart to perfuse the tissues leads to stimulation of the SNS and RAAS in an attempt to increase CO.

The most successful drugs for the treatment of CHF modulate this neurohormonal response by angiotensin blockade, beta receptor blockade and aldosterone blockade.

Diuretics

These drugs treat and control fluid retention but do not prevent progression of HF. Symptoms improve and exercise tolerance is increased.

- Given to control pulmonary and peripheral symptoms and signs of congestion.
- Only rarely used on their own as the fluid loss can stimulate RAAS and so accelerate progression of the disease. This was shown in the SOLVD trial in 1991 (see Table 5.9).
- Should be combined with an ACEI and sometimes a beta blocker.
  Loop diuretics (e.g. *furosemide*) are usually used because:
  - there is superior fluid loss for same degree of sodium loss (natriuresis)
  - they work even in the presence of renal impairment that often accompanies severe HF
  - there is high ceiling (i.e. increased diuretic effects with increased dosage)
  - they produce some arteriolar vasodilation.

Adverse effects
- Potassium loss occurs. This may be counterbalanced by ACEIs.
- Digitalis toxicity may be precipitated by over-diuresis and hypokalaemia.
- Metabolic alkalosis.
- Reduced levels of magnesium and calcium.
- In the elderly may lead to hypovolaemia, hypotension and increased risk of collapse. Must ensure that dehydration does not occur.

In mild HF, thiazides (***bendroflumethiazide*** or ***metolazone***) may be preferred, especially if hypertension is present.

Diuretic doses are higher than those used in hypertension. Thiazides do lose potency as renal function falls.

In severe HF, loop diuretics can be combined with thiazide diuretics producing a diuresis of up to 5−10 L/day.

Angiotensin converting enzyme inhibitors (ACEIs)

(***E.g. cilazapril, enalapril, fosinopril, lisinopril, perindopril, quinapril and ramipril)***The evidence base for the use of this group of drugs is very strong. Several large trials (e.g. CONSENSUS, SOLVD, AIRE, TRACE; see Table 5.9) have established their benefit in HF.

- ACEIs improve both symptoms and prognosis.
- They slow down the development of HF and are beneficial in asymptomatic HF following a MI.
- Risk of death, HF and recurrent MI are all reduced and the improvement in mortality is seen within the first few days of their use post MI.
- ACEIs are now the cornerstone of HF management.

Mechanism of action A neurohormonal intervention that works by blocking the RAAS (see Section 5.2).

- Reduce the generation of angiotensin II from angiotensin I by ACE.
- Angiotensin II is a powerful vasoconstrictor. It also has detrimental effects on ventricular remodelling and renal function in CHF.
- It stimulates aldosterone release from the adrenal cortex and this hormone has detrimental effects in HF.
- ACEI vasodilate and also reduce aldosterone production. This gives a diuretic effect and causes the loss of sodium and the retention of potassium.
- Reduce the breakdown of bradykinin. Bradykinin may augment nitrous oxide production and so this could also be beneficial (vasodilatory).
- Decrease cardiac preload and afterload.
- Prevent ventricular remodelling and decrease LVH.

Seventy per cent of patients with CHF respond to ACEI symptomatically.

They have been shown to reduce mortality in HF by up to 35%. For the patient this means:

- dyspnoea reduced
- exercise tolerance increased
- hospital admissions reduced
- life expectancy increased.

All patients with low left ventricular ejection fraction (LVEF), CHF should be treated with an ACEI, no matter how mild or severe their symptoms.

Other properties of potential value include the reduction in incidence of arrhythmias post MI. They may improve coronary blood flow at the same time as decreasing oxygen demand.

Adverse effects These are described in Section 5.2.

When severe hypotension occurs, it is usually in the over-diuresed and dehydrated patient. A reduction in BP will occur but is usually of little concern. If there is symptomatic hypotension, a reduction in dose of diuretic, other vasodilator or ACEI is required.

Regular monitoring of renal function is required. Extra caution is needed in those with atherosclerosis as they may already have clinically silent reno-vascular disease.

Angiotensin II receptor antagonists (ARBs)
(E.g. candesartan, valsartan)

Block the action of angiotensin II at its receptor (AT_1 receptor) and are also known as ARBs. The use of these drugs as an alternative to ACEIs for the treatment of hypertension is described in Section 5.2. They are effective in the treatment of CHF and are recommended for ACEI-intolerant patients.

May also have benefit when added to ACEIs in HF. This was demonstrated in the CHARM trial (see Table 5.9) where the addition of ***candesartan*** to an ACEI and other standard treatment reduced mortality by 17%.

Beta-adrenergic antagonists

Can precipitate HF in acute situations and it used to be assumed that beta blockers should not be given in CHF due to their negative inotropic effects (depress cardiac contractility). However, in 1999 two major trials (CIBIS-II using ***bisoprolol*** and MERIT-HF using ***metoprolol***; see Table 5.9) demonstrated that these beta blockers improve survival in patients with stable, mild to moderately symptomatic low LVEF CHF. The drugs were added to full conventional therapy, including an ACEI.

- Quality of life improved and hospital admissions were reduced.
- Significant reduction in mortality.

Dual neurohormonal blockade of both RAAS and SNS has resulted in halving 1-year mortality in patients with CHF.

The COPERNICUS trial in 2003 using *carvedilol* showed significant reduction in mortality in severe HF. The CAPRICORN trial added *carvedilol* to post-MI care if LV dysfunction was present with or without symptoms (see Table 5.9). A significant reduction in mortality occurred and effects are additive to ACE inhibition. *Bisoprolol* is another betablocker that is licensed for use in stable HF.

- Beta blockers need to be used with caution. Sudden intense neurohormonal inhibition is potentially dangerous. Have a period of gradual dose titration over several months.
- Only prescribed by specialists in HF because of the risk of acute deterioration.
- The only absolute contraindication is asthma.
- Major adverse effect is early worsening of HF. Normally transient and can be treated by temporary increase in diuretic use.
- Occasionally bradycardia can occur and is important if symptomatic or if use is in those under 50 years of age even if asymptomatic.

Beneficial effects in CHF include a reduction in heart rate that improves coronary blood flow and a decrease in the force of cardiac contraction that adds to the decrease in myocardial oxygen demand. Automaticity is reduced and this lessens cardiac arrhythmias. There is also less renin production.

Aldosterone antagonists

Spironolactone, eplerenone Spironolactone is a synthetic competitive aldosterone antagonist and competes with aldosterone for intracellular aldosterone receptors in the cells of the renal distal tubule.

- Aldosterone is a hormone produced by the adrenal cortex that increases sodium retention and potassium loss.
- Blockade of the receptors leads to increased sodium loss and hence water loss with some retention of potassium.
- *Spironolactone* is thus a potassium-sparing diuretic and is used in combination with loop diuretics in HF. It is particularly useful in resistant oedema.

Research has shown that in addition to the above, aldosterone has adverse effects on structure and function of the heart in HF. It appears able to produce endothelial dysfunction which may increase coronary events. It also produces LV dysfunction and fibrosis (Struthers, 2005).

- The RALES study in 1999 (see Table 5.9) showed that *spironolactone* reduced progressive HF and sudden death.
- The reduction in cardiac deaths observed is probably related to both reduction in new coronary events and reduction in LV dysfunction and fibrosis (Struthers, 2005).

- Used when patients remain symptomatic despite optimal therapy.
- May also be used in hepatic cirrhosis where aldosterone cannot be metabolized efficiently and in hyperaldosteronism (over-secretion of aldosterone).

Adverse effects

- Risk of hyperkalaemia especially if given with ACEI and blood potassium levels must be monitored. Creatinine levels must be monitored to check renal function.
- May act on steroid receptors other than the kidney and give gynaecomastia (breast enlargement in males) in about 10% of patients. Menstrual disorders and testicular atrophy may occur.
- *Eplerenone* has fewer hormonal side effects and can be used when *spironolactone* cannot be tolerated.

Potassium supplements must not be given with aldosterone antagonists due to the risk of hyperkalaemia.

Inotropes and digitalis

Positive inotropic agents increase contractility and so improve cardiac function and increase CO. However, they are potent drugs and may have serious side effects:

- increased myocardial oxygen requirements
- vasoactive effects
- arrhythmogenesis.

Digoxin is the only inotrope with a role to play in the treatment of CHF.

Mechanism of action

- Inotropes increase the concentration of calcium in the cardiac muscle cell by a variety of methods.
- The force generated by cardiac muscle is proportional to the amount of intracellular calcium present during contraction.

There are three such classes of drug important at present:

- *Sympathomimetics* that stimulate the β_1 receptor (e.g. *dobutamine*). These increase the formation of cyclic adenosine monophosphate (cAMP), which increases calcium in the muscle cell.
- *Phosphodiesterase inhibitors* (PDEIs; e.g. *milrinone*). These inhibit the enzyme that destroys cAMP so that it builds up in the cell, increasing calcium concentration.

- *Cardiac glycosides* (e.g. *digoxin*). These block the $Na^+/K^+/ATPase$ pump in the cell membrane. The decreased expulsion of Na^+ from the cell decreases the activity of a sodium—calcium exchange pump also in the membrane. The result is that calcium is not extruded from the cell and so builds up, increasing contractility.

Use of inotropic agents
- To improve CO and maintain tissue oxygenation for patients in shock.
- To provide support for the heart to maintain adequate organ perfusion. This can be achieved in low output or CHF for short periods only.
- Long-term beneficial effects are difficult to demonstrate.
- PDEIs have been associated with increased mortality during chronic treatment, probably due to the development of arrhythmias.
- Sympathomimetics are associated with tolerance to their effects and an increased incidence of arrhythmias.
- *Digitalis* remains the only inotropic drug recommended for general use.

Cardiac glycosides

Digitalis from the foxglove was first used by William Withering in 1775 for 'dropsy' (fluid retention). It is now usually administered in the form of *digoxin* that is eliminated renally but is also available as *digitoxin* that is metabolized by the liver and used if renal function is impaired.

It is an inotrope that also inhibits the SNS and augments parasympathetic activity.

Uses
- Strongest indication is when CHF is combined with AF. Sometimes used alongside a beta blocker that improves exercise tolerance and ejection fraction.
- Is sometimes used to control ventricular rate in AF.
- Reduces symptoms and hospitalization in CHF but does not have an effect on overall mortality.
- Benefits in CHF are greatest in those with severe symptoms so may be used as symptoms become more severe.

Actions on the heart
Inotropic effects
- Increases the availability of calcium in the muscle cell. Inhibits the $Na^+/K^+/ATPase$ pump and this leads to a rise in intracellular calcium.
- Increases the force of cardiac contractility.
- Increases the excitability and automaticity of contractile and pacemaker cells. This is a toxic effect and leads to ectopic beats.

Parasympathomimetic effects
- Sinus bradycardia.
- Increased refractory period in AV node, promoting better ventricular filling.
- Slowed AV conduction is beneficial in AF.
- Heart block in toxic concentrations.

Other effects
- Reduced sympathetic activity.
- Increased baroreceptor sensitivity.
- Increased renal perfusion that leads to a decrease in oedema formation.

Pharmacokinetics
- Half-life of *digoxin* is 36−48 hours, which means it takes about a week to obtain a stable plasma level.
- A loading dose is not usually necessary in CHF. A satisfactory plasma level can be obtained in a week.
- Therapeutic index is approximately 2. This means that the patient should be monitored for digoxin toxicity.
- Mostly excreted unchanged in the urine at about one-third of the body stores daily.
- Does not cross the placenta.
- 70%−80% oral bioavailability in modern preparations.
- 10% of population harbours the enteric bacterium *Eubacterium lentum*, which can inactivate about 30%−40% of the available digoxin.

Contraindications Heart block, WPW syndrome, ventricular tachycardia or VF and certain myopathies. Not usually used following a recent MI.

Administration Administered orally.

A loading dose of 0.75−1 mg may be given in divided doses over 24 hours if rapid digitalization is needed in atrial fibrillation or flutter. This dose is reduced in the elderly. A loading dose is rarely necessary.

Maintenance dose is 62.5−250 micrograms daily or on alternate days according to heart rate and response.

Plasma digoxin levels must be monitored at first but this is not necessary once the maintenance dose is established. Plasma levels alone do not define toxicity as this is dependent on the response also. Current thinking is towards lower plasma levels being effective in CHF (0.5−1.0 micrograms/L). Toxicity becomes likely as the levels increase from 1.5 to 3 micrograms/L.

Adverse effects In excessive doses produces a variety of arrhythmias.

- Partial or complete AV block.
- Excessive bradycardia.
- Ventricular extrasystoles due to direct effects on ventricular muscle. Partly due to increased calcium-coupled beats (pulsus bigeminus) and then ventricular tachycardia and VF may follow.

Extracardiac effects include:

- loss of appetite
- nausea and vomiting
- abdominal pain and diarrhoea
- visual disturbances
- headache, fatigue, drowsiness, confusion.

Digoxin activity is greatly enhanced by hypokalaemia, which may occur with the use of potent loop diuretics.

- Unwanted effects depend on not only the plasma concentration of the drug, but also the sensitivity of the conducting system of the myocardium, which is often increased in myocardial disease.
- Renal function should be monitored. Digoxin toxicity may occur if reduced.

In the elderly, signs of digoxin toxicity may be less specific and include confusion, falls and reduced mobility.

Treatment of digoxin toxicity Serious cases of overdosage should be discussed with the National Poisons Information Service.

- Reduce dose or withdraw the drug.
- Raise plasma potassium if low.
- *Atropine* if heart block present.
- Digoxin-specific antibody fragments are indicated if severe acute toxicity that is life-threatening. Given as an intravenous infusion.
- Antiarrhythmic drugs if needed for ventricular arrhythmias. *Amiodarone* should be avoided as it increases plasma digoxin levels.

Other inotropic agents

Intravenous inotropic drugs are used to support the heart in CS and following cardiac surgery. They may be used in end-stage HF to bridge until transplantation. All inotropes used in an acute situation increase cAMP availability and thus increase calcium levels. The drug used depends on whether vasodilation or temporary vasoconstriction (***noradrenaline***) is required.

Sympathomimetic drugs

Adrenergic agonists include **adrenaline, noradrenaline, dobutamine** and dopamine.

Dopamine Dopamine is a precursor of adrenaline but in certain cells within the brain and interneurons of the autonomic ganglia dopamine is not converted to noradrenaline and is released as a neurotransmitter.

Uses. Severe HF and CS I infarction or cardiac surgery.

Mechanism of action. As well as action on alpha and beta adrenoreceptors, dopamine also acts via dopamine (D_1 and D_2) receptors via G-protein-coupled receptors to lead to increased or decreased levels of cAMP.

Effects. Cardiovascular effects depend on rate of infusion and vary between patients. The dose should be kept as low as possible to get the desired effects.

At lower rates (up to 10 µg/kg per min), β_1 effects predominate:

- Increased cardiac contractility.
- Increased heart rate.
- Increased CO.
- Increased coronary blood flow.
- Also stimulates release of endogenous noradrenaline (norepinephrine).

At higher rates (>10 µg/kg per min), alpha effects tend to predominate leading to:

- increased SVR and venous return
- fall in renal blood flow.

As with all inotropes an adequate preload is essential to help to control tachycardia.

Less likely to cause arrhythmias than adrenaline (epinephrine).

Inactive orally and only administered intravenously, usually via a central line.

- Acts within 5 minutes and has a duration of action of 10 minutes.
- About 25% is converted to noradrenaline (norepinephrine) in the peripheries.
- Half-life is about 3 minutes.

α_1 Agonists

Phenylephrine is a direct-acting sympathomimetic amine with potent α_1 agonist actions.

- Rapid rise in SVR and BP.
- No effect on beta adrenoreceptors.
- Used to increase a low SVR in spinal anaesthesia.
- Intravenous administration produces a rapid rise in BP which lasts 5–10 minutes.

Dobutamine

- Synthetic analogue of dopamine.
- β_1 Effects predominate but does have small effect at β_2 receptors.
- Potent inotrope but β_2 stimulation may lead to hypotension.
- Long-term mortality may be increased following its use and so is now less popular.
- Sometimes is given combined with dopamine to counteract vasodilatory effects.

Metaraminol Synthetic drug that acts mainly via α_1 receptors, but retains some β-adrenoreceptor activity. It is used to correct hypotension associated with spinal or epidural anaesthesia where an intravenous bolus is given. It reduces uterine blood flow and is not used in obstetrics.

Phosphodiesterase-III inhibitors

Enoximone, milrinone Inhibition of phosphodiesterase inhibits the breakdown of cAMP in cardiac and smooth muscle, increasing cardiac contractility and giving peripheral vasodilation. 'Inodilators' is a term that has been used to describe them. There is little change in heart rate or BP but increased risk of ventricular arrhythmias. The drugs give sustained haemodynamic benefit but there is no evidence of any benefit on long-term survival.

In the OPTIME-CHF trial (see Table 5.9) **milrinone** was associated with no extra benefit than placebo in CHF but with more new developments of AF and hypotension.

Milrinone may be used in severe orthostatic hypotension due to autonomic dysfunction when other forms of treatment are not adequate.

Glucagon

- Secreted by alpha cells in the islets of Langerhans in the pancreas.
- Activation of glucagon receptors, via G-protein-mediated mechanisms, stimulates adenylate cyclase and increases intracellular cAMP.

- Occasionally used in beta blocker overdose for cardiogenic shock that does not respond to atropine.
- Hyperglycaemia and hyperkalaemia may complicate its use.

Calcium

Intravenous calcium salts often improve BP for a few minutes but use should be restricted to circulatory collapse due to hyperkalaemia and calcium channel antagonist overdose.

5.7 ANTITHROMBOTICS

Haemostasis is the arrest of blood loss from damaged blood vessels and is essential to life. It involves three main stages:

- Contraction of blood vessels.
- Adhesion and activation of platelets − formation of a 'platelet plug'.
- Formation of fibrin and an insoluble blood clot.

Thrombosis is the unwanted formation of a haemostatic plug or thrombus within the blood vessels or the heart. It is a pathological condition usually associated with arterial disease or stasis of blood in the veins or atria of the heart.

The clotting cascade

- Blood coagulation takes place by two routes − the extrinsic pathway and the intrinsic pathway.
- Both lead to the formation of prothrombin activator, which converts prothrombin to thrombin which then converts fibrinogen to fibrin.
- The whole process is an accelerated enzyme cascade and has to be very closely controlled by inhibitors. If it were not, the whole blood in the body would solidify within minutes of clotting starting!
- The endothelium of the blood vessels releases heparin sulphate. This is an example of an inhibitor. Heparin is needed for the activity of antithrombin-III, which prevents the binding of fibrinogen to thrombin.
- Once fibrin is thrombin bound, heparin is not active because anti-thrombin III no longer interacts with thrombin.
- Vitamin K is a fat-soluble vitamin that occurs in plants and is synthesized by bacteria in the gut. It is needed for the synthesis of several clotting factors.
- Unwanted coagulation in the vascular system results in thrombus formation.
- The commonest form of thrombus is in the deep veins of the legs (deep vein thrombosis [DVT]).

A thrombus is a solid mass of blood products formed within the circulation during life. It differs from a blood clot, which occurs in non-flowing blood.

Thrombogenesis

The process of thrombus formation is known as thrombogenesis and may occur in the arterial or the venous sides of the circulation.

- Arterial thrombosis is the most common cause of MI, stroke and limb gangrene.
- Deep venous thrombosis in the leg veins may lead to pulmonary embolism (PE) (when a portion of the thrombus travels in the bloodstream and becomes lodged in the pulmonary circulation).
- AF is associated with thrombogenesis around the heart valves. The thrombi may break away and travel in the bloodstream, lodging in blood vessels in the brain. This is a cerebral embolus (stroke).
- Venous thrombosis is a problem in various cancers (e.g. breast, lung, prostate, pancreas and bowel) and after surgery, especially orthopaedic surgery.
- Oestrogens are associated with raised levels of some clotting factors and an increased risk of venous thrombosis.

Three factors may be involved in the formation of a thrombus. These were recognized by Virchow over 150 years ago and are known as **Virchow's triad**.

- Vessel wall abnormalities and injury (e.g. atheroma deposition, trauma).
- Changes in blood constituents such as clotting factors (hypercoagulability).
- Changes in blood flow (e.g. sluggish circulation; important in venous thromboembolism).

Antithrombotic therapy A thrombus consists of platelets adhering together and enmeshed by insoluble fibrin threads.

The treatment and prevention of thrombosis involves three classes of drugs:

- anticoagulants (e.g. *heparin*)
- antiplatelets (e.g. *aspirin*)
- thrombolytics (fibrinolytics) (e.g. *alteplase*).

Anticoagulants and antiplatelet drugs are used to prevent thrombosis occurring. When a thrombus has already formed, as in MI, it may be broken down by thrombolytic drugs.

Anticoagulants

Anticoagulants inhibit the clotting cascade and their main use is to prevent thrombus formation or extension of an existing thrombus in the slower-moving venous side of the circulation.

Heparin

Heparin was discovered in 1916 by a second-year medical student and is present in our bodies in the granules of mast cells and in plasma. Currently it is prepared from beef lung or pig intestine, and is a mixture of polysaccharides of varying molecular weights (average 15,000 daltons). Each molecule has a mean of 45 polysaccharide units. This form of heparin is called standard or UFH to differentiate it from the more widely used LMWHs (e.g. *enoxaparin*), which are heparin fragments. They have a longer duration of action and other advantages over UFH (see below).

Mechanism of action The main action of heparin is on the coagulation cascade. Heparin inhibits blood clotting by stopping the formation of fibrin.

- UFH combines with and activates an anticoagulation factor, **antithrombin III**, naturally found in the plasma. The complex thus formed neutralizes activated clotting factors, especially **factor Xa**, and inhibits thrombin.
- Heparin also has some inhibitory effect on platelet aggregation and reduces adhesiveness of platelets.
- LMWHs increase the action of antithrombin III on **factor Xa** but not its action on thrombin (molecules too small to bind).

Pharmacokinetics and administration
- Heparin is not absorbed from the gastrointestinal tract because it is too large a molecule and is heavily charged (ionized).
- Has to be given intravenously or subcutaneously and must not be given intramuscularly as it could cause haematoma formation.
- UFH acts immediately following intravenous administration but has a short duration of action (3–6 hours). The onset of action is delayed to approximately 60 minutes if given subcutaneously.
- Dosage is expressed in terms of units of biological activity.
- Heparin does not cross the placenta and so may be used in pregnancy as an anticoagulant.
- LMWHs have a more predictable anticoagulant effect and at least twice the duration of action. Their half-life is 3–4 hours and they may be given by subcutaneous injection once or twice daily.

Monitoring heparin therapy UFH has a low therapeutic index and, when used to treat thromboembolism, monitoring, preferably daily, is necessary.

The **activated partial thromboplastin time** (APTT) is the blood test that is used and the dose of heparin is adjusted to keep the APTT within a target range (e.g. 1.5–2.5 times the control for full anticoagulation).

The effect of LMWHs is much more predictable and so does not usually need monitoring. LMWHs cannot be monitored using APPT and a more complex test for factor Xa inhibition has to be used, but this is only rarely necessary.

Main therapeutic uses

- Treatment of DVT and PE. An oral anticoagulant (usually warfarin) is started at the same time as the heparin.
- May be used alongside other therapies in the management of acute MI, unstable angina and acute peripheral artery occlusion.
- Prophylaxis in patients undergoing general surgery, to prevent post-operative DVT and PE in high-risk patients such as those with obesity, malignant disease, previous history of DVT or PE, aged over 40 or undergoing large or complicated surgical procedures.
- Prophylaxis in orthopaedic surgery.

LMWHs are used in most cases but UFH is still given intravenously in some patients; for example, those with mechanical valves undergoing surgery or in those at high risk of bleeding because it can be discontinued abruptly.

Adverse effects

Bleeding. This is the chief side effect. It may occur at any site and may be life-threatening.

It is usually sufficient to withdraw heparin, but if rapid reversal of the effects of heparin is required, **protamine sulphate** is the antidote. It only partially reverses the effects of LMWHs.

Risk factors for bleeding include old age, any clotting defect (commonly drug induced; e.g. by aspirin or fibrinolytic therapy), recent trauma or renal biopsy, lumbar puncture or epidural and recent eye surgery. The risk of bleeding is calculated as unacceptable in certain instances; for example, following a recent cerebral bleed.

Heparin-induced thrombocytopenia

- This is a severe drop in platelet count and is a rare reaction. It is due to antibody formation and does not usually develop for 6–10 days but can occur between 2 days and 2 weeks following the start of treatment. It is associated with thrombotic as well as haemorrhagic complications.
- Platelet counts are recommended for patients receiving heparin (including LMWHs) for longer than 5 days.
- A small decrease in platelet count in the first 2 days of therapy is common (approximately one-third of patients) but clinically unimportant.
- Heparin should be stopped immediately, and not repeated, in those who develop a 50% reduction of platelet count.

- Patients requiring continued anticoagulation should be given *hirudin*, *lepirudin* or a heparinoid such as *danaparoid*.

Osteoporosis and vertebral collapse. This is a rare complication described in young adult patients receiving heparin in doses of 10,000 units or more daily for longer than 10 weeks (usually longer than 3 months). Osteoporosis is due to enhanced reabsorption of bone.

Hypoaldosteronism and hyperkalaemia
- Inhibition of aldosterone synthesis by heparin (including LMWHs) may result in hyperkalaemia.
- The most susceptible are patients with diabetes mellitus, chronic renal failure, acidosis, raised serum potassium and those taking potassium-sparing diuretics.
- The risk does appear to increase with duration of therapy and plasma potassium levels should be taken in those at risk before they commence heparin and monitored regularly, especially if heparin is to be continued for more than 7 days.
- Skin necrosis very rarely may occur at the site of subcutaneous injection after several days of treatment and is usually associated with thrombocytopenia.
- Hypersensitivity reactions including chills, fever, urticaria, bronchospasm and anaphylactoid reactions occur rarely.

Contraindications for heparin use
- Haemophilia and other haemorrhagic disorders.
- Thrombocytopenia (including history of heparin-induced thrombocytopenia).
- Peptic ulcer.
- Recent cerebral haemorrhage.
- Severe hypertension.
- Severe liver disease.
- Following major trauma or recent surgery (especially eye or nervous system).
- Hypersensitivity to heparin.

Low-molecular-weight heparins

A number of drugs are available with similar mechanisms of action but different molecular weights. This leads to differences in the extent to which they bind to plasma proteins, their inhibition of factor Xa and their plasma half-lives.

Current LMWHs available in the UK include *dalteparin, enoxaparin, tinzaparin*.

Box 5.5 lists the advantages of LMWHs.

BOX 5.5 Advantages of low-molecular-weight heparins.

- Haemorrhagic complications may be reduced
- Have a longer duration of action and can be given once or twice daily by subcutaneous injection
- As effective and as safe as the unfractionated form and may be more effective in orthopaedic practice
- Bioavailability is around 90% while that of UFH increases with dose but is only about 10%–30% at prophylactic doses when given subcutaneously
- Predictable dose–response due to better bioavailability and dose–independent clearance
- Monitoring not usually necessary
- Patients can be taught to administer LMWHs at home
- Osteoporosis with long-term treatment may be less

LMWHs, Low molecular weight heparins; UFH, unfractionated heparin.

Other parenteral anticoagulants

Danaparoid is a heparinoid that contains no heparin. It can be used in the prevention of DVT prior to surgery. It is derived from pig intestine and works in a similar way to LMWHs. It is useful when heparin cannot be given due to side effects.

Hirudin This is a 65 amino acid anticoagulant purified from the medical leech, *Hirudo medicinalis*, which binds thrombin with high specificity and sensitivity.

Bivalirudin is a hirudin analogue and a thrombin inhibitor, licensed for use in PCI.

Fondaparinux This is a synthetic drug with no animal components, which inhibits activated factor X. It may be used as an alternative to heparin and is licensed for prophylaxis of thromboembolism in medical patients and those having orthopaedic surgery. According to some research, it reduces the risk of thromboembolism after orthopaedic surgery by more than half compared with LMWH. It is given once daily by subcutaneous injection.

Oral anticoagulants

Warfarin A change in agricultural policy in Canada in the 1920s led to sweet clover being used as cattle food. It was soon discovered that the cows were bleeding after minor injury. This was due to coumarin in the clover and warfarin has been developed from this compound. It was first used as rat poison but became the most used oral anticoagulant in the western world. It is gradually being replaced by direct acting oral anticoagulants (DOACs) which are safer alternatives with fewer side effects and less requirement for monitoring.

Mechanism of action

- Warfarin prevents the reduction of vitamin K which is needed for the clotting process.
- It inhibits the enzyme needed to reduce vitamin K in the liver and thus interferes with the formation of vitamin K-dependent clotting factors including prothrombin.
- Warfarin and vitamin K are similar structurally and the inhibition is competitive.
- This means that excess vitamin K will compete with warfarin and prevent its action, enabling vitamin K to be used as an antidote if too much warfarin is given.
- There is a delay of 2—7 days in the onset of action of warfarin. This is because there are already clotting factors present in the blood that have to be degraded before the warfarin will have an effect.
- Heparin has to be used for immediate anticoagulation and needs to be continued for at least 5 days until the international normalized ratio (INR; see later) has been in the therapeutic range for 2 consecutive days.

Pharmacokinetics

- Warfarin is given orally and is absorbed quickly and totally from the gastrointestinal tract.
- It is almost totally bound to plasma albumin (>95%) with a half-life of approximately 37 hours.
- Protein binding and half-life vary in individuals, meaning the dose has to be tailored to the patient according to their INR.
- Although the peak concentration in the blood occurs 1 hour after administration, the peak pharmacological action is 36—48 hours later.
- The effect on prothrombin time does not begin to appear for 12—16 hours and lasts 4—5 days.
- Metabolized in the liver by cytochrome P450 enzymes to inactive metabolites excreted in urine and stool. Other drugs are also metabolized by this enzyme system and this may lead to drug interactions (see later).
- Warfarin crosses the placenta and is not given in the first months of pregnancy because it is teratogenic. It is not given in the later months of pregnancy as it may cause an intracerebral haemorrhage in the baby during delivery.
- Warfarin does appear in breast milk but does not usually put the baby at risk.
- Maintenance doses can vary from 1 to 20 mg daily but are usually between 3 and 9 mg daily, with 4—5 mg the most usual.

It is important that the daily dose of warfarin be taken at the same time each day.

Monitoring of warfarin action. There is considerable variability in the effect warfarin has on coagulation in different patients. Its effectiveness is influenced by:

- age
- racial background
- diet
- co-medication such as antibiotics.

The action of warfarin is monitored by its effect on the **prothrombin time**. This will be prolonged if there is a deficiency of clotting actors.

The results are reported as a ratio of the patient's prothrombin time to that of a control − INR − and dosage is adjusted to give a ratio of between 2 and 4, dependent on the condition the drug is prescribed for.

The INR has to be determined daily or on alternate days when the warfarin is first prescribed. Monitoring may then be reduced to longer intervals, depending on the patent's response, and eventually up to every 12 weeks.

Therapeutic uses
- Treatment and prevention of DVT.
- Treatment and prevention of PE.
- In AF to reduce the risk of embolization.
- To reduce risk of emboli developing on prosthetic heart valves.
- May also be used in MI or transient ischaemic attacks (TIAs) but an antiplatelet drug is first line here.

The optimal duration for anticoagulant therapy for DVT and PE is undetermined. Research is showing that those who are anticoagulated for longer periods have less risk of recurrence of DVT. Benefits of months over weeks of treatment have been shown. More research is needed.

Adverse effects. Haemorrhage is the main adverse effect of all anticoagulants.

- The antidote for warfarin is vitamin K (***phytomenadione***), which may be given by slow intravenous injection in major bleeding. The patient also may require prothrombin complex concentrate or fresh frozen plasma.
- Action does depend on the severity of the bleeding and the INR. In cases where the INR is between 6.0 and 8.0 and there is no bleeding, the warfarin may be stopped and restarted when the INR is <5.0.
- The higher the INR, the higher the risk of bleeding.
- Risk of bleeding with warfarin is highest at the start of treatment, the risk during the first month being 10 times the risk at 12 months.
- Commonest sites are the gastrointestinal tract, the urinary tract, the soft tissues and the oropharynx.
- Intracranial bleeding is comparatively rare; about 2% of all anticoagulation bleeding, but it is the commonest cause of fatal bleeding.

BOX 5.6 Risk factors for bleeding with anticoagulant therapy.

- Serious co-morbid disease, especially liver disease and renal disease
- Previous gastrointestinal bleeding
- Erratic or excessive alcohol misuse
- Immobility
- Uncontrolled hypertension
- Poor-quality monitoring
- Limited understanding of anticoagulation by patient

Box 5.6 shows the principal risk factors for bleeding with anticoagulant therapy.

Other rare adverse reactions include hypersensitivity and skin rashes, diarrhoea, alopecia, jaundice and skin necrosis.

Interactions with other drugs, herbal medicines and diet

- Vitamin K is found in the diet but is also manufactured in the large bowel by bacteria there. Dietary sources high in vitamin K include green vegetables such as broccoli, spinach, cabbage and lettuce, as well as beetroot, soya beans and beef liver.
- Consistency in diet is important and the patient on warfarin should not suddenly increase their intake of green vegetables and vitamin K as this will reduce the effectiveness of the warfarin. Likewise, if they suddenly reduce their intake, anticoagulation will be greater.
- Broad-spectrum antibiotics may suppress the action of gut bacteria and thus reduce vitamin K and increase anticoagulation.
- Warfarin is highly bound to plasma albumin and some dugs may compete for this binding. Examples are aspirin and some NSAIDs. They displace warfarin from its binding site and thus increase the amount of 'free' warfarin. This will briefly increase its effects.
- Some drugs, herbal remedies and dietary substances inhibit the liver enzymes that metabolize warfarin and so lead to increased anticoagulation. Examples are cranberry juice, ***amiodarone*** and ***cimetidine***.

The safest rule is to tell the patient on oral anticoagulants not to take any over-the-counter medications, including herbal medicines, without medical advice.

- Others stimulate liver enzymes and so decrease the effectiveness of the warfarin. Examples are Brussels sprouts, St John's wort and *rifampicin*.
- Antiplatelet drugs such as *aspirin* may potentate the risk of bleeding with big interindividual variations. Low combinations of aspirin 75 mg and warfarin 3 mg daily are often safe.

Table 5.11 shows some of the other factors that affect coagulation when taking warfarin.

TABLE 5.11 Factors enhancing or reducing coagulation when taking warfarin.

Factors that enhance anticoagulation	Factors that reduce anticoagulation
Weight loss	Weight gain
Increased age (>80 years)	Diarrhoea
Acute illness	Vomiting
Impaired liver function	Relative youth (<40 years)
Heart failure	Asian or Caribbean background
Renal failure	Excess alcohol ingestion

It can be seen that warfarin is not an easy drug for the patient to have to take but before DOACs were licensed, many patients had to take warfarin (be warfarinized) for the rest of their lives (e.g. those with AF). Now any patient newly diagnosed is prescribed a DOAC.

Phenindione is an alternative anticoagulant that is an oral vitamin K antagonist but there are concerns regarding hepatotoxicity, nephrotoxicity and blood dyscrasias. Only given in those hypersensitive to warfarin.

Direct acting anticoagulants

Apixaban, *dabigatran*, *edoxaban* and *rivaroxaban* are newer anticoagulants that may be prescribed instead of warfarin. Dabigatran is a direct thrombin inhibitor and the other three drugs inhibit factor Xa, which catalyses the conversion of prothrombin to thrombin. They thus decrease clot formation induced by thrombin.

Dabigatran

This is a **thrombin (factor IIa) inhibitor** with a rapid onset of action. It binds to the active site of the thrombin molecule and prevents it activating other coagulation factors in the clotting cascade. It can inactivate thrombin even when the thrombin is fibrin-bound and may enhance fibrinolysis.

It has a much better safety profile than warfarin and a much more reliable pharmacokinetic profile.

Dabigatran was licensed the UK in 2008 and is now on the WHO's list of Essential Medicines which lists the safest and most effective medicines needed in a healthcare system (WHO, 2019).

Pharmacokinetics

- Dabigatran has a half-life of approximately 12—14 hours and exerts its maximum effects within 2—3 hours of ingestion.
- Fatty foods delay absorption.
- It is given orally twice a day, usually 110—150 mg.
- Dabigatran is 80% eliminated by the kidneys and so is unsuitable in renal insufficiency.
- Its use is not recommended in pregnancy due to toxicity in animal studies.

In its early years, unlike warfarin, there was no antidote. In 2015 an antidote, *idarucizumab*, to be given in cases of severe bleeding, was licensed.

It has far fewer interactions with other medication than warfarin.

It does not require regular routine anticoagulant monitoring which is a big advantage for both patients and healthcare staff. INR tests are unreliable.

A large study in 2011 (Wann et al. 2011) with 134,000 patients compared dabigatran with warfarin and concluded that dabigatran has a lower risk of overall mortality ischaemic stroke and bleeding in the brain than warfarin. Gastrointestinal bleeding was more common in those treated with dabigatran.

A large comparative study (196,061 people) of warfarin and DOACs in the UK (Vinogradova et al. 2018) assessed the risk of major bleeding with DOACs and warfarin. The primary outcome was major bleeding leading to hospital admission or death. In those with AF, dabigatran and apixaban were associated with a lower risk of intracranial bleeding than warfarin. None were associate with a difference in risk of ischaemic stroke compared to warfarin.

Uses

Prophylaxis of stroke in non-valvular AF.

Prophylaxis of venous thromboembolism following knee or hip replacement

Treatment of DVT and prophylaxis of PE.

Side effects

These may include abnormal liver function, anaemia, nausea, gastrointestinal disorders and bleeding.

Apixaban

Inhibits factor Xa in the clotting cascade and thus prevents the formation of thrombin from prothrombin.

Its uses are similar to dabigatran but it has an advantage in that it can be used in those with renal insufficiency.

Edoxaban and *rivaroxaban* are two other factor Xa inhibitors. Their use in the UK as recommended by NICE is summarized in Box 5.5.

Although monitoring is not appropriate for DOACs, regular follow up is still needed to assess compliance and make sure the patient has no adverse effects, especially bleeding. NICE emphasizes three safety issues relating to all anticoagulants.

1. Information and awareness. Those who are prescribed anticoagulants and those involved in their care should have the necessary information to use them safely and effectively. All health and social care workers should be aware that DOACs are anticoagulants. Some may still not recognize the generic or brand names.
2. Care with dosage and administration. Doses of DOACs should not be delayed or omitted as their half-lives are much shorter than warfarin.
3. Interactions. Warfarin has many drug—drug interactions and drug-food interactions as highlighted above. The use of an anticoagulant with other drugs that increase the risk of bleeding such as antiplatelets may increase the risk of bleeding.

Antiplatelet drugs

Platelets are essential for haemostasis and a low platelet count results in purpura with spontaneous bleeding into the skin and other tissues. Platelets aggregate following activation and this is an essential part of haemostasis; however, platelet adherence to an injured arterial endothelium may be the start of thrombus formation on the arterial side of the circulation.

The endothelium of the blood vessels produces a substance called **prostacyclin** that lessens platelet stickiness. It is a prostaglandin. The platelets themselves produce a substance called **thromboxane A$_2$** that increases their stickiness. This is also a prostaglandin.

When an atherosclerotic plaque ruptures, this is associated with endothelial damage that induces platelet adherence and initiates the release of adenosine diphosphate (ADP) and thromboxane, stimulating platelet aggregation. ADP also induces the activation of the fibrinogen binding sites on the platelet surface.

This process is a common feature in CHD, PVD and cerebrovascular disease. **Antiplatelet drugs** decrease platelet aggregation and so may inhibit the formation of thrombi in the arterial side of the circulation. They are used as prophylaxes and may be enzyme inhibitors or receptor antagonists.

Enzyme inhibitors

Aspirin Aspirin can prevent about one quarter of serious vascular events in a wide range of high-risk patients. The drug is playing an increasing role in prevention of cardiovascular disorders and unstable angina trials have shown it to decrease the incidence of MI by up to 50%.

Mechanism of action. The actions of aspirin are described fully in Section 3.3. Only action relevant to antiplatelet activity is given here.

- Aspirin alters the balance between thromboxane, which promotes platelet aggregation, and prostacyclin, which inhibits it.
- Aspirin irreversibly inhibits the enzyme **cyclo-oxygenase** (COX). This enzyme (COX-1) is found in platelets and needed for the manufacture of prostaglandins including thromboxane which increases the stickiness of platelets.

- Platelets cannot manufacture new proteins such as enzymes; therefore they are unable to make thromboxane for their entire lifespan of 7−10 days.
- The blood vessel walls that manufacture prostacyclin are only inhibited temporarily because they can synthesize more enzyme.
- Aspirin reduces platelet aggregation but does not totally abolish it as other pathways are involved.
- Some patients appear not to respond to aspirin for reasons unknown and those with high cholesterol levels often do not show significant platelet inhibition with aspirin.
- A low dose of aspirin is sufficient; 75 mg daily is recommended by NICE.
- Absorption is over 80% with extensive presystemic metabolism to salicylic acid.

Therapeutic use. To inhibit thrombus formation, especially on the arterial side of the circulation.

- In ischaemic cardiac chest pain such as angina or MI, a single dose of aspirin 150−300 mg is given as soon as possible. It should be chewed or dissolved in water for rapid absorption. This is followed by aspirin 75 mg daily.
- In a low dose (75 mg daily) as secondary prevention of CVD. Unless there are contraindications, aspirin is given to everyone at risk. This includes those with angina, intermittent claudication and following MI. High BP must be controlled before aspirin is given due to the risk of intracranial bleeding.
- Following coronary bypass surgery.
- Sometimes in AF instead of other anticoagulants if the patient is young with no other risk factors.

Adverse effects. Up to 25% of patients may not tolerate regular and prolonged use of aspirin. Table 5.12 shows contraindications to aspirin. Even 10 mg daily reduces gastric mucosal prostaglandins to 40% of baseline level. Aspirin can aggravate asthma in aspirin-sensitive asthmatics. Can aggravate gout because of impaired urate excretion.

Dipyridamole

This drug is also an enzyme inhibitor. It inhibits phosphodiesterase, an enzyme needed for the uptake of adenosine into platelets and other cells. Widely used before the advent of aspirin.

TABLE 5.12 Contraindications to aspirin.

Absolute	Relative
Active gastrointestinal ulceration	History of ulceration or dyspepsia
Hypersensitivity	Children
Thrombocytopenia	Bleeding disorders
	Warfarin treatment

TABLE 5.13 Contraindications to thrombolysis.

Absolute	Relative
Recent or recurrent haemorrhage, trauma or surgery	Previous peptic ulceration
Active peptic ulceration	Warfarin
Coagulation defects	Liver disease
Oesophageal varices	Heavy vaginal bleeding
Coma	
Recent or disabling cerebrovascular accident	
Hypertension	
Aortic dissection	

- Reduces platelet adhesiveness and may be used in combination with low-dose aspirin for secondary prevention of ischaemic stroke and TIAs. Trials as to its effectiveness are ongoing.
- Its effect is relatively short lasting, and repeated dosing or slow-release preparations are needed to achieve 24-hour inhibition of platelet function.

TABLE 5.14 Recommended uses of oral antithrombotic drugs — factor Xa inhibitors and direct thrombin inhibitors.

Apixaban — factor Xa inhibitor	Dabigatran — direct thrombin inhibitor	Edoxaban — factor Xa inhibitor	Rivaroxaban — factor Xa inhibitor
Prevention of VTE after knee or hip surgery	Prevention of VTE after knee or hip surgery		Prevention of VTE after knee or hip surgery
Treatment of DVT and/or PE. Prophylaxis of recurrent DVT or PE	Treatment of DVT and/or PE. Prophylaxis of recurrent DVT or PE	Treatment of DVT and/or PE. Prophylaxis of recurrent DVT or PE	Treatment of DVT and/or PE. Prophylaxis of recurrent DVT or PE
Prevention of stroke with one risk factor and non-valvular AF	Prevention of stroke with one risk factor and non-valvular AF	Prevention of stroke with one risk factor and non-valvular AF	Prevention of stroke with one risk factor and non-valvular AF
			Prevention of antithrombotic events following ACS in certain circumstances.

ACS, Acute coronary syndrome; *AF,* atrial fibrillation; *DVT,* deep vein thrombosis; *PE,* pulmonary embolism; *VTE,* venous thromboembolism.
Table adapted from information within the BNF (2019).

- Given with oral anticoagulation in those with prosthetic heart valves, to prevent thromboembolism.
- It vasodilates, and side effects include throbbing headache, dizziness, hot flushes and tachycardia.

Platelet adenosine diphosphate receptor antagonists

Clopidogrel

Mechanism of action

- Clopidogrel is a prodrug that when converted to its active form in the liver irreversibly inhibits ADP binding to its receptors on the platelet surface. This helps to prevent the platelet binding fibrin and thus forming a thrombus.
- The site of action is different to that of aspirin and the two drugs are used together in acute coronary syndrome without ST elevation. They are given for at least 1 month but no longer than 9−12 months.
- Does not work fully in up to 14% of the population who have a deficiency of the liver enzyme required to convert clopidogrel to its active form.
- Its uses include:
  - In combination with aspirin in AF if other anticoagulants are unsuitable.
  - To prevent atherothrombotic events in patients with a history of ischaemic stroke.
  - In combination with aspirin in PCI and for at least 1−6 months afterwards depending on the type of stent.
  - In TIAs if aspirin not suitable
  - Prevention of atherothrombotic events in ACS
- Onset of action on platelets occurs in hours but steady-state inhibition only occurs in 3−7 days.
- Loading dose may be given to ensure maximal inhibition of platelets in 2 hours.

Adverse effects

- Increased incidence of bleeding when used with aspirin.
- May cause indigestion, abdominal discomfort and diarrhoea.
- Blood disorders such as neutropenia (drop in white blood cells − neutrophils) and thrombocytopenia (fall in platelets).
- Thrombocytopenia usually occurs within 2 weeks of initiation of therapy and responds to plasma exchange.

Contraindications

- Active bleeding and breastfeeding are contraindications.
- Caution should be taken if patients are at risk of bleeding from trauma, surgery or other conditions.
- The drug should be discontinued 7 days before planned surgery unless antiplatelet effect is needed.

Prasugrel. This works in a similar way to clopidogrel and is an irreversible antagonist of one type of ADP receptor on the platelet thus preventing platelet aggregation.

It inhibits the aggregation more rapidly than clopidogrel and more consistently.

It is sometimes used in combination with aspirin in patients with ACS undergoing PCI and is usually continued for 12 months.

Ticagrelor. This is another ADP receptor antagonist that is licensed for the prevention of atherothrombotic events in those with ACS.

Recommended, as one treatment option, by NICE in combination with low dose aspirin for up to 12 months in ACS.

Cangrelor. This is a direct ADP receptor antagonist in platelets that blocks ADP induced platelet aggregation.

It is used in combination with aspirin in PCI when other forms of antiplatelet therapy have not been given.

Glycoprotein IIb/IIIa inhibitors

Compete with fibrinogen to occupy the glycoprotein IIb/IIIa receptor on platelets so preventing platelet aggregation by blocking the binding of fibrinogen to the platelet receptors. This is the final pathway leading to platelet aggregation and allows platelets to interact with other components of the clotting cascade. The receptor binds circulating von Willebrand factor and fibrinogen, which crosslinks adjacent platelets, leading to thrombus formation.

Abciximab

- This is a monoclonal antibody made by recombinant DNA technology that binds to the receptors.
- It is given to prevent complications in patients at high risk during PCI.
- Also used in patients with unstable angina if they are not responding to other treatments and are due to have PCI.
- Dose-dependent antiplatelet effect. Correlation between percentage of receptors blocked and the inhibition of platelet aggregation. To be effective, 90% of receptors have to be blocked.
- Should be used once only. After intravenous administration platelet aggregation is 90% inhibited within 2 hours, but function recovers over a period of 2 days.

Tirofiban and eptifibatide

- These are **synthetic antagonists** specific for glycoprotein IIb/IIIa.
- *Eptifibatide* is a synthetic derivative of a substance purified from the pygmy rattlesnake.
- These drugs are only used in specialized coronary care units.
- They are given by intravenous infusion in patients with unstable angina or non-ST segment elevation MI when the chest pain has been present in the past 24 hours.

Fibrinolytic drugs

A clot is formed from insoluble fibrin threads and will be removed very slowly by the body in nature. The fibrinolytic substance that dissolves the clot is called plasmin and it is formed from an inactive precursor (plasminogen) by the action of tissue plasminogen activator (tPA).

Drugs may break up and remove a pre-existing thrombus either by potentiating the body's own fibrinolytic pathway (e.g. *streptokinase*) or by mimicking natural thrombolytic molecules such as **tPA**.

The first agent, *streptokinase*, was derived from bacterial products which was highly antigenic making allergic reactions more likely.

Fibrinolytic agents are indicated for any patient with acute MI for whom the benefit is likely to outweigh the risk of treatment. Benefits are shown to be greater in an ST-elevation infarct.

Primary coronary angioplasty may be carried out immediately and a stent inserted to hold the walls of the coronary artery open. This procedure has been shown to give better overall outcomes than thrombolysis if fast access is available.

The drugs are used in cases of MI where PCI is not available within the 120 minutes that a fibrinolytic drug can be administered. They are also used in ischaemic stroke and may be used to treat a large pulmonary embolus.

The newer drugs are less antigenic than streptokinase and more thrombus specific, which increases efficacy and specificity.

Drugs used are alteplase, reteplase, tenecteplase and streptokinase.

- Lack of site specificity with these drugs means there is a risk of haemorrhage (gastrointestinal, intracranial, etc.).
- Hypersensitivity, especially with streptokinase, is important − manifests as flushing, breathlessness, rash, urticaria and hypotension. Severe anaphylaxis is rare.

Streptokinase

- Converts plasminogen to plasmin, the main fibrinolytic enzyme, and thus potentiates fibrinolysis.
- Not site-specific, lysing a thrombus anywhere in the body.
- Derived from haemolytic streptococcal bacteria and therefore **antigenic**− repeated administration results in neutralizing antibodies and allergic reactions.
- A single injection of 1.5 MU for acute MI results in neutralizing antibodies that have been shown to persist for up to 4 years. They neutralize a repeat administration of the same dose in approximately half of cases.
- Should not be used again beyond 4 days of administration.

Alteplase (rt-PA)

- Produced by recombinant DNA technology. *Alteplase* is recombinant tPA and mimics the endogenous molecule that activates the fibrinolytic system.
- Does not elicit an allergic response and is more clot specific.
- Has a **short half-life** and needs continuous infusion to achieve greatest efficacy.
- Used in acute MI, PE and acute ischaemic stroke.
- In acute MI treatment should be initiated within 6 hours of symptom onset.
  - Dose calculated according to approximate body weight.
  - Given by intravenous injection followed by intravenous infusion over a period of 90 minutes.
- In stroke treatment must begin within 4−5 hours of symptom onset.
  - Intracranial haemorrhage must be discounted first by the use of computed tomography
  - Given by IVI over 60 minutes
- In PE a smaller dose is used by intravenous infusion. For more detail, see the current BNF (2019) and the NICE guidance.

Tenecteplase

- Developed on animal models from snake venom and the vampire bat.
- Does not bind to liver receptors and this prologues half-life to 22 minutes.
- Fibrin specificity is 10 times greater than natural tPA.
- Given as a single weight-adjusted bolus of 30−50 mg.
- *Tenecteplase* was the first thrombolytic agent to match the efficacy of tPA with a single bolus.

  This means it could be given in the prehospital environment.

- **'Time is muscle'** and every minute counts so this was a big move forward.
- Only used in acute MI.

Side effects

Table 5.12 shows contraindications to thrombolysis.

The main adverse side effects of thrombolytics are nausea, vomiting and bleeding.

- If used following an MI, reperfusion arrhythmias may occur.
- Hypotension.
- Bleeding − usually at the site of injection but also from other sites and rarely intracerebral haemorrhage may occur.
- Streptokinase may cause allergic reactions and anaphylaxis.

Haemostatics

These are drugs that stop bleeding.

Tranexamic acid

Prevents clot breakdown by inhibiting fibrinolysis.

Clinical use

- To prevent excessive bleeding in certain operations and in dentistry if the patient has haemophilia.
- In significant haemorrhage following trauma (unlicensed use).
- Epistaxis.
- Menorrhagia (extremely heavy menstrual bleeding) and severe epistaxis (nose bleed).
- Thrombolytic overdose.

Etamsylate

Reduces capillary bleeding by correcting abnormal platelet adhesion. It used to be used in menorrhagia but is less effective than other agents, and its use is no longer recommended (BNF, 2019).

Emicizumab

This is a monoclonal antibody that bridges activated factor IX and factor X to restore the function of missing activated factor VIII, which is needed for haemostasis.

It is used for the prophylaxis of haemorrhage in patients with haemophilia.

Respiratory, renal and gastrointestinal systems

Section Outline

6.1 RESPIRATORY SYSTEM

The main function of the airways is to transport air containing oxygen into the lungs and to remove carbon dioxide. The oxygen diffuses from the alveoli into the bloodstream, attaches to haemoglobin and is transported round the body to all cells and tissues. Survival depends on these processes being reliable, sustained and efficient. To accomplish this, a number of processes are required:

- Pulmonary ventilation: the lungs have to expand and contract using the diaphragm and intercostal muscles.
- External respiration: there has to be movement of oxygen and carbon dioxide across the respiratory membrane from the lungs to blood.
- Transport of respiratory gases:
  - The blood carries oxygen in two ways: dissolved in plasma and attached to haemoglobin.
  - Carbon dioxide is carried in blood in three ways: dissolved in plasma, bound to haemoglobin or converted to bicarbonate ions and transported in plasma.
- Internal respiration: gaseous exchange has to take place between the systemic capillaries and the tissue cells.

There is autonomic innervation of the airways, which regulates some aspects of respiration.

- Parasympathetic innervation predominates and maintains smooth muscle tone in the airways. Postganglionic fibres innervate airway smooth muscle, vascular muscle and glands. Muscarinic receptors present in ganglia are embedded in the walls of bronchi and bronchioles, and stimulation

A Nurse's Survival Guide to Drugs in Practice. https://doi.org/10.1016/B978-0-7020-7658-9.00006-8

287

increases mucous production as well as leading to bronchoconstriction and bronchial vasodilation.

- Although there is no evidence of sympathetic innervation of bronchial smooth muscle, there are many β_2 adrenergic receptors in airways smooth muscle; stimulation of these by circulating adrenaline causes relaxation of bronchial smooth muscle and therefore bronchodilation.

Common symptoms of pulmonary disease include:

- cough, haemoptysis (coughing up blood)
- wheeze
- sputum production (not always present)
- shortness of breath, orthopnoea (breathlessness when lying flat).

The effect of drugs on the respiratory system:

- Respiratory depression can be caused by drugs that suppress the central nervous system (CNS) such as opioids, barbiturates and alcohol.
- Respiration can be stimulated by analeptic drugs, such as *doxapram*, which are respiratory stimulants. Their use has declined and been replaced by ventilatory support. These drugs are still occasionally used for patients in ventilatory failure when ventilatory support is contraindicated. They are given intravenously and have a short duration of action. Their use must be combined with active physiotherapy and they are only given under expert supervision in hospital.
- Ventilation can be improved by drugs such as *salbutamol*, which relax smooth muscle and widen the airways leading to improved air entry and oxygenation. These drugs do not actually stimulate respiration.

Cough mixtures and decongestants

A cough is a common symptom of respiratory disease and the underlying cause should be found where necessary. A cough also may be a side effect of another drug (e.g. ACE-inhibitors) or it may be associated with pollution or smoking. The cough mixture will only treat the cough and not the cause.

A **cough suppressant** may be used if the cough is dry and unproductive. This is useful if sleep is disturbed but can cause retention of sputum in chronic obstructive pulmonary disease (COPD) where cough suppressants should not be used.

- **Opiates** are powerful cough suppressants.
- *Codeine phosphate* may be used and is available as codeine linctus but it is constipating and may cause dependence if given over a period of time. Large doses may also cause some respiratory depression. *Pholcodine or dextromethorphan* are considered safer.

Cough suppressants containing codeine should not be given to children under 12 years of age and the Medicines and Healthcare Products Regulatory Agency (MHRA) guidance is not to give children under the age of 6 any cough preparations containing bromphe-niramine, chlorphenamine or other antihistamines, dextromethorphan, pholcodine, guaifenesin, ipecacuanha or ephedrine and derivatives.

- *Morphine* is used as a cough suppressant in terminal lung cancer. *Methadone linctus* is an alternative but may accumulate due to its long duration of action. These drugs are not used for other forms of cough as they cause opioid dependence in addition to sputum retention.
- Cough suppressants sold over the counter (OTC) usually contain sedating antihistamines as the cough suppressant and their main action will cause drowsiness.
- **Simple linctus** is a cheap and safe preparation that may soothe a dry and irritating cough. It contains citric acid and is safe to give in paediatric form to children.
- Inhalations containing volatile substances, such as menthol and eucalyptus, may be useful in coughs and for relieving nasal congestion. The inspiration of the moist, warm air is useful but boiling water should not be used because of scalding.

Expectorants are taken to aid the expulsion of secretions when coughing. There is no real evidence that they can actually do this (BNF, 2019).

- An *ammonia* and *ipecacuanha mixture* would cause vomiting in larger doses but in a small dose is taken as an expectorant. It has to be recently prepared.

Mucolytics are given to decrease the viscosity of the sputum and so enable it to be expectorated. They are helpful in some patients with COPD, cystic fibrosis or those with a chronic productive cough.

- *Carbocisteine*, *acetylcysteine* and *erdosteine* are used but should not be given to people with a peptic ulcer as they interfere with the mucosal barrier in the stomach.
- *Dornase alpha* is an enzyme that breaks up DNA in the sputum in cystic fibrosis, thus reducing viscosity and aiding clearance of secretions. It is produced by genetic engineering and is administered by inhalation of a nebulized solution. Optimizing lung function is a major aim in cystic fibrosis and intensive physiotherapy plays a vital role. Prevention and management of infection is also vitally important.

Nasal decongestants may be given orally for systemic action to prevent the rebound congestion that can occur following nasal administration.

- They contain *pseudoephedrine* and are stimulants of the sympathetic nervous system (SNS) so should be used with caution in a list of conditions including hypertension (see the British National Formulary [BNF, 2019] for details).
- Available preparations include *ephedrine hydrochloride* and *pseudoephedrine hydrochloride*.

Aromatic inhalations of volatile substances such as *menthol and eucalyptus* may be taken to relieve nasal congestion or in sinusitis. **Tincture of benzoin** (Friars' balsam) is also occasionally used. These substances are added to hot − not boiling − water and the vapour is inhaled.

Pulmonary surfactants

Neonatal respiratory distress syndrome (NRDS) occurs in newborn babies, usually premature, when their lungs are not fully developed. It is caused by a deficiency of pulmonary surfactant, which usually starts to be produced in the baby around 24−28 weeks' gestation. The immature lungs in a preterm baby cannot manufacture sufficient of their own surfactant to breathe adequately until around week 34 but sometimes NRDS occurs in full-term babies.

Surfactant is a substance made up of protein, lipids and carbohydrates that is needed to reduce surface tension in the alveoli and to prevent the lung collapsing following expiration. Replacement of natural surfactant has been available since the 1980s in the form of purified mammalian surfactant. Available are *beractant* and *poractant alfa*, both given via the endotracheal tube in specialized neonatal units or via minimally invasive methods if possible. They are used in neonates to prevent respiratory distress syndrome. Antenatal steroids may be given to the mother prior to delivery to aid the development of the baby's lungs.

Respiratory disorders

May be divided into:

- *Obstructive:* causes narrowing of the airways such as in asthma and bronchitis.
- *Restrictive:* when the actual ability of the lungs to expand is reduced, lessening the surface area and volume of air available for gas exchange such as that observed in pulmonary fibrosis and adult respiratory distress syndrome.

Asthma and chronic bronchitis are the two main obstructive disorders affecting the respiratory tract.

The effect of the autonomic nervous system on the airways

- The airways are constricted by acetylcholine, the transmitter of the para-sympathetic nervous system (PNS). They are relaxed by circulating adrenaline (epinephrine).
- Mucus secretion is inhibited by the SNS and stimulated by the PNS as well as inflammatory chemical mediators and cold air.
- Drugs that inhibit the action of acetylcholine relax the airways and reduce mucus secretion. One such drug is *ipratropium* (*Atrovent*), which is a cholinergic antagonist.
- Drugs that stimulate adrenergic receptors cause bronchodilation. *Salbutamol* (*Ventolin*) is one such drug.
- Bronchodilators such as *ipratropium* and *salbutamol* work on two different receptor sites in the lungs: *ipratropium* blocks cholinergic (muscarinic) and *salbutamol* stimulates adrenergic (β_2) to relax the smooth muscle of the airways when bronchoconstriction is present.

Asthma

Asthma is a common inflammatory respiratory condition that occurs in response to a wide range of stimuli. An asthma attack varies in severity from mild to fatal. Initially it is a reversible recurrent condition leading to airways obstruction caused by bronchospasm, increased secretion of sticky mucus and oedema. The bronchospasm observed in asthma is believed to be linked to the release of histamine, an inflammatory mediator.

The effect of histamine on the bronchioles during an asthmatic attack is that it contracts bronchial smooth muscle as strongly as a muscarinic receptor agonist would. It also causes plasma leakage from the postcapillary venules and increases the secretion of mucous. The airways in those with asthma are hyperresponsive to histamine and to other agents that contract smooth muscle. Research still continues into this hyperresponsiveness to histamine (Yamauchi and Ogasawara, 2019).

Symptoms include a cough, wheeze, chest tightness, difficulty with expiration and shortness of breath. These symptoms tend to be:

- variable
- intermittent
- worse at night
- provoked by triggers including exercise.

Asthma has three characteristics:

- airflow limitation, usually reversible with treatment
- airway hyper-responsiveness
- inflammation of the bronchi with oedema, smooth muscle hypertrophy, mucus plugging and epithelial damage.

During exacerbations the patient will have reduced peak flow rates and usually a wheeze. Outside acute episodes there may be periods of remission with no objective signs of asthma.

As a result of inflammation, the airways are hyper-reactive and narrow easily in response to a wide range of stimuli.

While initially reversible, the inflammation may lead to an irreversible obstruction of airflow. If the bronchospasm is frequent and prolonged, the bronchial muscle layer may become permanently thickened which results in long-term bronchoconstriction.

Extrinsic asthma
- There is a definite external cause. It commonly develops during childhood, often runs in families, and identifiable factors provoke wheezing. It is a hypersensitivity disorder and may be associated with hay fever and eczema that also occur in individuals who are atopic and have a high incidence of allergies due to increased levels of IgE antibodies in their blood.
- Precipitating factors include house dust mites, pollens and spores, pets, smoke, chemicals, certain foods and drugs (especially beta blockers and nonsteroidal anti-inflammatory drugs (NSAIDs) such as ibuprofen). In some, an asthma attack is brought on by exercise or even just cold air. Emotional factors may also be involved.
- Response to an allergen usually begins within minutes (early reaction), reaches its maximum in about 15−20 minutes and subsides within an hour.
- Following the immediate reaction, many, but not all, develop a more prolonged and sustained attack that is more resistant to drug therapy.

Intrinsic asthma
- No causative agent can be identified. This type of asthma begins in adult life and airflow obstruction is more persistent. Most exacerbations have no obvious stimuli other than a respiratory tract infection. Other triggers may be weather conditions, pollution, smoke or stress. Sometimes the trigger is not known.

It is now believed that the two types of asthma have much in common and involve the production of IgE locally in the airways in response to trigger factors.

Acute asthma

On assessment, the severity of the asthma is graded (British Thoracic Society, 2019).

Acute severe asthma

Can be life-threatening and must be treated promptly. Clinical features include:

- peak expiratory flow (PEF) 33%−50% of best normal
- breathlessness and inability to complete a sentence in one breath

- respiratory rate over 25 breaths/min
- tachycardia: heart rate over 110 beats/min
- wheezing: this may be absent early on but becomes more apparent as the asthma becomes worse.

The patient may be very anxious and a calm atmosphere is essential. It should be noted that speed of onset varies — some attacks come on over minutes; in some patients, deterioration occurs slowly over days.

Asthma can produce symptoms of all grades varying from very mild to life-threatening. Its danger should never be underestimated and several hundred people die each year from asthma.

Life-threatening asthma

In a patient with severe asthma, any one of the following features may be present:

- PEF < 33% of best or predicted best (approximately 150 L/min in adults)
- Saturation of peripheral oxygen (SpO_2) < 92%
- PaO_2 < 8 kPa
- Altered conscious level
- Exhaustion
- Arrhythmia
- Hypotension
- Cyanosis
- A silent chest
- Poor respiratory effort.

Patients are not always distressed and may not show all these features; any one of the features is significant.

If the patient deteriorates despite pharmacological interventions it may be necessary to use intermittent positive-pressure ventilation.

Medication in asthma

The British Thoracic Society, together with SIGN, has published revised guidelines in 2019: the British Guidelines on the Management of Asthma. There are guidelines for children, adolescents and adults, and the reader is referred to this document for details. These are found at https://www.brit-thoracic.org.uk.

The aim is to totally control symptoms and reduce medication to a level that will maintain this control.

Drugs are usually delivered directly into the lungs by **inhalation**.

Two major types of medication are used:

- **Relievers**: bronchodilators (e.g. *salbutamol*).
- **Controllers**: anti-inflammatory steroids.

Bronchodilators

Bronchodilators give relatively rapid relief of symptoms and are believed to work predominantly by relaxation of airway smooth muscle.

- β_2-adrenoreceptor agonists (e.g. *salbutamol*).
- Xanthines (e.g. *theophylline*).
- Muscarinic receptor antagonists (e.g. *ipratropium bromide*).

β_2 adrenoreceptor agonists

These relax the smooth muscle of the respiratory tract via the SNS whatever the cause of the bronchoconstriction and dilate the bronchi. They are antagonists of smooth muscle contraction and are usually administered via the inhalation of aerosol, powder or nebulized solution, but can be given orally or by injection.

- Short acting (e.g. *salbutamol*, *terbutaline*). These act immediately, peaking after 30 minutes and lasting for 3–5 hours. They are given as an aerosol on an 'as needed' basis to control symptoms. A nebulizer may be administered for more acute life-threatening attacks
- Longer acting (e.g. *salmeterol*, *formoterol*). These are given by inhalation and can last between 8 and 12 hours. They are given regularly twice a day but the patient must be using a corticosteroid inhaler already.

Short-acting β_2 agonists

Most frequently used is *salbutamol* and is often the first line of drugs in an asthmatic attack. It causes dilation of the bronchioles and thus helps breathing. It will also relax uterine muscle and may be used to delay the onset of premature labour (see Section 7.5).

Salbutamol has a direct action on the β_2 adrenergic receptor that:

- relaxes the smooth muscle
- inhibits mediator release from mast cells
- may inhibit vagal tone and increase mucus clearance by an action on the cilia
- has no effect on inflammation.

Salbutamol is the drug of choice in an emergency as well as in mild asthma, where it is given as needed.

- It does not reduce the underlying inflammation in the respiratory tract. If asthma worsens the patient should not rely on this drug but needs additional drug therapy such as anticholinergics or steroids.
- It has a rapid onset of action and starts to work within minutes. Its maximum effect is within 30 minutes and its duration of action is up to 4—6 hours.

Salbutamol is usually given **by inhalation**. This enhances selectivity by increasing concentration in the airways and reduces the chances of systemic side effects.

The inhalation may be in the form of a metered dose inhaler (MDI) or a dry powder device.

- 20% of the inhaled dose may be absorbed into the body. Only 10%—25% actually stays in the lungs; the rest is swallowed.
- The inhaler may be taken prior to an activity or stimulus that is likely to cause bronchoconstriction. Many patients can prevent exercise-induced bronchoconstriction if they inhale a short-acting β_2 stimulant 5—10 minutes before exercise starts.
- In a severe asthma attack the client will need higher doses of β_2 stimulant, which is given in the form of a **nebulizer.**

Salbutamol is available orally in the form of a syrup or tablets. A solution for intramuscular or intravenous administration is also available.

Side effects
- Tachycardia: reflex effect from increased peripheral vasodilation via β_2 receptor.
- In high doses it can also cause a muscle tremor; but this is more common in older patients.
- Dizziness and restlessness.
- Reduces the potassium level in the blood and may cause hypokalaemia, especially if xanthines and steroids are given as well.

β_2 stimulants do not control the inflammation in asthma.
- Some evidence that tolerance to salbutamol can develop in asthma as with intense prolonged use there may be a decline in the numbers of β_2 receptors in the lungs.
- Steroids can help here because they inhibit beta receptor downregulation.
- Patients with mild or moderate chronic asthma should take shorter-acting β_2 stimulants as needed to relieve symptoms. Regular fixed-interval use gives no additional benefit and may possibly cause harm.

If given to asthmatic patients, β$_2$ antagonists such as propranolol can precipitate a potentially serious asthma attack. This is because the bronchodilation normally occurring in response to stimulation of the β$_2$ receptor cannot occur if it is blocked.

Long-acting β$_2$ agonists (e.g. salmeterol, formoterol)

The longer-acting β$_2$ stimulants are not used in the immediate management of acute symptoms as they take time to work. They are designed for regular twice-daily administration and not for use prior to activities.

A single dose gives bronchodilation lasting 8–12 hours.

Used in asthma but only when the patient is already on inhaled corticosteroids (ICSs).

Salmeterol and *fluticasone* (a steroid) are available in one inhaler (*Seretide*).

Muscarinic receptor antagonists (anticholinergics)

The main drug in this class is **ipratropium bromide (Atrovent).** It is related to **atropine** and relaxes the bronchial constriction caused by increased tone due to parasympathetic stimulation.

This occurs in asthma produced by irritant stimuli and can occur in allergic asthma.

- Can provide short-term relief in chronic asthma but *salbutamol* acts more quickly and is preferred.
- Effective in COPD where *glycopyrronium, tiotropium* and *umeclidinium* are also licensed but are not suitable for the relief of acute bronchospasm.
- Inhibits mucus secretion and may increase mucociliary clearance of bronchial secretions.
- Has no effect on the later inflammatory stages of asthma.
- Given as an inhaled dose in an aerosol or nebulizer and is not absorbed from the gut.
- Has a powerful local action without causing systemic side effects.
- Maximum effect 30–60 minutes after inhalation and lasts approximately 3–6 hours.
- It has few unwanted effects and in general is safe and well tolerated.
- It can be given with β$_2$ agonists.

Side effects
These are due to the antimuscarinic effects.

- Dry mouth.
- Nausea, constipation.
- Headache.
- Tachycardia and occasionally atrial fibrillation.

Can cause worsening of glaucoma (as it dilates the pupils) and may cause retention of urine in prostatic hypertrophy.

Methylxanthines
Naturally occurring xanthines include *theophylline* and *caffeine* (contents of tea and coffee).

Aminophylline is the main therapeutic drug of this class and used as a bronchodilator, but the use of theophylline has declined due to the greater effectiveness of β$_2$ agonists. Aminophylline has many more side effects and a lower safety profile than salbutamol. It is necessary to monitor the levels of theophylline in the plasma as the drug has a narrow margin between the therapeutic and the toxic dose; 10–20 mg/L are usually needed for bronchodilation but adverse effects may occur even in this range. As the concentration increases so does the severity of the toxicity.

Plasma theophylline concentrations are increased in heart failure, liver disease and in the elderly. Concentrations are decreased in smokers and chronic drinkers.

Modified-release tablets of theophylline are available.

Theophylline, as *aminophylline* (theophylline mixed with ethylenediamine to give greater water solubility), is occasionally given by very slow intravenous injection (over 20 minutes) or in dextrose 5% as an infusion for severe asthma.

Modified-release tablets of aminophylline are available as *Phyllocontin Continus*. Usually given at night in COPD or to prevent nocturnal attacks of asthma. *Phyllocontin Continus Forte* tablets are available for smokers or those with increased metabolism of theophylline.

Mechanism of action

- Inhibits the enzyme phosphodiesterase and so prevents the breakdown of cyclic adenosine monophosphate. Produce direct smooth muscle relaxation.

- Does have some anti-inflammatory action.
- Relatively high doses are needed for airway smooth muscle relaxation but there is increasing evidence that theophylline has anti-inflammatory properties or immunomodulatory effects at lower plasma concentrations (5–10 mg/L).
- These drugs are weak respiratory stimulants, and caffeine has been used in neonates for this purpose.

Other actions and side effects

- Actions on CNS. Have a stimulant action causing increased alertness. Can cause tremor and nervousness and interfere with sleep.
- Actions on the cardiovascular system. All xanthines stimulate the heart. Have positive inotropic and chronotropic action. Cause vasodilation in most blood vessels but vasoconstriction in the cerebral blood vessels.
- Actions on the kidney. Have a weak diuretic effect.
- Increase adrenaline (epinephrine) secretion.
- Inhibit prostaglandins.
- Side effects include nausea, vomiting, nervousness, tremor, headache, restlessness, gastro-oesophageal reflux.
- In greater concentrations arrhythmias may occur that can be fatal.
- Epileptic seizures, especially in children (usually plasma concentration >3 mg/L).

Caffeine is very similar to *aminophylline* and is a mild central stimulant. It is not used therapeutically in adults.

Histamine antagonists

Although mast cells are thought to play a part in the immediate phase of allergic asthma, histamine antagonists have been disappointing in the treatment of asthma. Some of the newer, nonsedating antihistamines, such as *cetirizine*, have been shown to be effective in mild atopic asthma such as that due to pollen allergy.

Glucocorticoids

The most effective drugs to prevent inflammatory changes in adults and older children are inhaled *steroids*. Steroids are used for their anti-inflammatory action and must be taken regularly. They are not bronchodilators, but prevent inflammation and make the airways less hypersensitive to trigger factors. Regular use reduces the risk of exacerbation of asthma.

It is important to prevent chronic inflammation of the airways and airway remodelling from occurring in asthma. These changes are due to the release of chemical mediators, such as leukotrienes, prostaglandins and bradykinin, which are produced by inflammatory cells including eosinophils (a type of white blood cell). Histamine produces immediate bronchoconstriction, whereas leukotrienes act more slowly. They attract large white blood cells — called macrophages — to the area and these release more chemicals that can be damaging to the lining of the airways, causing loss of epithelial cells and increased hyper-reactivity. Growth factors are released that cause thickening of the basement membrane and the smooth muscle layer in the bronchioles. These changes are shown in Fig. 6.1.

Mechanism of action

- They are not bronchodilators. They reduce inflammation and allergic re-actions and a clear improvement should follow within 3—7 days of administration. They do not work immediately and this has led to some patients not taking them, as they do not immediately feel relief from their symptoms.
- Bind to **glucocorticoid receptors** in the cytoplasm that regulate the expression of multiple genes.
- Inhibit the generation of chemicals by white blood cells, particularly the leukotriene IL-5. This reduces the recruitment of inflammatory cells such as eosinophils.
- Inhibit other leukotrienes including the spasmogens LTC_4 and LTD_4, as well as the prostaglandins PGE_2 and PGI_2.

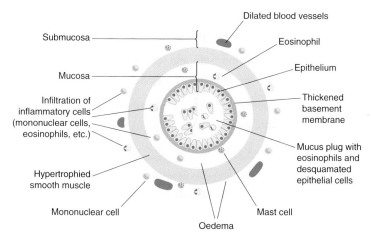

FIG. 6.1 Schematic diagram of a cross-section of a bronchiole showing the changes that can occur with severe chronic asthma. The individual elements depicted are not, of course, drawn to scale. *Reproduced with permission from Rang, H.P., Dale, M.M., Ritter, J.M. et al. 2007. Rang & Dale's Pharmacology, sixth ed. Churchill Livingstone, Edinburgh.*

- Long-term use eventually reduces the early phase response to allergens and prevents exercise-induced asthma. This may be because they reduce the synthesis of the cytokine that regulates mast cell production.
- They inhibit the downregulation of the beta-receptor and so prevent tolerance to β_2 agonists. *Salmeterol* should not be prescribed unless the patient is already receiving a steroid by inhalation.
- They do have side effects over a period of time and are given in an inhaled form to prevent systemic action as much as possible.
- Effective in virtually all patients, irrespective of age and severity of asthma.
- Reduce airway hyper-responsiveness. Improvement occurs slowly over several months.
- They suppress inflammation but do not cure the underlying cause.

Administration

The exact threshold for the introduction of steroids is still open to debate but the asthma guidelines say they should be considered if the patient has had exacerbations of asthma in the last 2 years, or the salbutamol inhaler is being used more than twice a week, or the patient has asthma symptoms three times a week or is waking 1 night a week.

Five ICSs are licensed for the treatment of patients with asthma. These are beclometasone dipropionate (*Becotide*), budesonide (*Pulmicort*), ciclesonide (*Alvesco*), fluticasone propionate (*Flixotide*) and mometasone furoate (*Asmanex*). The steroids are also available combined with a long-acting β_2 agonist such as salmeterol or formoterol. This makes it more likely that the two drugs will be taken regularly.

Each is available for administration via an MDI, with or without a spacer, or as a dry powder from a range of different devices.

The reader is referred to the BNF and asthma guidelines for the doses of different inhaled steroids and their equivalency.

Most inhaled steroids are more effective if taken twice daily, except *ciclesonide*, which is once daily. When control is good, once-daily steroids may be given at the same time of day.

Side effects

These are less than occur with the systemic use of steroids but are a major issue in the long-term use of inhaled steroids. They are mainly related to the size of the inhaled dose, but some people do appear more susceptible. High doses of inhaled steroid should only be used when smaller doses are less effective and the large dose is clearly beneficial.

Local side effects Due to deposition of inhaled steroid in the oropharynx.

- *Candida* infections (thrush) of the mouth may occur in about 5% of patients. This is due to local lowering of resistance by the steroid and a spacer helps to prevent this. It can be treated by antifungal lozenges without discontinuing the steroid inhaler.
- Hoarseness (dysphonia) develops in up to 40% of patients taking high doses.
- Throat irritation and cough may be due to additives in the MDI − rarely with dry powder inhalers (DPIs). The salbutamol inhaler should be taken first to prevent this.

Systemic side effects These are due to absorption both from the respiratory tract and the gastrointestinal (GI) tract (GIT). Absorption from the GIT is greatly reduced by the use of a spacer and mouthwashes.

- **Adrenal suppression** can occur with high doses over a prolonged period, and a steroid card should be carried. Patients may need corticosteroid cover when having an operation or at other times of stress. Excessive doses should be avoided in children where adrenal crisis and coma have been seen.
- **Reduced bone density** and osteoporosis can occur with high doses over a long period.
- **Growth** should be monitored in children as slowing may occur. With normal doses this does not appear to affect the growth achieved in adulthood.
- Small risks of **cataract** and **glaucoma** have been reported.

In 2018 the MHRA published advice that there is a rare risk of chorioretinopathy with inhaled administration of steroids and with systemic administration. Patients should be advised to report any blurred vision or visual disturbances.

Oral steroids

- A severe acute asthma attack is treated with a short course of oral steroids. *Prednisolone* is given for a few days only. It can usually be stopped abruptly but should be tailed off if asthma control is poor.

- Regular oral steroids (at the lowest possible dose) are only indicated in the most severe asthmatic patients who cannot be controlled with high-dose inhaled steroids and additional bronchodilators. The inhaled steroid is continued to allow the smallest dose of oral steroid to be given.
- The oral steroid should be given once daily in the morning as this upsets the body's own rhythm of secretion less.
- Enteric-coated tablets cause less GI disturbance.

Parenteral steroids

Hydrocortisone is sometimes given intravenously in a severe asthma attack.

Chromates

Sodium cromoglicate (Intal), nedocromil sodium (Tilade)

The mode of action of these drugs is not totally understood but they stabilize the mast cell and prevent the release of histamine.

- Little used now but are alternatives if steroids cannot be used. They need to be given regularly and do reduce both immediate and late-phase asthmatic responses, reducing bronchial hyper-responsiveness in some cases of allergic asthma.
- Of benefit in some adults but more effective in children aged 5−12 years. Not easy to predict who will benefit from their use. They can be given for 4−6 weeks and the response assessed.
- They are not of benefit in an acute asthma attack but can sometimes prevent exercise-induced asthma.
- Very poorly absorbed orally and given by pressurized aerosol or rotahaler.
- The usual dose is three to four inhalations daily.
- Bitter taste: now available in menthol aerosols to mask the taste.
- Burning sensation due to activation of thermoreceptors.

Leukotriene receptor antagonists

Montelukast (Singulair)

The cysteinyl leukotrienes LTC_4, LTD_4 and LTE_4 are important chemical mediators in asthma. They are released by eosinophils, basophils and mast cells. Activation of leukotriene receptors results in contraction and proliferation of smooth muscle, oedema, eosinophil migration and damage to the mucous layer in the lung. Leukotriene receptor antagonists block the receptor for leukotrienes and were first manufactured in the 1990s.

- They are taken regularly, not as needed, to prevent asthma attacks, and are not for use in acute asthma attacks.

- These drugs were expected to revolutionize the treatment of asthma but have not been shown to be more effective than a steroid inhaler, although the two drugs together do appear to have an additive effect.
- They successfully treat some asthmatics, especially asthma — which is aspirin sensitive — and exercise-induced asthma, but not so effective in those with severe asthma who are already on high doses of other drugs.
- Trial of therapy (4 weeks) should be given and objective improvement documented before continuing as regular therapy.
- May be used alone or with an inhaled steroid. The two drugs appear to have an additive effect.
- These drugs are available as tablets and rapidly absorbed after oral administration; they may improve compliance with long-term therapy. Peak plasma concentration after swallowing a tablet is at 3 hours and at 2 hours for the chewable paediatric form of montelukast.
- Taking with food reduces bioavailability by about 40% in 75% of people.

Side effects
- Include GI symptoms and headaches.
- Some have developed abnormalities in liver function; they need to be checked regularly.
- Treatment does not allow a reduction in existing corticosteroid treatment.

Monoclonal antibodies
Mepolizumab

This is a monoclonal antibody that reduces the production and survival of eosinophils. It is licensed as an add-on in those with severe refractory eosinophilic asthma, under specialist care. The blood eosinophil count has to be 300 cells/μL or more during the past 12 months and the patient should have had at least four acute asthma exacerbations needing systemic steroids within the past 12 months (https://www.nice.org.uk/guidance/ta431).

Omalizumab

This is a monoclonal antibody that binds to free IgE in the blood and on the surface of B-lymphocytes. It does not bind to IgE that is already bound to the IgE receptor on mast cells and antigen presenting cells.

It is used in the prophylaxis of severe, persistent, allergic asthma and is given by subcutaneous injection.

Hypersensitivity reactions and anaphylaxis occur in approximately 1–2 patients per 1000 and it may be more than 24 hours after the first injection that the reaction occurs.

The National Institute for Health and Care Excellence (NICE) guidance is available for this drug (https://www.nice.org.uk/guidance/ta278).

Reslizumab

This is a humanized monoclonal antibody that interferes with the interleukin-5 receptor binding and therefore reduces the survival and activity of eosinophils. It is prescribed only by specialists when high-dose steroids with another treatment are not effective. Again, NICE guidance is available (https://www. nice.org.uk/guidance/ta479).

Inhalers and nebulizers

Inhalation is the preferred route for drugs aimed at the respiratory tract. The drug is administered directly to the bronchioles; therefore smaller doses are required. Compared with oral administration there should be more rapid relief with fewer side effects.

In asthma, patients usually have two types of inhaler, a reliever such as salbutamol and a corticosteroid preventer. Sometimes a steroid and a long-acting beta-2 agonist are combined in one inhaler.

- Asthma UK have a UK helpline on 0300 222 5800 where patients can get advice on their inhaler from an expert asthma nurse. Their website is also very useful at https://www.asthma.org.uk/advice/inhalers-medicines-treatments/.

Inhalation devices

Inhalation devices include pressurized MDIs, breath-actuated inhalers (BAIs) and DPIs. Greater Glasgow and Clyde NHS have produced a useful inhaler identification chart that can be found at: http://www.ggcprescribing.org.uk/ media/uploads/prescribing_resources/inhaler_id_chart_-_1701.pdf

- The choice of device is vitally important as incorrect use leads to suboptimal treatment.
- The choice is dependent upon several different factors including the severity of the disease, the patient's age, co-ordination of movement and manual dexterity.
- Patient preference is also important.
- Many can be taught to use pressurized MDIs but there are groups such as the very young and the elderly who find this difficult.
- Spacer devices help here as there is no need to co-ordinate actuation with inhalation. Spacers are effective even in children under 5 years.
- Alternatives are BAIs or DPIs. BAIs are activated by the patient's inhalation and eliminate the need for correct co-ordination. They may cause coughing and are less suitable in children.
- There is an optimum peak inspiratory flow for any inhaler device. The MDI uses a propellant, and to get the best lung deposition, inhalation should be slow. In comparison, DPIs work better when inhalation is faster.

Metered dose inhalers

- Most commonly used type of inhaler.
- Suspension of the active drug with particle size of 2–5 μm, in a liquefied propellant.
- The inhaler releases the drug in a droplet size of 35–45 μm. The propellant (responsible for the increased particle size) evaporates on expulsion from the inhaler.
- Older inhalers were chlorofluorocarbon propellants and damaged the ozone layer. These have changed to hydrofluoroalkanes which do not cause this damage.

Advantages

- Widely available.
- Easy to carry around.
- Multidose.

Disadvantages

- Not easy to use well; a good technique is required and patient education is vitally important. The actuation of the inhaler must be co-ordinated with the beginning of inspiration. The inhaler should only be prescribed after tuition and the patient demonstrating a satisfactory technique.
- Only deliver about 10% of the drug to the lungs and deposit about 80% in the nasopharynx.
- They irritate the back of the throat and this may inhibit the continuation of inspiration.
- Studies do show that personal tuition improves technique. This is time-consuming and may be complemented by video material and instructions available on the asthma UK website (see above).

Using metered dose inhalers Box 6.1 shows a stepwise checklist for patients using an MDI.

Spacers

A spacer is a large plastic or metal container, with a mouthpiece at one end and a hole for the aerosol MDI at the other. The drug is administered by repeated single actuations of the MDI into the spacer, each followed by inhalation, which should occur as soon as possible after actuation.

Large-volume spacers (750 mL) with a one-way valve are more efficient than smaller spacers and have been shown to provide better bronchodilation. They have been used instead of a nebulizer in acute severe asthma attacks. The spacer prescribed needs to be compatible with the MDI used.

BOX 6.1 Patients can be given a stepwise checklist for using a metered dose inhaler

- Remove inhaler cap and check mouthpiece is clean
- Shake inhaler well
- Hold inhaler upright with thumb on base, below mouthpiece
- Gently breathe out
- Place inhaler in mouth and grip gently between the teeth. Ensure tongue is underneath inhaler then seal lips around mouthpiece
- Start inhaling – slowly and deeply – then press the canister to release aerosol. Keep inhaling until the lungs are full
- Hold breath and count to 10 (or as long as comfortable)
- Breathe normally
- If another dose is required, wait 30 s before repeating

Advantages

- Allow greater evaporation of the propellant and thus reduce particle size. They also reduce the velocity of the aerosol.
- Decrease deposition in the throat and back of the mouth (reduces the incidence of thrush with steroid inhalers).
- Useful if co-ordination is poor.
- Compliance is better, especially in children.

Disadvantage

- Larger to carry around.

Spacers need to be washed monthly in mild detergent. More frequent washing reduces the coating that prevents electrostatic charge. This affects drug delivery.

Nebulizers

Nebulizers convert a solution of the drug into an aerosol for inhalation. They do this by blowing air or oxygen through the solution. Higher doses of the drug are easily administered by this route and nebulizers are often used in the acute setting. They have decreased the need for drugs to be given intravenously in severe asthma.

The percentage of the solution reaching the lungs may still be as low as 10% with the rest remaining in the nebulizer, tubing or mouthpiece, but because much higher doses are given the patient receives many times more drug than through an MDI.

Many drugs are available for nebulization including salbutamol and ipratropium.

Peak flow meters and self-management plans in asthma:

- All patients with asthma should have an individual self-management plan made by the doctor or nurse in conjunction with themselves. As the patient is more involved in the care of their asthma, they gain in both knowledge and confidence. The plan is reviewed at least annually in adults and 6-monthly in children.

- The patients are allowed to change their medication within set limits, to gain better control of their asthma. Peak flow monitoring is an important part of this process and a peak flow diary is encouraged. These readings enable patients to detect deterioration in their asthma very early, as there will be a fall in peak flow rate. Clear guidance is given as to what the patient should do if their peak flow falls.

Nonpharmacological management

This is a book on drugs, so we have concentrated on medicine management. However, there are other factors important in the management of asthma and these include allergen avoidance, measures to control levels of dust in the home surroundings (removal of carpets and soft toys, etc.), and if allergic to animals, not to have these in the house. Parents should not smoke and should be offered support to stop smoking if necessary.

Dietary manipulation may have a role in some cases as may weight loss if obese.

Chronic obstructive pulmonary disease

This is the term used to describe chronic airflow obstruction that is not fully reversible by bronchodilators and is commonly due to:

- Chronic bronchitis: a productive cough for most days of 3 consecutive months for more than 1 year and characterized by excessive mucous production.
- Emphysema: permanent enlargement of the air sacs within lung tissue and destruction of pulmonary tissue loss leading to continued increase loss of elastic recoil.

Cigarette smoking predominantly causes COPD in this country, although other factors — particularly some occupational exposures and pollution — may contribute to its development. An estimated 3 million people have COPD in the UK, 2 million of whom are undiagnosed (NICE, 2018c). Most people are diagnosed in their 50s.

Obstruction is the result of chronic inflammation within the respiratory tract and develops slowly and progressively over a period of many years, but rarely before middle age.

- There is a morning cough, and little sputum may be present; breathing difficulties do not change markedly over many months; and the person may not be aware of any problem until there is significant airflow obstruction and a wheeze present.

- Eventually symptoms, such as breathlessness on exertion with gradual increase in dyspnea at rest and use of accessory muscles of respiration occur, leading to extreme anxiety during very breathless periods, disability and reduced quality of life.
- The disease is preventable but once developed there is no cure, and symptoms can be reduced only with the use of medication.
- Forced expiratory volume in 1 second (FEV_1) is used as a measure of airway obstruction. In obstruction, there is a reduced FEV_1/forced vital capacity (FVC) ratio. Normally with a forced expiration, about 80% of the total air expelled from the lungs is expelled in the first second of forced expiration (giving a ratio for FEV_1/FVC of >0.8). In airway obstruction FEV_1/FVC is < 0.7.
- Changes occur to acid base balance to maintain body pH:
  - Respiratory acidosis ($PCO_2 > 5.7$ kPa; pH < 7.4).
  - Metabolic alkalosis ($HCO_3^- > 26$ mmol/L; pH > 7.4).

The Medical Research Council Dyspnoea Scale (shown in Table 6.1) is used to measure breathlessness. Questions were originally devised from data collected from Welsh miners with pneumoconiosis and became the Dyspnoea Scale in 1959 (Williams, 2017). The latest version was published in 1986 and is recommended by NICE in their latest guidelines as an aid to diagnosis.

NICE produced detailed guidelines for the treatment and management of COPD in 2019. These are available on the website (www.nice.org.uk). The importance of encouraging the patient to stop smoking is emphasized and is put forward as one of the most important components of management.

Reviews of those with COPD should be at least annually and twice a year if the disease is severe.

TABLE 6.1 Grades of breathlessness using the MRC Dyspnoea Scale.

Grade	Degree of breathlessness related to activities
1	Not troubled by breathlessness, except on strenuous exercise
2	Short of breath when hurrying or walking up a slight hill
3	Walks slower than most people on level ground because of breathlessness or has to stop for breath after a mile or so or after 15 minutes, when walking at own pace
4	Stops for breath after walking about 100 yards or after a few minutes on level ground
5	Too breathless to leave the house or breathless when undressing

Used with permission of the Medical Research Council (https://mrc.ukri.org/research/facilities-and-resources-for-researchers/mrc-scales/mrc-dyspnoea-scale-mrc-breathlessness-scale/).

The main principles of treatment are as follows:

- Bronchodilators are used to control symptoms and also to increase exercise capacity. Short-acting β_2 agonists (*salbutamol*) or antimuscarinics (*ipratropium*) are used as needed for the initial treatment.
- If the patient is still symptomatic, a long-acting bronchodilator — either a β_2 agonist or antimuscarinic — is added.
- Combination therapy in the form of a long-acting antimuscarinic, a long-acting β_2 agonist and sometimes an ICS may be used. There are specific guidelines issued by NICE as to which categories of patient should be offered these drug combinations.
- If an ICS is added, the patient should be reassessed after 3 months and the steroid discontinued if symptoms have not improved.
- Theophylline is considered next if the patient is still symptomatic by mouth but is of uncertain benefit.
- Mucolytic drugs may be given for those with a chronic cough and sputum production. They should be discontinued if they do not improve symptoms.
- Sometimes long-term prophylactic antibiotics are needed and guidelines are given by NICE (2018c). Azithromycin is the antibiotic recommended by NICE, but sputum should be collected for organisms and sensitivity before the antibiotic is started.
- Long-term oxygen therapy (LTOT) at home may prolong life in patients with severe progression of the disease and hypoxaemia. There are guidelines given by NICE as inappropriate oxygen therapy may cause respiratory depression in COPD.

Compound bronchodilator preparations of salbutamol and ipratropium are available. Flexibility is lost, but for patients on stable doses, compound inhalers may be useful.

It is important in patients with COPD to prevent exacerbations. Annual influenza vaccination and pneumococcal vaccination should be encouraged, and antibiotics may be needed to treat chest infections. If there is a chronic productive cough, a trial of mucolytic therapy should be instigated.

Pulmonary hypertension and cor pulmonale (right-sided heart failure, secondary to lung disease) may occur in chronic COPD. There is salt and water retention with peripheral oedema, and this is treated with diuretics. Optimal COPD treatment should be given.

Although not within the scope of his book, pulmonary rehabilitation involving a multidisciplinary programme of care is a vital part of the treatment regimen.

Oxygen in respiratory disorders

Oxygen is useful when there is hypoxia. This is likely to occur in asthma, COPD, pneumonia, pulmonary oedema, pneumothorax and pulmonary embolism.

In the air, oxygen is present at a concentration of approximately 21%. It can be added to inspired air to produce concentrations ranging from 24% to 60%–80% depending on mask and flow of oxygen available. Oxygen levels in the blood are best measured by an arterial blood gas measurement (PO_2); however, measuring the concentration needed does not only depend on the degree of hypoxia, but also on the level of carbon dioxide in the blood. Arterial blood gas analysis includes the measures of:

- pH 7.35–7.45
- Carbon dioxide (PCO_2) 4.6–5.6 kPa (35–42 mmHg)
- Oxygen (PO_2) 12–14.6 kPa (90–110 mmHg)
- Bicarbonate (HCO_3^-) 22–26 mmol/L
- Base excess 0
- Oxygen saturation 94%–98%.

A combination of these measurements can determine a patient's metabolic and respiratory status:

- Metabolic acidosis HCO_3^- < 22 mmol/L; pH < 7.4
- Metabolic alkalosis HCO_3^- > 26 mmol/L; pH > 7.4
- Respiratory acidosis PCO_2 > 5.7 kPa; pH < 7.4
- Respiratory alkalosis PCO_2 < 5.7 kPa; pH > 7.4.

Other methods:

- The haemoglobin saturation with oxygen using a pulse oximeter is an alternative that is not invasive and frequently used.
- End tidal carbon dioxide ($ETCO_2$) monitoring is also noninvasive and monitors exhaled carbon dioxide. The normal range is 4.5–5.7 kPa, which reasonable reflects partial pressure of arterial CO_2. In the presence of airway narrowing or other lung disease associated with respiratory changes there is:
    - a decrease in $ETCO_2$ early in the condition (respiratory alkalosis) associated with type I respiratory failure
    - an increase in $ETCO_2$ as the disease progresses (respiratory acidosis) associated with type II respiratory failure.

At a normal P_AO_2 haemoglobin is about 95% saturated with oxygen. This falls to 90% when the P_AO_2 falls to 8 kPa. Below this level cerebral hypoxia occurs.

Concentrations of oxygen required

- High concentrations of oxygen:
  - These are usually not required and can be unsafe if PO_2, oxygen saturation or $ETCO_2$ are within normal limits, but combining these measures with other patient parameters (e.g. blood pressure, heart rate, temperature, respiratory rate, level of consciousness) is necessary to determine patients' overall condition before a decision regarding oxygen administration is made.
  - In type I respiratory failure when there is hypoxia with normal or low carbon dioxide levels, such as occurs in acute asthma, pulmonary oedema (left ventricular failure) or pulmonary embolus, oxygen should be given.
  - If type I respiratory failure progresses to type II respiratory failure (e.g. worsens [hypoxia with high levels of carbon dioxide; with the exception of COPD]) high concentrations of oxygen can continue to be given but usually this type of deterioration requires additional respiratory support such as noninvasive ventilation or intermittent positive pressure ventilation.
- Low concentrations of oxygen:
  - Chronic high levels of carbon dioxide occur in COPD. This is type II respiratory failure with hypoxia and a raised carbon dioxide level.
  - In COPD a carbon dioxide level above 6.6 kPa would make it dangerous to give high concentrations of oxygen (see below).

Oxygen therapy is a topic that has been long debated, and there is a lack of randomized controlled trials on which to base treatment. The reader is directed to the current NICE guidelines (2019f) for full current recommendations. Only a brief summary of the potential problems is given here.

Background to the debate

The respiratory centre in the brain stem controls our respiratory rate and depth, and responds to the concentration of hydrogen ions and the partial pressure of carbon dioxide in body fluids. If the body increases its production of carbon dioxide, this increases the production of carbonic acid, which dissociates to form hydrogen ions resulting in a fall in pH (increased acidity) of the cerebrospinal fluid. This is detected by the central chemoreceptors in the respiratory centre. The rate and depth of respiration is increased to get rid of excess carbon dioxide via the lungs and thus reduce carbonic acid and return the blood pH to normal.

In respiratory disease, when breathing is affected, there is difficulty in expiration and in eliminating carbon dioxide. This may cause respiratory acidosis (increased acidity of the blood due to respiratory problems) as the number of hydrogen ions in the blood increases (and hence acidity increases). The hydrogen ions cannot be eliminated adequately as excess carbon dioxide cannot be removed by increased rate and depth of breathing.

Low oxygen levels in the blood do not affect the central chemoreceptors but are picked up by peripheral chemoreceptors in the aortic arch and carotid sinuses. The oxygen level is very low before these are triggered. The response is to increase rate and depth of respiration.

- In a small proportion of patients with COPD, gradual adaptation to high concentrations of carbon dioxide has occurred and they are more reliant on low oxygen levels to stimulate breathing.
- The administration of high concentrations of oxygen to these patients may cause a rise in carbon dioxide levels and increased acidosis by decreasing respiratory drive. It is not easy to predict which patients will be affected.
- Uncontrolled oxygen in these patients can result in reduced respirations, carbon dioxide necrosis and ultimately respiratory arrest.
- Worsening breathlessness in an exacerbation of COPD may be associated with severe hypoxia and oxygen is commonly used, especially in pre-hospital care, to relieve symptoms and raise the levels of oxygen in the blood. As can be seen, this may be dangerous in those with raised carbon dioxide levels (hypercapnia).

NICE recommendations for oxygen use in COPD

- In hospital, arterial blood gases should be measured.
- Oxygen saturation should be measured if there are no facilities to measure arterial blood gases.
- It must be remembered that pulse oximetry gives no information about carbon dioxide levels or pH.
- Oxygen should be given to maintain oxygen saturation above 90%.
- Patients with pH < 7.35 should be considered for ventilatory support.

Transfer to hospital by the emergency services

- An oxygen saturation > 93% is not desirable.
- Oxygen therapy should be started at 40% and titrated upwards if the saturation falls below 90% and downwards if the patient becomes drowsy or saturation is above 93%.
- Extra caution should be applied to patients with known type II respiratory failure.

The aim of supplemental oxygen therapy in exacerbations of COPD is to maintain oxygen saturation above 90% without precipitating respiratory acidosis or worsening hypercapnia.

NICE also recommends that long term oxygen therapy (LTOT) is beneficial in some patients with a low partial pressure of oxygen in arterial blood (<7.3 kPa when stable). The patient breathes low flow supplemental oxygen for at least 15 hours a day.

Ambulatory oxygen therapy should not be offered to manage breathlessness in those with COPD who have mild or no hypoxaemia, but it should be offered if exercise desaturation occurs and there is an improvement in exercise capacity with oxygen (NICE, 2018c).

Short-burst oxygen therapy should only be considered if other treatments in an episode of severe breathlessness do not work (NICE, 2019f).

Other areas where the administration of prescribed oxygen is important

The emergency administration of oxygen is required to increase the content in the air when a patient is suffering from hypoxia. Hypoxia is oxygen deficiency in the body cells and may be caused by:

- Deficient oxygenation of the blood: due to respiratory disease or chest injuries.
- Inadequate transport of oxygen by haemoglobin: as in anaemia or haemorrhage.
- Circulatory inadequacy: as in heart disease or emergency situations (e.g. cardiac arrest).
- Inability of cells to use oxygen: rare, an example is cyanide or carbon monoxide poisoning.

Oxygen therapy is a specific medical treatment and is given as prescribed by medical staff who will write the percentage of oxygen and the method of administration on the prescription sheet. The concentration given depends upon the condition being treated (BTS, 2018):

1. Critical illness requiring high levels of supplemental oxygen; a reservoir mask at 15 L/min it should quickly become possible to reduce the oxygen dose while maintaining oxygen saturation between 94% and 98%.
2. Serious illness requiring moderate levels of supplemental oxygen if the patient is hypoxaemic with a target range of 94%−98%:
   - Nasal cannulae 2−6 L/min
   - Simple face mask 5−10 L/min.
3. Conditions for which patients should be monitored closely but oxygen therapy is not required unless the patient becomes hypoxaemic as in a serious illness with a target oxygen saturation range of 94%−98%.
4. COPD and other conditions requiring controlled or low-dose oxygen therapy aiming for oxygen saturation of 88%−92%:
   - Use a Venturi mask at 2−3 L/min
   - 28% Venturi mask at 4 L/min
   - Nasal cannulae at 1−2 L/min.

Oxygen concentration

An inappropriate concentration of oxygen may have lethal effects.

- Low concentrations of oxygen (24%–28%) are used to treat patients with chronic obstructive airways disease (COPD). A higher concentration in these patients may lead to a respiratory arrest as their respiratory centre is being stimulated by the low oxygen concentration in the blood.
- High concentrations of oxygen are prescribed in severe asthma attacks and in pneumonia, but may also be seen in shock or haemorrhage. If high concentrations of oxygen are used, some form of humidification will be needed or the oxygen will have a very drying effect on the mucosa. If the patient's own airways have been bypassed, as when oxygen is given via an endotracheal tube, humidification is essential.
- Oxygen toxicity may follow prolonged periods (over 24 hours) of administration of high (over 50%) concentrations of oxygen. The end result of this may be pulmonary fibrosis. Thus, oxygen should be reduced/stopped as soon as there is indication from the patient's observations, oxygen saturation and arterial blood gases that they are stable.

There are some clinical studies that provide evidence showing conflicting data on the effects of oxygen treatment and calling for the potential harmful effects of oxygen to be considered (Shuvy et al. 2013).

Oxygen is an inflammable gas and great care must always be taken because of this.

6.2 RENAL SYSTEM

The kidney has a prime role in maintaining normal healthy life. It maintains many of the body's major homeostatic functions:

- Regulates:
  - Body fluid volume
  - The composition of urine
  - Electrolyte balance such as calcium, sodium and potassium.
- Maintains acid base balance by regulating H^+ concentration of body fluids. Acid or alkaline urine is excreted according to the body's needs.
- Excretion of waste products from body metabolism such as urea and creatinine.

- Secretion of hormones that regulate:
  - Red blood cells (RBCs) production − erythropoietin
  - Renin that maintains blood pressure and glomerular filtration rate (GFR)
  - Prostaglandins used in the inflammatory immune response and to enhance GFR.
- Metabolism of vitamin D.

Many early changes that occur in the body may be reflected in the urine well before they become clinically obvious. Three processes are involved in the production of urine:

- Glomerular filtration (GF), which takes place in the glomerulus, determined by the net filtration pressure and the GFR (regulated by the renin-angiotensin-aldosterone mechanism and the stress response).
- Tubular re-absorption occurs as most of the contents of GF are quickly reclaimed and returned to the blood; water and many other ions are continuously regulated in response to hormonal signals.
- Tubular secretion is re-absorption in reverse, as contents that require excretion are filtered from blood into the renal tubules such as some drugs (penicillin and phenobarbital), undesirable substances (urea and uric acid), potassium ions and excessive acids to maintain acid base balance.

The kidney filters about 100 L of fluid per day. Most of this is reabsorbed in the renal tubules leaving only the amount needed to maintain fluid balance within the body; the rest is lost as urine. This means that a very small percentage decrease in reabsorption can lead to a marked increase in excretion. A 1% decrease in water reabsorption will result in a doubling of urine output.

Diuretics

Diuretics are drugs that increase the production of urine by the kidneys. They produce their effect by decreasing the reabsorption of water and electrolytes (mainly Na^+) in the renal tubules. Diuretics decrease the reabsorption of Na^+ and an accompanying anion (usually Cl^-) from the filtrate; water loss follows as a result of the increased excretion of NaCl (natriuresis). This can be achieved:

- by direct action on the cells of the nephron
- indirectly, by modifying the content of the filtrate.

Their main uses are in heart failure and in lower doses to control hypertension.

Diuretics reduce salt and water retention and are used to treat oedema in:

- pulmonary oedema, left ventricular failure and heart failure
- nephrotic syndrome
- chronic renal insufficiency
- cirrhosis of the liver.

Causes of sodium and water retention

- A low cardiac output as in heart failure results in underfilling of the arterial system, which causes the kidney to excrete less sodium and water.
- Raised pressure in the veins and capillaries leads to fluid movement from the blood to the tissue spaces.
- Low levels of protein in the plasma, as in the nephrotic syndrome due to protein loss, and cirrhosis of the liver due to a failure to make sufficient proteins.
- Increased secretion of aldosterone by the adrenal glands causes sodium and water retention.
- Excessive activity of the SNS and thus the renin-angiotensin-aldosterone system as in chronic heart failure (CHF).

The action of diuretics on the renal tubule is shown in Fig. 6.2. Diuretics may be classed as:

- osmotic diuretics
- thiazide diuretics
- loop diuretics
- potassium-sparing diuretics.

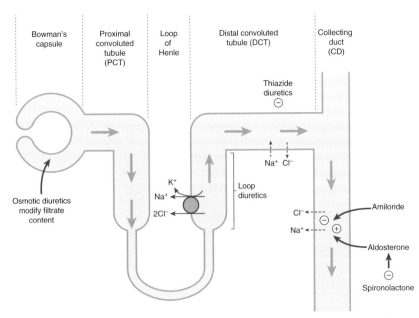

FIG. 6.2 **Action of diuretics on the kidney tubule.** Loop diuretics inhibit the $Na^+/K^+/2Cl^-$ cotransporter in the ascending limb of the loop of Henle. Thiazides inhibit Na^+/Cl^- transport in the distal convoluted tubule. Amiloride inhibits Na^+/Cl^- transport in the collecting duct. Spironolactone inhibits the action (sodium and water retention) of aldosterone.

Osmotic diuretics

These are substances that filter through the glomeruli but are not reabsorbed in the renal tubules. This increases the osmotic pressure of the filtrate and causes more water to be excreted. They are not used in heart failure where the reverse can happen and they can expand the blood volume thus putting more strain on the heart.

They can be used to reduce cerebral oedema and reduce raised intracranial pressure as in head injury or cerebral tumour. Long term use is not recommended in head injury; as dehydration occurs the osmotic pressure increases in the blood and cerebral oedema can be made worse. They may be used in cardiac surgery to maintain urinary function and in glaucoma to reduce intraocular pressure prior to surgery.

Mannitol is an example, which is given intravenously as a 10% or 20% solution.

Thiazides and related diuretics

Bendroflumethiazide, hydrochlorothiazide, metolazone, chlortalidone, xipamide. This group of diuretics act on the distal tubule where they inhibit the sodium-chloride symporter and prevent sodium and chloride − and therefore water − leaving the tubule to re-enter the cells. They are used to relieve modest oedema due to CHF and, in lower doses, to reduce blood pressure. They may be used in combination with loop diuretics in severe heart failure. They are less powerful than loop diuretics, but are better tolerated. Together with the vasodilator effect, this group of drugs is preferred in the treatment of uncomplicated hypertension. In small doses they are unlikely to cause dehydration or electrolyte imbalance.

Mechanism of action

- Act on the cortical segment of the nephron and decrease sodium reabsorption in the distal tubule by inhibiting action of Na^+/Cl^- cotransporter pump. Do not have any action on the loop of Henle.
- Moderate diuresis produced leading to the excretion of a maximum of 5%−10% of filtered sodium since over 90% is reabsorbed before reaching the distal tubule.

Pharmacokinetics

Absorbed well from the intestine so can be given orally.

Action begins in 1−2 hours, most peak at about 4 hours and last 12−24 hours. *Bendroflumethiazide* lasts up to 24 hours. This means the drugs only need to be taken once daily.

Chlortalidone, a thiazide-related diuretic, has a longer duration of action, so it can be taken on alternate days for oedema.

Uses of thiazide diuretics

- Cardiac failure: once daily. In mild cardiac failure these drugs are less fierce than loop diuretics and so may be better tolerated by the patient. They are less likely to increase incontinence or lead to retention of urine in the patient with an enlarged prostate. In hypokalaemia they may precipitate arrhythmias.
- Hypertension — no longer used as first line therapy but when prescribed, a small dose of *bendroflumethiazide* 1.25—2.5 mg is given daily. This small dose is not likely to cause problems with hypokalaemia. The response in hypertension is not dose dependent and increasing the dose will not further reduce blood pressure. Higher does may cause changes in plasma potassium, sodium, uric acid, glucose and lipids with very little further effect on lowering blood pressure. The full antihypertensive action may take up to 6 weeks to achieve.
- Cirrhosis with ascites. Use with caution, as may cause mental changes due to K^+ loss. Potassium is already low due to increased aldosterone levels.
- Prevention of renal stones in hypercalciuria.
- Nephrotic syndrome but often needs more powerful diuretic.

Adverse effects

Thiazides are usually well tolerated, especially in low doses.

Hypokalaemia may occur with higher doses or following change in diet or bout of diarrhoea.

- This is less of a problem when combined with an angiotensin converting enzyme (ACE) inhibitor or angiotensin receptor blocker (ARB).
- Induced hypokalaemia may cause ventricular arrhythmias and contribute to torsade de pointes and sudden death. This is only usually important with high doses.
  - Hypomagnesaemia may occur and could contribute to arrhythmias.
  - Hypercalcaemia may lead to a decreased risk of hip fractures in the elderly.
  - Hyponatraemia can be potentially serious, especially in the elderly.
  - May provoke diabetes especially if combined with a beta blocker.
  - Increase total blood cholesterol. May increase low-density lipoprotein and lower high-density lipoprotein. The cholesterol may return to baseline levels within a year and the increase in lipids is greater with higher doses.
  - Decrease uric acid excretion. This may lead to gout especially if there is a family history.
  - Impotence found in several trials. Even on low doses the rate of impotence is twice that found in most antihypertensive treatments.

Thiazide-like diuretics

Metolazone differs from other thiazides in that it is a powerful diuretic that will sometimes produce a diuresis when others fail. It is particularly effective when combined with a loop diuretic even in renal failure. The patient should be monitored as a profound diuresis may occur.

Chlortalidone has a longer duration than thiazides and may be given on alternate days to control oedema and may be useful if acute retention is likely to be caused by a sudden diuresis.

Indapamide is related to *chlortalidone* and used in hypertension. It claims to reduce blood pressure with less metabolic disturbance, especially in diabetes. Vasodilates and has some class I and class III antiarrhythmic effects (see Sections 5.2 and 5.5).

Loop diuretics

Furosemide, bumetanide, torasemide

These are the most powerful of all diuretics and are capable of causing 15%−25% of filtered sodium in the filtrate to be excreted. They are called high-ceiling diuretics because, as the dose is increased, the diuresis increases. The main example is *furosemide*, which is the one most commonly used. *Bumetanide* and *torasemide* are alternatives with similar action.

Mechanism of action

- Act on the thick part of the ascending loop of Henle and inhibit the transport of sodium out of the loop of Henle.
- Inhibit the $Na^+/K^+/2Cl^-$ cotransporter concerned with the transportation of chloride across the lining cells of the ascending limb of the loop of Henle.
- Increased excretion of potassium occurs and also some magnesium and calcium are lost.
- Hydrogen ions are also lost − possibility of alkalosis.
- Compared with thiazides there is relatively less sodium and potassium loss for the volume of water loss. Hypokalaemia is still a danger.
- There is an increase in renal blood flow and also in venous capacitance that leads to a reduced left atrial pressure.
- Venodilation reduces the preload in acute left ventricular failure within 5−15 minutes; this mechanism is not well understood. Active vasoconstriction may follow.

Uses of loop diuretics

- Acute pulmonary oedema due to left ventricular failure. Relieves breathlessness and preload faster than would be expected due to their diuretic effect.
- Oedema due to CHF. May be combined with a thiazide in resistant oedema.

- Oliguria in renal failure if unresponsive to less powerful diuretics.
- Nephrotic syndrome.
- Cirrhosis of the liver complicated by ascites.
- Occasionally to reduce blood pressure.

Pharmacokinetics

- Intravenously act almost immediately: within 5—10 minutes. The diuresis is over within 2 hours.
- Orally act within an hour, peak in 1.5 hours and duration of action is 4—6 hours.
- Can be given twice a day and still not interfere with sleep.
- Plasma half-life is 1.5 hours for *furosemide*.

Adverse effects

- Loss of potassium may lead to hypokalaemia. Avoided by the addition of a potassium-sparing diuretic.
- Diuretic-induced hypokalaemia can contribute to torsade de pointes and hence to sudden death. Low levels of magnesium may contribute to this.
- Loss of hydrogen ions may lead to metabolic alkalosis.
- Hypovolaemia and hypotension may follow the 'torrential diuresis' that can occur.
- In heart failure, *digitalis* toxicity may be precipitated by over diuresis and hypokalaemia.
- Ototoxicity leading to deafness rarely occurs. It is dose dependent thus intravenous furosemide should be given at no more than 4 mg/min in an infusion to reduce this.
- The large diuresis may lead to retention of urine if there is an enlarged prostate.
- Rarely skin rashes.

Box 6.2 shows some differences between thiazides and loop diuretics.

BOX 6.2 Some differences between thiazides and loop diuretics

Loop diuretics:
- have a shorter duration of action
- have a different site of action
- are high-ceiling diuretics: response increases with dose. At least 2.5 times more potent than thiazides
- have increased capacity to work in renal failure

Potassium supplements combined with loop diuretics

Low levels of potassium with high doses of diuretics should be avoided but most patients taking diuretics do not need potassium supplements and patients on permanent diuretic therapy are in more danger. Potassium-sparing diuretics are used in combination with stronger diuretics to conserve potassium and are the recommended solution where possible. This is because the use of potassium supplements may lead to a dangerous hyperkalaemia.

Potassium-sparing diuretics

These are weak diuretics and their main use is alongside thiazides or loop diuretics to prevent excessive potassium loss. The main drugs in this group are *amiloride* and *triamterene*.

Mechanism of action

- Work on the distal tubule and the collecting ducts and inhibit sodium reabsorption and potassium excretion.
- Cause excretion of about 5% of the sodium in the filtrate.
- Main importance is their potassium-sparing ability.

Potassium supplements must NOT be given alongside potassium-sparing diuretics! Potassium-sparing diuretics administered alongside ACE inhibitors or ARBs may result in severe hyperkalaemia.

Aldosterone antagonists

Spironolactone, eplerenone

This group of drugs are potassium-sparing diuretics but up to 5% of sodium can be excreted. They potentiate the action of loop or thiazide diuretics by antagonizing aldosterone with a resultant reduction in the sodium retained and the potassium lost. The onset of action is slow and takes several days to develop. If given without other diuretics, hyperkalaemia can result.

Uses

- Congestive cardiac failure: increasingly used for its aldosterone-blocking ability (see Section 5.6). Reduces the damage caused by aldosterone release.
- Hepatic cirrhosis and other forms of hyperaldosteronism.
- Nephrotic syndrome.

ACE inhibitors and ARBs also inhibit aldosterone and so are weak potassium-sparing diuretics.

Carbonic anhydrase inhibitors

These drugs act as a diuretic by preventing the reabsorption of bicarbonate.

Acetazolamide (*Diamox*) is weak and not recommended as a diuretic, but is still useful for its effect in suppressing carbonic anhydrase in the eye. Reduces the formation of aqueous humour and its main use now is in glaucoma. It is not strong enough to be used for its diuretic action alone. It is also used as prophylaxis for mountain sickness (unlicensed indication) but should not be used as a substitute for acclimatization (BNF, 2019).

Combination diuretics

Fixed combination tablets are most useful when compliance is a problem. This is especially the case if the patient is elderly and taking many different medications. Various combinations of potassium-sparing and other diuretics are available.

Diuretics should be administered early in the day so that diuresis does not interfere with sleep.

Urine output

When a patient is receiving diuretics, urine output is significant and may need to be measured in the early days following prescription to ensure the desired action is being achieved. Urination generally occurs when about 200 mL of urine has collected in the bladder, activating stretch receptors. Monitoring is necessary when the minimum urine output is equal to or less than 30 mL/h, although some practitioners prefer 50–70 mL/h.

Monitoring urine output

The significance of documenting fluid intake and urine output is to:

- Determine fluid intake (intravenous [IV], oral, enteral feeding).
- Measure fluid output (urine, wound/chest drains, vomiting, diarrhoea, insensible loss).

A balance between the two can be either negative or positive over a 24-hour period and has implications for the patient's response to diuretic therapy and the potential for complications:

- Positive fluid balance can imply fluid overload, heart failure and the need for or increase of diuretic therapy or renal failure.
- Negative fluid balance can imply dehydration, hypovolaemia or bleeding.

Fluid balance is not a diagnostic tool when used alone, and other measures need to be taken into account before a diagnosis can be made. These include blood results, the presence of pulmonary or peripheral oedema (positive balance), and changes in blood pressure and heart rate (negative balance).

Fluid overload is an increase in circulating volume which can occur for many reasons:

- Circulation problems prior to admission; for example, heart failure, peripheral vascular disease leading to a primary defect in the pumping activity of the heart.
- Kidney problems (e.g. renal failure)
- Cirrhosis of the liver
- Following IV fluid replacement therapy (FRT) given after surgery or shock:
  - Too much salt and/or water overload due to crystalloid fluid
  - Too much colloid fluid increasing colloid oncotic capillary pressure
  - Blood transfusion
- Sluggish arterial and venous circulation caused by a stagnant flow of blood through the circulation due to continued bed rest or immobility.

The immediate intervention for fluid overload due to any cause is a diuretic to reduce circulating volume. Furosemide is the most effective as it is potent and quick acting; it is a nonpotassium-sparing loop diuretic that if used in high doses or long term (not recommended) requires that blood levels of potassium need to be strictly monitored.

Fluid resuscitation

The administration of prescribed fluid resuscitation is required following loss of circulating volume whether whole blood (trauma), plasma (burns), fluid loss (dehydration) or fluid movement (excessive inflammation).

Blood transfusion may be necessary when the body loss is so great that homeostatic mechanisms can no longer maintain blood pressure. The human cardiovascular system is designed to minimize the effects of blood loss. The body can compensate for only so much blood loss. Losses of 15%–30% cause pallor and weakness; a loss of more than 30% of blood volume results in severe shock and can be fatal. To treat haemorrhage, whole blood should be used as routine especially when blood loss is substantial.

Blood transfusion

A blood transfusion of whole blood is prescribed:

- to replace blood lost during an operation or after an accident
- to treat anaemia; for example, iron deficiency, vitamin B_{12} deficiency (pernicious anaemia) or folate deficiency anaemias
- for other medical conditions:
  - haemophilia: affects the bloods ability to clot
  - sickle cell anaemia, thalassaemia: disruption of the normal production of RBCs
  - leukaemia: RBCs are produced at a reduced rate
  - malaria: RBCs are destroyed
  - renal failure: reduction in the production of erythropoietin, which plays a key role in the production of RBCs.

Blood transfusions can cause serious reactions – some of which arise from the changes that occur in stored blood. Because the administration of blood and blood products is an area of nursing practice, the nurse has to be vigilant, both in checking the correct blood group and RhD antigen factor and in observing for any signs of transfusion reactions. Frequent observations will enable the nurse to detect any reaction at an early stage; these include discomfort, flushing, rash or pain.

Blood products are any therapeutic substances prepared from human blood:

- **Packed red cells** (whole blood from which most of the plasma has been removed) are generally only used to treat anaemia.
- **Fresh frozen plasma** (FFP) should never be used as a volume expander. It is better to use FFP for patients with bleeding disorders, where there is a deficiency in platelets or clotting factors; for example, in disseminated intravascular coagulation, warfarin overdose, trauma or thrombotic thrombocytopenia.
- **Preparations from human plasma**:
  - cryoprecipitate
  - coagulation factors
  - immunoglobulin
  - albumin (e.g. human albumin solution).

For a more detailed account of blood products, see Table 6.2.

Volume expanders

Volume expanders are used when it is necessary to increase the circulating fluid volume. There are two main types of volume expanders: **crystalloids** and **colloids**.

Crystalloids are solutions of water-soluble molecules such as mineral salts. They include commonly used IV fluids such as normal saline and 5% Dextrose.

Colloids contain much larger molecules that are not soluble in water and therefore maintain the osmotic pressure in the blood. Plasma itself is a colloid, and other colloids include gelatine as in gelofusine and starch as in tetrastarch.

TABLE 6.2 Current blood products.

Blood product	Constituents	Uses
Whole blood (510 1/2 45 mL)	Use is restricted to circumstances where red blood cells as well as plasma proteins are needed; i.e. where large amounts of blood are lost	Ideal in hypovolaemic shock, since it both increases oxygen carrying capacity and expands circulating volume
Packed cells (280 1/2 60 mL)	This is whole blood, but the majority of the plasma has been removed. It contains half the volume of whole blood, less sodium, potassium, albumin and citrate. Does contain some white blood cells and platelets	Ideal in chronic anaemia, sickle cell disease, thalassaemia and renal disease. It is not recommended in iron deficiency and vitamin B_{12} or folate deficiency, as these should be treated with the appropriate vitamin; e.g. iron tablets
Washed packed cells	These are packed cells with all the white blood cells, platelets and plasma removed	Indicated for patients who have a long history of transfusion reactions
Fresh frozen plasma (FFP) (200–300 mL)	This is blood product, which is nearly always frozen and contains all the coagulation factors	Used for the treatment of coagulation deficits. It is not recommended as a volume expander, except in certain neonatal conditions
Cryoprecipitate (20 1/2 5 mL)	Prepared from FFP and contains mainly clotting factors (factor VIII and fibrinogen)	Used to treat haemophilia or AIDS patients
Platelets (50 1/2 10 mL)	Produced from the residue left over from the production of plasma and leukocyte-depleted red blood cell concentrates	Indications for use are thrombocytopenia, when platelet content of blood is reduced due to bleeding or diluted following massive transfusion, in acute leukaemia, aplastic anaemia, disseminated intravascular coagulation or sepsis

Colloids

Colloids are sometimes called plasma expanders and are used in emergency states, such as trauma, shock, and burns, where the objective is to restore the circulating circulatory volume, and therefore improve or maintain oxygen transport. The result of their administration is:

- haemodynamic stability, achieved by increasing the blood volume to maintain and restore cellular function
- improved oxygen availability, oxygen consumption, circulating volume, haemodynamic status and tissue perfusion.

Colloids work as they contain large molecules. In the body this is mostly albumin which gives blood its colloidal oncotic pressure (COP). This determinant pressure in capillaries holds fluid within the circulation (see Fig. 6.3). Increasing the COP in the blood will draw fluid into the circulation from the intracellular spaces, increasing circulating volume. The problems with giving too much colloid is that these large molecules are not excreted via the renal tubules and so the effect of colloids can go on longer than the actual depletion of the circulation, giving rise to fluid overload (see above). Despite the use of diuretics in this situation, albumin and some other large molecules are still not excreted in the renal tubules leading to continued fluid overload episodes.

Table 6.3 includes a list of all colloid fluids.

Crystalloids

Crystalloids are solutions that contain small molecules and electrolytes. They will influence fluid movement and the most powerful is sodium.

- 0.9% normal saline is an isotonic solution. This will maintain sodium at a normal level, and have no effect on fluid movement. An infused solution of 0.9% normal saline will stay in the circulation and increase/maintain circulating volume and thus blood pressure.

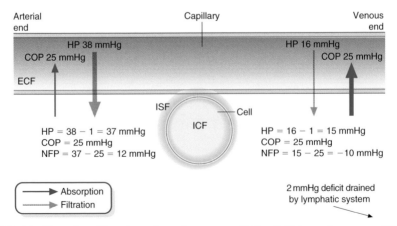

FIG. 6.3 Normal capillary dynamics and pressures. *COP*, colloidal osmotic pressure; *ECF*, extracellular fluid; *HP*, hydrostatic pressure; *ICF*, intracellular fluid; *ISF*, interstitial fluid; *NFP*, net filtration pressure.

TABLE 6.3 Colloid infusions available.

Colloid	Constituents	Uses
Human albumin solution (HAS) — manufactured from human blood plasma	20% solution 50 and 100 mL bottles osmotic pressure of 100 −200 mmHg; 4.5% solution 50 mL, 100 mL, 250 mL and 500 mL bottles osmotic pressure of 26−30 mmHg	Used in cases of hypoalbuminaemia due to renal disease, liver disease, acute pancreatitis and sepsis. Used as a plasma expander
Haemaccel	3.5% solution of gelatine, more stable and has a longer shelf life than HAS. Generally, no adverse reactions or adverse effect on coagulation	Contains calcium and should not be given in the same line as blood as it will cause coagulation in the line. Plasma expander
Gelofusine	Similar to Haemaccel	Does not contain calcium and can be run through the same line as blood. Plasma expander
Isoplex 4% solution	Similar to Gelofusine	Contains gelatine 20 grams in 500 mL of water, contains sodium, potassium and chloride. Plasma expander
Dextran	Two solutions of 40 and 70 kDa. A polysaccharide, stable; a nontoxic and nonpyrogenic artificial colloid	Uses are limited as it has several problems: interferes with haemostasis by reducing platelet adhesiveness, can cause disseminated intravascular coagulation, anaphylactic reactions, blockage of the renal tubules leading to acute renal failure
Hespan	6% starch solution produced from corn hydrolysis, similar to Dextran 70 kDa	A synthetic colloid, with similar uses and problems to Dextran
Voluven	Is starch in sodium chloride	A plasma volume substitute used to restore blood volume

Continued

TABLE 6.3 Colloid infusions available.—cont'd

Colloid	Constituents	Uses
Volulyte	Is starch in sodium chloride, sodium acetate trihydrate; potassium chloride; magnesium chloride hexahydrate	Same use as Voluven
Perfluorocarbons (synthetic blood derivatives)	Unrelated to blood, but are able to transport oxygen in solution	Used as an oxygen-carrying substitute. Valuable in patients who refuse human blood transfusion, and in those with carbon monoxide poisoning and sickle cell crisis

- 5% Dextrose contains no electrolytes, just glucose in water. When administered intravenously it dilutes the sodium in the extra cellular fluid compartment. There is an increase in sodium in the intracellular fluid and fluid moves into the cells. It is good for rehydration but not for low circulating volume states.

Monitoring of vital signs and fluid balance is essential during fluid resuscitation of all types, as over administration can lead to fluid overload or haemodilution; both can be life threatening.

Table 6.4 includes a detailed list of crystalloid solutions. Those requiring further detail may refer to the latest Cochrane review (2018) on the use of crystalloids and colloids. This can be found at https://www.cochranelibrary.com/cdsr/doi/10.1002/14651858.CD000567.pub7/epdf/full.

6.3 GASTROINTESTINAL TRACT

Nutrients are required to carry out vital functions to sustain life, to form new body components or to assist in the functioning of various body processes, such as breathing and physical activity. The GI tract is subject to many disease conditions, some of which are very common, and there is a multitude of drugs used to treat these.

TABLE 6.4 Crystalloid infusions.

Crystalloid	Constituents	Uses
0.9% Normal saline	Contains sodium and chloride, no calories, has approximately the same osmolality as both intracellular and extracellular fluid	Increases mainly extracellular volume with no significant increase in intracellular volume
5% Dextrose (not a true crystalloid as it contains no electrolytes)	Contains only 200 cal/L, adds water to the extracellular compartment and reduces osmolality of extracellular fluid	The water will pass into the intracellular fluid to reach equilibrium, does not stay in the circulation, good for dehydration
4% Dextrose 0.18% normal saline	Contains a combination of both of the above	
Hartmann solution (compound sodium lactate IV infusion or Ringer solution)	Mixture of sodium chloride; sodium lactate; potassium chloride and calcium chloride in water	Used to replace fluids and electrolytes due to low circulating volume or blood pressure
Plasma-Lyte	Is similar to Hartmann's; contains sodium, potassium, magnesium, chloride, acetate and gluconate	A crystalloid solution used as a source of water and electrolytes

The GIT is under both neural and endocrine control. Also, the fact that a proportion of patients in hospital and in the community suffer from stress and malnutrition has an impact.

The effects of stress on the GIT

These are initiated by the nervous and endocrine systems.

- Stress stimulates the SNS, promoting:
  - Suppression of reproduction, growth and thyroid hormones.
  - The medulla of the adrenal gland releases catecholamines into the blood stream, adrenaline and noradrenaline.

- It is noradrenaline that has the major effect on the GIT as it leads to relaxation, inhibition of GIT activity and absorption, which can be significant to cause ischaemia to the stomach and duodenal mucosa.
- The adrenal cortex is also activated in long-term stress, leading to the release of cortisol, which affects carbohydrate, protein and fat metabolism resulting in an increase in blood glucose. Cortisol maximizes the action of catecholamines. The GIT effect of cortisol is to increase gastric secretion, which may be enough to cause ulceration of the gastric mucosa.

The effects of malnutrition

- Increased post-surgical complications (e.g. pneumonia)
- Impaired immune response
- Delay in wound, pressure ulcer healing and tissue viability:
  - Protein, carbohydrates and fats
  - Iron and zinc
  - Vitamin K, A, C and E
- Decreased muscle strength, resulting in immobility.

Stress and malnutrition can also lead to complications such as ulceration and/or GIT hypoxia. These can compound to prevent the replenishment of energy sources and can impact on a patient's illness and recovery and delay, prevent the absorption of drugs.

Drugs and the gastrointestinal tract

The commonest route for drug administration in the UK is orally and they are absorbed during their passage through the GIT.

Some drugs have an effect on the GI tract that is unwanted. They may cause side effects such as constipation, diarrhoea or they may be gastric irritants.

Other drugs are required for interventions to cure or reduce symptoms of GIT disease: to suppress gastric acid secretion; to relieve nausea or prevent vomiting; to increase or reduce gut motility and defecation; and to effect the formation and excretion of bile.

Gastric secretion

The stomach secretes 2.5 L of gastric juice a day. This production of acid is important for the digestion of food, absorption and prevention of infection. A protective layer of mucous protects the stomach from this acidic environment. Disruption to these protective mechanisms can lead to gastric damage such as gastric-oesophageal reflux disease and peptic ulcer. NSAIDs may have a negative impact on the protection given by the gastric mucosa. Drugs that are used to treat disorders affecting both the upper and lower GI tract are described.

Drugs used to suppress or neutralize gastric acid secretion

If acid enters the oesophagus, a burning sensation is felt: 'heartburn'. This is **gastro-oesophageal reflux,** and if there is continuous presence of acid in the lower oesophagus, **oesophagitis** may occur. One cause is a hiatus hernia. Treatment includes lifestyle changes such as reducing alcohol intake, reducing fat intake and losing weight, as well as drug therapy and occasionally surgery.

Normally, the aggressive acid in the stomach is balanced by the defensive mechanisms of the stomach mucosa. When this equilibrium is disturbed, an **ulcer** may develop.

- Peptic ulcers may be gastric (in the stomach) or duodenal. Duodenal ulcers are much more common as the duodenum is not so protected.
- On average, patients with duodenal ulcers produce about twice as much acid as normal subjects. About half those with a duodenal ulcer have normal acid secretion.

The stomach mucosa is normally protected due to its impermeability to gastric acid, its ability to secrete mucus and bicarbonate and its capacity to replace worn out epithelial cells. Prostaglandins are involved in all the above.

The mucosa of the stomach is unfavourably affected by the following factors. Their presence leads to an increased incidence of peptic ulcer.

- Use of NSAIDs: these drugs block the synthesis of prostaglandins (see Section 3.3) and are associated with the development of gastric ulcers.
- Cigarette smoking.
- Heredity (male sex, blood group O).
- Presence of *Helicobacter pylori* in the stomach (Box 6.3).

Drugs that aid the healing of ulcers may work by interfering with acid secretion in the stomach.

Drug treatment is usually with antacids, alginates and drugs to reduce acid secretion in the stomach such as H$_2$ receptor antagonists and proton pump inhibitors. Sometimes a drug to increase peristalsis, such as *metoclopramide*, may help by increasing the speed with which the stomach empties.

Antacids

Antacids are simple chemicals that counteract the acid in the stomach. They use salts of magnesium (cause diarrhoea) and aluminium (cause constipation). Thus, a mixture of the two is often used (e.g. *magnesium trisilicate*).

Mechanism of action

- Weak bases that readily combine with hydrochloric acid and neutralize it.
- Effective, well tolerated, inexpensive; useful for occasional symptoms.
- They provide **rapid symptom relief**, especially in liquid formulations, but tablets may be more convenient.

BOX 6.3 *Helicobacter pylori*

- *Helicobacter pylori* is a bacterium that survives by burrowing into the stomach lining. It can stand brief exposures to acid by using the enzyme urease to produce ammonia from urea and thus briefly neutralize the environment around itself. It is present in the mucosa of about 40% of the population in the UK and up to 90% in other countries
- *H. pylori* is implicated in gastritis and both peptic ulcer and gastric cancer. It is found in approximately 95% of patients with gastric ulcer and 80% with duodenal ulcer (Waller and Sampson 2017)
- If infection with *H. pylori* is confirmed it must be eradicated to enable long-term healing of peptic ulcers. If the bacteria are not eradicated, approximately 80% of ulcers will recur within 1 year of treatment and initial healing
- Antibacterial drugs are combined with those to inhibit stomach acid; reinfection is rare
- 1-week triple therapy regimens are successful in over 90% of cases and include a proton pump inhibitor; for example, **omeprazole** or **lansoprazole**, **amoxicillin** and either **clarithromycin** or **metronidazole** (See BNF, 2019 for all recommended regimens). If this fails it is possible that there may be resistance to one of the antibiotics used or that there is noncompliance with medication
- Alternative regimens for resistant cases are to be found in the BNF, and quadruple therapy may be used with **bismuth** included
- Following eradication of the bacteria, the proton pump inhibitor does not need to be continued unless there is haemorrhage or perforation of the ulcer

---

Indications

- They should be taken when symptoms are expected, such as between meals and at bedtime: about four times daily.
- Occasionally they may need to be taken more frequently: up to one dose an hour.
- If they are taken on an empty stomach their action is short — up to an hour — because of stomach emptying.

Preparations used

There are many indigestion preparations available OTC to the public and a full list is provided in the BNF.

Sodium bicarbonate Used to be popular but is not much used nowadays as it can result in a secondary rise in acid secretion. It should not be taken in patients who have to restrict their salt intake and should not be taken long term because of the risk of alkalosis. It is one of the preparations that may cause excessive belching.

Aluminium hydroxide

Tablets (500 mg): one or two should be chewed four times daily and at bedtime.

Suspension — tastes of peppermint — 5–10 mL at same time intervals. *Aludrox*, *Maalox* and *Mucogel* are all examples.

Magnesium carbonate (magnesium trisilicate)

May cause belching and diarrhoea. Comes as tablets or suspension and may be combined with sodium bicarbonate. **Hydrotalcite (*Altacite*)** contains a mixture of magnesium and aluminium and comes as a suspension.

Adverse effects

- Belching can be a problem due to the formation of liberated carbon dioxide when carbonate preparations react with the stomach acid.
- Magnesium-containing formulations tend to be laxative, whereas aluminium tends to constipate. Some preparations contain both in an attempt to reduce these side effects.
- As long as kidney function is normal, the accumulation of aluminium in the body does not appear to be a problem.
- They may impair the absorption of other drugs (e.g. tetracycline) and may destroy the enteric coating on tablets such as aspirin.
- Those formulations with high sodium content should be avoided in those with renal or cardiac impairment.
- Systemic alkalosis may occur if extremely large doses are taken (not magnesium as it is poorly absorbed from the gut).

Alginates

These are **inert substances** that float on the surface of the stomach contents and provide a mechanical barrier against reflux events.

They are combined with an antacid.

Examples are Algicon, Gastrocote, Gaviscon, Rennie Duo and Topal.

Histamine H₂-receptor antagonists

This group of drugs *cimetidine, famotidine, nizatidine* and *ranitidine* are used to inhibit gastric acid secretion. All except *cimetidine* are available OTC to the general public for the short-term treatment of heartburn and indigestion. They reduce the symptoms of gastritis or reflux oesophagitis but diagnosis should always be confirmed first as they can mask the symptoms of gastric cancer.

Cimetidine was the first to be manufactured but it slows down the metabolism of many other drugs, including warfarin, resulting in an enhancement of their effects.

There is accumulative evidence to suggest that some Ranitidine (Zantac) contains high levels of possible cancer-causing substances, and there are increasing demands for specific companies to recall their version of the drug from the counters.

Mechanism of action
● Block the histamine receptor on the gastric parietal cells and reduce gastric acid and pepsin secretion by about 60%.

Adverse effects
● Diarrhoea.
● Headache, dizziness and tiredness.
● Confusion in the elderly.
● *Cimetidine* inhibits P450 drug-metabolizing enzymes and effects the metabolism of other drugs such as anticoagulants and tricyclic antidepressants.

Uses
● To relieve gastro-oesophageal reflux disease.
● To aid healing of gastric and duodenal ulcers by reducing acid secretion.
● Not used for Zollinger–Ellison syndrome where proton pump inhibitors are more effective.

Proton pump inhibitors

The first drug of this type was *omeprazole*, which inhibits the end stage of the acid secretory pathway. Other proton pump inhibitors include *esomeprazole, lansoprazole, pantoprazole* and *rabeprazole*.

Mechanism of action
● Acid is secreted from gastric parietal cells by a 'proton pump'. These drugs inhibit acid secretion by blocking the proton pump and thus preventing the addition of hydrogen to chloride to make hydrochloric acid.
● They are more powerful than H_2-receptor antagonists.
● Profound and prolonged acid suppression occurs with a single daily dose and this relieves symptoms rapidly in most patients and helps to achieve healing.

Indications
● Short-term treatment and acid reduction in gastric and duodenal ulcers.
● As part of a regimen to eradicate *Helicobacter pylori* infection in conjunction with combination antibacterial therapy such as *amoxicillin* and *metronidazole* or *clarithromycin* (other combinations are also used).
● Prevention and treatment of gastric ulceration in those taking NSAIDs.
● Reduction of acid secretion in Zollinger–Ellison syndrome (rare gastrin-producing tumour).

Adverse effects
● May increase the risk of infection in the GI tract as they reduce the acid secretion.

- May mask symptoms of gastric cancer.
- Dry mouth.
- GI disturbances: nausea, vomiting, diarrhoea, constipation, flatulence, abdominal pain.
- Liver dysfunction.
- Hypersensitivity reactions: rashes, oedema, anaphylaxis.
- *Omeprazole* induces P450 liver enzymes and may interact with warfarin and phenytoin.
- Adverse consequences of hypoacidity:
  - Acid suppressants may increase the risk of acquiring enteric infections. This is especially true in the elderly and in those travelling to developing countries.
  - Predisposition to infection with *Salmonella, Shigella, Klebsiella* and *Pseudomonas* has been demonstrated.
  - Effects of this will be worse in those who are immunosuppressed, elderly or frail.
  - Threefold increase in the risk of developing bacterial diarrhoea with an acid suppressant.

Treatment of undiagnosed dyspepsia with drugs is to be discouraged as the symptoms of gastric carcinoma may be concealed. Gastric malignancy should be ruled out in those with probable symptoms.

- NICE (2019e) have produced a surveillance report of gastro-oesophageal reflux disease and dyspepsia in adults. This follows a systematic review on the effectiveness of proton-pump inhibitors (PPIs), H$_2$RAs and prostaglandins (Scally et al. 2018) used for a range of disorders. There were 849 trials included, 580 assessed the prevention of ulcers, 233 assessed healing and 36 assessed the treatment of acute upper GI bleeding. The average length of treatment was 1.4 months. The drugs did reduce upper GI tract bleeding (PPIs the most effective) and increased ulcer healing (PPIs most effective). There was a possible association between PPIs and cardiovascular events but no adverse effects when combined with aspirin rather than clopidogrel. The evidence did suggest an increased occurrence of community-acquired pneumonia and infection with *Clostridium difficile* in people taking PPIs. PPIs were very occasionally associated with adverse effects on the kidney. Four systematic reviews found an association between the risk of fractures and PPIs.

Drugs that protect the mucosa

These are called 'cytoprotective' and form a barrier over the surface of the ulcer.

Bismuth chelates

- May be used as part of combination therapy in resistant cases of *Helicobacter* infection. It has toxic effects on the bacillus and also protects the mucosa.
- May be combined with ***ranitidine*** as ranitidine bismuth chelate (***Pylorid***).

Adverse effects

- Nausea and vomiting.
- Blackening of the tongue and faeces.
- Bismuth is toxic if it accumulates. It is normally excreted by the kidneys but in renal impairment its accumulation can lead to encephalopathy.

Sucralfate

This is aluminium hydroxide combined with sucrose. In an acid environment it forms a gel with mucus and binds to the ulcer base to form a protective barrier to pepsin and acid. It has minimal antacid properties. It is not absorbed, and 3 hours after taking the mixture, 30% is still in the stomach.

Adverse effects

- Reduces the absorption of several other drugs (some antibiotics, theophylline, tetracycline, digoxin and amitriptyline).
- Antacids will reduce its action.
- Constipation in approximately 15% of patients.

Misoprostol

- This is a synthetic prostaglandin analogue. Prostaglandins have a generally homeostatic protective action in the GIT. NSAIDs inhibit the formation of prostaglandin E_2 that is needed for the production of the mucosal lining in the stomach. ***Misoprostol*** may be used to prevent ulcers in those who are old and frail but need to have NSAIDs.

Adverse effects

- Diarrhoea and abdominal pain in approximately 10%−20% of patients.
- Uterine contractions (avoid in pregnancy).
- Postmenopausal bleeding.

Antiemetic drugs

These are drugs that prevent or treat nausea and vomiting, which is an un-wanted side effect of many clinically used drugs. Vomiting is preceded by a feeling of 'queasiness' or nausea and can be accompanied by retching. It is protective in certain circumstances, such as the ingestion of toxic substances or large amounts of alcohol, and may be life-saving in these circumstances.

The vomiting centre in the brain stem may be stimulated by:

- Gastric distension or irritation.
- The labyrinth of the inner ear in vertigo or motion sickness.
- The chemoreceptor trigger zone (CTZ) close to the vomiting centre:
  - Lies in the fourth ventricle of the brain but is outside the blood–brain barrier.
  - It is sensitive to chemical stimuli by man drugs such as morphine, the cardiac glycoside digoxin and some anticancer drugs, which can cause unendurable nausea and vomiting.
  - Transmitters that are important in the CTZ include acetylcholine, histamine, dopamine and serotonin.
  - Drugs that block their receptors are useful in controlling nausea and vomiting.

Higher centres: pain, repulsive sights and smells, emotion and fear. The drugs used will vary according to the cause of the vomiting and should only be prescribed when the cause is known or they may mask symptoms and thus delay diagnosis.

Categories of drug used to stop vomiting

- Acetylcholine (muscarinic) receptor antagonists (antimuscarinics).
- Antihistamines.
- Dopamine receptor antagonists.
- Phenothiazines.
- $5-HT_3$ receptor antagonists.
- Other antiemetics.

Antimuscarinic agents

Hyoscine *(scopolamine)* The action of acetylcholine on the vomiting centre is blocked by this drug.

- It is used in motion sickness and is given either orally or as a transdermal patch, which is applied 6 hours before the start of the journey to allow maximum absorption.
- It may cause some drowsiness and blurring of vision and is contraindicated in glaucoma.

Antihistamines *(e.g. Cinnarizine, cyclizine, meclizine, promethazine)*

- Block histamine and acetylcholine receptors in the CTZ.
- All appear to be equally effective but length of action and incidence of side effects such as drowsiness vary.
- They are used to treat nausea and vomiting, especially in motion sickness and vestibular disorders which include vertigo, tinnitus and Meniere disease.
- Some are available OTC to prevent motion sickness (e.g. *Sea-legs* is *meclizine*) in 12.5 mg tablets.
- All are given orally but only *cyclizine* is commonly used intramuscularly or intravenously.
- *Promethazine* may be used short term for vomiting in pregnancy if a drug is absolutely necessary. It does not appear to be teratogenic.

In pregnancy, morning sickness may be a problem, especially in the first 3 months, but it is inadvisable to take any drugs as there is the greatest potential for damage to fetal development during this period. One drug is now licensed for sickness in pregnancy (2018) and this is a combination of the antihistamine *doxylamine*, which binds with the H$_1$ receptors in the brain, and *pyridoxine* (vitamin B6). The drug is *Xonvea* and it is a delayed release formulation. There is a risk of sleepiness and dizziness that may impact on driving.

Dopamine receptor antagonists

Domperidone (Motilium), metoclopramide (Maxolon)
Phenothiazines are in this category but are also antimuscarinic (e.g. *chlorpromazine* [Largactil], *haloperidol, perphenazine, prochlorperazine, trifluoperazine*).
Mechanism of action
  Block the action of dopamine on the CTZ.

  Pure dopamine antagonists such as *domperidone* are not effective in motion sickness. They are mostly used to reduce vomiting induced by drugs or surgery.

MHRA – risk of cardiac side effects with domperidone. This drug is contra-indicated where there are or could be cardiac conduction defects and with drugs that prolong the QT interval. Should be used at the lowest dose possible for the shortest period of time.

Metoclopramide
- Commonly used as an antiemetic.
- Available orally and by intramuscular or intravenous injection.
- Often used postoperatively, in opioid-induced vomiting and in migraine.

- It may be used intravenously in vomiting induced by cytotoxic drugs such as *cisplatin*, and at higher doses it has enhanced efficacy because it also blocks 5-HT receptors.
- It has antiemetic actions on the gut due to enhancing the action of acetylcholine here. It reduces vomiting by increasing the tone of the gastro-oesophageal sphincter and increasing the speed of stomach emptying (prokinetic). It causes dilation of the duodenum as well as increasing peristalsis in the small intestine.
- May be used before emergency anaesthesia to aid emptying of the stomach.

Adverse effects

- Metoclopramide crosses the blood−brain barrier and blocks dopamine receptors. This occasionally results in **extrapyramidal dystonia** especially of the neck and facial muscles (facial spasms, torticollis, oculogyric crises).
- This is commoner in children and young people and may occur even with normal doses in some patients. It can be quite frightening. The spasms pass off in a few hours but can be controlled by *diazepam*.
- Use in those under 20 years is restricted.
- Should only be prescribed short term (maximum of 5 days).
- Long-term use in the elderly may lead to tardive dyskinesia.

Phenothiazines

- Nonspecific in action and do have side effects such as sedation.
- They may be useful in nausea and vomiting caused by the administration of other drugs such as opioids, general anaesthetics and cytotoxics.
- Also helpful in radiation sickness or vomiting in advanced cancer and may be used to treat vestibular disorders and motion sickness.
- *Prochlorperazine* is the drug most frequently used. Other drugs more commonly used as antipsychotics, such as *chlorpromazine* and *haloperidol*, may be used if the vomiting is not responding to other medication, and for intractable hiccups.
- *Prochlorperazine* is available orally as syrup or tablets, rectally as suppositories, as a buccal preparation or by deep intramuscular injection.

Adverse effects

- As with metoclopramide above, *prochlorperazine* may **induce facial and skeletal muscle spasms** and oculogyric crises due to its antidopaminergic effects on the CNS.
- As these effects are more common in young people, its use is not recommended in children.

5-HT₃ antagonists

Dolasetron, granisetron, ondansetron, tropisetron

Mechanism of action

- Block the **5-HT₃ receptors** in the CTZ and in the GI tract.

Indications

- Very effective antiemetics that are being frequently used since their price decreased.
- They are used to prevent vomiting in patients receiving highly emetic **anticancer** drugs, such as cisplatin, which cause the release of 5-HT.
- Also given to prevent or relieve postoperative nausea and vomiting.

Route of administration

- They may be given by mouth or rectally 1 hour before the administration of a cytotoxic drug or by intravenous injection or infusion.
- Only some of these drugs may be given to children (see BNF).

Adverse effects

- Constipation.
- Headache.
- Following intravenous administration there may be seizures, chest pain and bradycardia.

Some common antiemetics, their uses and side effects are shown in Table 6.5.

Neurokinin receptor antagonists

Aprepitant, fosaprepitant, rolapitant

These drugs block the activity of neurkinin-1 and boost the activity of 5-HT₃ antagonists.

They are especially important in nausea associated with emetogenic chemotherapy.

Cannabinoids

- These are derivatives of marijuana (*Cannabis sativa*). **Nabilone** is a synthetic cannabinoid used for nausea and vomiting in cytotoxic therapy where there is little response to other drugs. Side effects of drowsiness and dizziness may frequently occur.

Histamine analogues

Betahistine is an analogue of histamine. It is used in Meniere disease for vertigo and tinnitus and is believed to lower the pressure inside the inner ear.

TABLE 6.5 Common antiemetic drugs, their uses and side effects.

Target receptor and drugs	Main indications	Main side effects
Dopamine receptor *Prochlorperazine* *Metoclopramide*	Postoperative nausea and vomiting (PONV) Gastrointestinal-induced vomiting Mild chemotherapy induced	Extrapyramidal side effects, abnormal movements, oculogyric crisis
5-HT receptor (serotonin) *Ondansetron* *Granisetron*	Chemotherapy induced PONV Radiotherapy	Mild headache Constipation Dizziness
Acetylcholine (muscarinic) *Hyoscine*	Motion sickness	Blurred vision Constipation Dizziness
Histamine (H_1) *Cyclizine*	Hyperemesis gravidarum Motion sickness Opioid-induced vomiting PONV	Sedation
Corticosteroid *Dexamethasone*	Chemotherapy induced PONV	Mood changes Insomnia
Cannabinoid *Nabilone*	Chemotherapy induced PONV	Dysphoria Sedation Hypotension

Dexamethasone is a steroid with antiemetic properties, which is used in cancer chemotherapy. It can be used alone or combined with metoclopramide, prochlorperazine or a 5-HT_3 antagonist.

Gastrointestinal motility

The rectum is normally empty and faecal material is stored in the descending and pelvic colon. When stimulated by food or drink, usually at approximately the same time or times each day, the colon contracts and faeces enter the rectum. The sensitive nerve endings here are activated and there is an urge to defaecate. Within the healthy population there is a wide variation in bowel habit from those who have their bowels opened three times each day to those who only go every 2−3 days. It does not mean that these people are suffering from diarrhoea or constipation unless there is an abnormality in the texture of the stool (Box 6.4).

BOX 6.4 Constipation

- Constipation is the passage of hard stools less frequently than is normal for that person
- Important to establish what the patient actually means when they say they are constipated
- Dietary advice may be needed: increasing fibre in diet, drinking sufficient fluids, etc.
- In the general population laxatives are among the most abused drugs
- Some patients believe laxatives are cleansing and this belief can be dangerous
- Abuse may lead to an atonic nonfunctioning colon and hypokalaemia
- Need to ensure there is no disease causing the constipation, and any laxative should be avoided in undiagnosed abdominal pain

---

Drugs that effect GIT motility include drugs that:

- Accelerate the passage of food through the intestine. The movement of food through the intestine can be hastened by several different kinds of drugs such as laxatives, faecal softeners and stimulant purgatives. These agents can be used to relieve constipation or to clear the bowel prior to surgery or examination.
- Increase the motility of the GIT smooth muscle without causing evacuation of the bowel or inducing bowel movement.
- Decrease bowel motility such as in diarrhoea.
- Decrease smooth muscle tone such as antispasmodic drugs.

Causes of constipation

- Neglecting the urge to defaecate.
- Pain when passing stool.
- Diet low in fibre or with insufficient fluid intake.
- Slow gut transit.
- Drugs: for example, opioids; calcium antagonists such as verapamil, antacids, antimuscarinic drugs and some antidepressants.
- Immobility.
- Old age.
- Hypotonic colon as in laxative abuse and sometimes in the elderly.
- Weak abdominal muscles.
- Depression.
- Disease: for example, cancer of the colon, myxoedema (underactive thyroid gland).

Laxatives

These are drugs, which accelerate the passage of food through the intestine.

Different types of laxatives work in one of several different ways.

- **Bulk laxatives** increase the volume of nonabsorbable solid residue.
- **Stimulant laxatives** increase motility and secretions.
- **Osmotic laxatives** increase the water content of the faeces.
- **Faecal softeners** alter the consistency of the faeces (Box 6.5).

Bulk-forming laxatives

High-residue foods contain a high proportion of indigestible cellulose, which increases the faecal bulk. Fruit, green vegetables and wholemeal bread are examples. Unprocessed wheat bran, taken with food, is most effective, but other examples that may be used if the patient cannot tolerate bran include *methylcellulose* (*Celevac*), ispaghula husk (*Fybogel*, *Isogel*) and sterculia (*Normacol*).

Mechanism of action

Depends on the amount of fluid that is taken with them. They work by the absorption of fluid from the gut.

- If given with a lot of fluid they will increase the size of the faecal mass and lessen the viscosity ('stickiness'), thus making small, hard stools larger, softer and bulkier.
- If given with no fluid or minimal fluid in cases where the stool is very runny, they will absorb water and so increase the viscosity of the stool, decreasing its fluidity. This may be useful in an ileostomy.

Adverse effects

- Flatulence and abdominal distension.
- If too little fluid is taken when there is not a fluid stool, obstruction of the colon may occur.
- Should not be taken immediately before going to bed because adequate **fluid intake** has to be maintained to prevent the possibility of obstruction with these preparations.

BOX 6.5 Laxatives

Laxatives should be avoided except:
- in drug-induced constipation — morphine and its derivatives especially
- when straining may exacerbate a condition such as angina
- when constipation may increase the risk of bleeding (e.g. haemorrhoids)
- for expulsion of parasites such as worms after treatment
- to clear the GIT prior to surgery or radiological investigations
- occasionally in the elderly where prolonged treatment may be needed

---

GIT, Gastrointestinal tract.

Stimulant laxatives

This group includes bisacodyl, senna, dantron, rhubarb and cascara.

- Any stimulant laxative causes increased intestinal motility and may cause abdominal cramp.
- They should be avoided in intestinal obstruction.

Senna (*Senokot*) may be used if increased fibre and bulk-forming laxatives are not tolerated.

Sodium picosulfate (*Dulcolax*) is a powerful stimulant used for bowel evacuation and not routinely for constipation.

Osmotic laxatives

These act by retaining fluid in the bowel by osmosis.

- *Lactulose* is a semi-synthetic disaccharide, which is not absorbed from the GI tract and holds water osmotically. It may take up to 48 hours to work. As it also discourages ammonia-producing micro-organisms it is useful in liver failure. Side effects include flatulence, cramps and abdominal discomfort.
- **Magnesium salts** are also in this category but are contraindicated in any acute condition of the GI tract. *Epsom salts* are magnesium sulphate.
- **Glycerol**, as a suppository, has an osmotic action.

Faecal softeners

- This type of laxative is most useful in haemorrhoids and anal fissure.
- *Liquid paraffin* is the best known but with prolonged use can interfere with the absorption of fat-soluble vitamins (A, D, E and K) and may cause a granulomatous reaction that could be related to the development of carcinoma of the colon.

Enemas and suppositories

- *Glycerol suppositories*, one or two moistened with water before insertion into the rectum, are given for constipation.
- *Phosphate enemas* may be used when bowel evacuation is needed before surgery or investigative procedures and may be used in constipation.
- *Sodium citrate* is given rectally in constipation as a **micro-enema**. It is combined with glycerol and sorbitol in a 5 mL viscous solution.
- Enemas containing *arachis oil* (ground nut oil, peanut oil) lubricate and soften impacted faeces and aid achievement of a bowel movement. Must not be given to patients allergic to nuts.
- *Steroid enemas* are used to treat bowel conditions, such as ulcerative colitis, and are not given to promote a bowel movement. They need to be retained if possible, for at least 1 hour.

Bowel cleansing solutions

These are used before colonic surgery or radiological examination to ensure there are no solid contents in the bowel. They are combined with a low-residue diet for several days before surgery and are not treatments for constipation. *Sodium picosulfate* (*Picolax*) is commonly used but others are available (e.g. *Klean-Prep*).

Antidiarrhoeal agents

Diarrhoea is an increase in volume, fluidity or frequency of bowel movements. In many instances drug intervention is not required. There are many causes of diarrhoea, which leads to an inflammation of the GIT/stomach termed gastroenteritis. This can be a mild inconvenience to a medical emergency requiring hospitalization and FRT. In gastroenteritis the diarrhoea serves to flush out the pathogens. In this instance the approaches to treatment are:

- Prevention of fluid and electrolyte depletion is essential, especially in the elderly and the very young.
- **Oral rehydration** preparations such as *Dioralyte* and *Rehydrate*. They are given according to the fluid loss and full instructions are included with the products. After reconstitution with water, any unused preparation must be discarded after 1 hour unless stored in a refrigerator where it may be kept for up to 24 hours.
- In most cases of simple gastroenteritis, antibacterials are not needed even where there may be a bacterial cause as most clear up quickly with no treatment; in the UK infective diarrhoea is usually viral.
- Some infections do require antibacterials. These include campylobacter enteritis, shigellosis and salmonellosis.

Antimotility drugs

- Slow down the motility of the gut and decrease transit time.
- Relieve the symptoms of uncomplicated acute diarrhoea but are not recommended in children.

    Opioids act as antimotility drugs.

- *Codeine phosphate* activates **opioid receptors** on the smooth muscle of the bowel, which **reduces peristalsis** and increases segmentation contractions so that passage of contents is delayed and more water is absorbed. Tolerance may develop with prolonged use and occasionally dependence has been known. If the client is also in pain then this drug may be useful as a dual-purpose preparation.

- *Co-phenotrope* (*Lomotil*) is a mixture of diphenoxylate hydrochloride and atropine sulphate. The former is a drug similar in structure to pethidine that has a similar effect on the bowel to morphine. The amount of atropine added is very small and is there partly to discourage abuse. Side effects include nausea, vomiting and abdominal cramps. In overdose, respiratory depression may occur.
- The action of these two antimotility drugs can be reversed by *naloxone*, which is the antidote to all opioid drugs.
- *Loperamide* (*Imodium*) impairs propulsion in the gut by an action on the longitudinal and circular muscles whereby it antagonizes peristalsis perhaps due to preventing the release of acetylcholine in the nerve plexus of the gut.
- Possible side effects include nausea, vomiting and abdominal cramps.

MHRA Warning (2017) that there are some serious cardiac adverse reactions seen with high doses of loperamide associated with abuse. Naloxone can be used if symptoms of overdose are apparent.

Antimicrobial-induced diarrhoea

Usually rapidly resolves when the drug is discontinued.

Occasionally broad-spectrum antibiotic therapy is associated with super-infection of the large intestine (pseudomembranous colitis) by toxin-producing *C. difficile*.

- This is particularly likely to occur in elderly and debilitated patients but can affect any age group.
- Once present, it may be transmitted between patients; therefore, in hospital, isolation is necessary.
- Within a few days of starting the antibiotic, watery diarrhoea occurs with abdominal pain and fever. In some cases, the infection may occur 4–6 weeks after commencing the antibiotics.
- It is responsible for severe systemic toxicity and the infection may be lethal in the frail.

Drugs that increase gastrointestinal motility

Metoclopramide, which is also an antiemetic, causes marked acceleration of gastric emptying and so is used sometimes in gastro-oesophageal reflux.

Domperidone is a dopamine antagonist also used as an antiemetic.

Cisapride stimulates acetylcholine release in the upper GI tract and is useful in reflux oesophagitis. It may be dysrhythmogenic in some patients.

Diverticular disease

A diverticulum is a pouch that forms at a weak point in the large bowel. Diverticula tend to occur in those eating a low-fibre diet and may cause lower abdominal pain and constipation or diarrhoea. It is treated with a high-fibre diet, bulk-forming drugs and bran supplements.

If they become infected (diverticulitis) there is increased abdominal pain and sometimes abscess formation. There is danger of perforation in acute diverticulitis.

Irritable bowel syndrome

Irritable bowel syndrome (IBS) is a motility disorder that occurs in approximately 15% of the population and is characterized by abdominal pain and alterations in bowel habit. These vary from diarrhoea to constipation. It is a chronic condition that may be lifelong. No cause can be found but symptoms may be precipitated by certain foods such as wheat flour. Some patients may respond to dietary changes that involve eliminating certain foods and increasing the fibre in the diet. There may be a psychological component to the disorder and counselling may help.

Adults with symptoms of IBS are offered tests for inflammatory markers (e.g. C-reactive protein and faecal calprotectin) as first-line treatment, to exclude inflammatory markers (NICE, https://www.nice.org.uk/guidance/qs114). These tests are useful to exclude inflammatory causes and therefore exclude inflammatory bowel disease.

Advice on dietary and lifestyle management is given. Fluid intake should be increased to at least 8 cups a day and the intake of caffeine and alcohol reduced.

Drug treatment is symptomatic and includes the use of antispasmodics such as *alverine citrate, mebeverine* or *peppermint oil*. These are available OTC and can be taken in addition to the advice on diet. It may be necessary to treat constipation or diarrhoea if these are present.

Linaclotide is a guanylate cyclase-C receptor agonist, which is used as a laxative in moderate to severe IBS with constipation.

Eluxadoline is an antimotility drug that acts locally on opioid receptors in the gut and can be used under NICE guidance in certain cases of IBS. It has to be started in secondary care and stopped at 4 weeks if there is no satisfactory relief of symptoms. There is a risk of pancreatitis and some cases have resulted in hospitalization or death; therefore this drug is only started by a specialist (MHRA, 2017). NICE guidance is available at www.nice.org.uk/guidance/cg61.

Antispasmodics

These drugs promote relaxation and reduce peristalsis in the intestine and are used to relieve the pain associated with spasm of the muscles in the gut. They may be useful in diverticular disease and in IBS.

Include antimuscarinic (anticholinergic) drugs and drugs that directly relax the intestinal smooth muscle.

Antimuscarinics

Dicycloverine, hyoscine (Buscopan), propantheline

- Reduce intestinal motility by decreasing the effects of the parasympathetic transmitter acetylcholine on the smooth muscle of the intestine. Acetylcholine normally promotes peristalsis and contraction of smooth muscle in the GI tract.
- *Atropine* is not used just for this action any more as the side effects caused by the blockage of cholinergic transmission are much greater than with other drugs.
- *Dicycloverine* has fewer side effects and may have additional direct action on the smooth muscle.
- *Hyoscine* is used for relaxation of smooth muscle in renal colic as well as spasm in the GI tract and is sold OTC as *Buscopan*. It may be given by intramuscular and intravenous injection in acute spasm and to promote relaxation in endoscopy.

Side effects

Antimuscarinic and include constipation, urinary urgency and retention, tachycardia and palpitations, dry mouth and occasionally giddiness, especially in the elderly.

Other antispasmodics

Alverine (Spasmonal), mebeverine (Colofac), peppermint oil (Mintec)

All are believed to be direct relaxants of the smooth muscle in the wall of the intestine. They have no serious side effects and may be useful in IBS, although response varies and is sometimes disappointing. They relieve spasm and distension. Peppermint oil is taken as capsules and is used to relieve flatulence. *Mebeverine* is sold OTC.

Chronic inflammatory bowel disease

This includes ulcerative colitis and Crohn's disease. The cause of these diseases is still not understood but they are chronic and relapsing in nature and are most commonly diagnosed between the ages of 15 and 40 years. Ulcerative colitis is limited to the large bowel and the mucosa, whereas Crohn's disease commonly affects the ileum (small intestine) but can affect any part of the GI tract. Drug therapy and nutrition are important in treatment. Surgery may be necessary in severe cases.

Drug treatment

This is aimed at relieving the inflammation and promoting a remission.

Chemicals that are involved in the inflammatory process in the bowel include kinins and prostaglandins, which induce ion secretion and diarrhoea. The anti-inflammatory drugs used are aminosalicylates and steroids.

Glucocorticoids (steroids)

Prednisolone, budesonide, hydrocortisone These are anti-inflammatory (see Section 7.2). If the rectum or sigmoid colon is affected, steroids may be given using **foam preparations** and **suppositories**. If the disease is diffuse, an oral steroid may be needed for short periods of 4—8 weeks.

Budesonide is less well absorbed and therefore has fewer side effects but may not always be as effective.

In severe cases, hospitalization is needed and the steroids may be given intravenously.

Aminosalicylates

Sulfasalazine (Salazopyrin), mesalazine, balsalazide, olsalazine

- The oldest drug is *sulfasalazine* and it has been used for many years in maintaining a remission in ulcerative colitis. It is available as **suppositories** if disease is limited to the rectum.
- Action is only partly understood but these drugs do interfere with prostaglandin synthesis and are therefore anti-inflammatory.
- Only mild acute symptoms will respond and this may take 6—8 weeks initially.
- Oral steroids produce a remission more rapidly and then aminosalicylates can be used to maintain this.
- *Sulfasalazine* has also been used to treat rheumatoid arthritis.

All aminosalicylates are associated with **blood dyscrasias** and patients should report any unexplained bleeding or bruising.

Drugs affecting the immune response. Methotrexate is sometimes used and folic acid is given to prevent methotrexate toxicity. Folic acid is usually given once a week on a different day to the methotrexate.

Cytokine modulators. Infliximab, adalimumab and *golimumab* are monoclonal antibodies that inhibit tumour necrosis factor alpha, which is a cytokine and a pro-inflammatory mediator. They are only used under specialist supervision.

Haemorrhoids

There are soothing preparations available that may give symptomatic relief by their astringent action. These include bismuth and zinc oxide preparations such as *Anusol* cream, ointment or suppositories.

Local anaesthetics may be used for severe pain and ***lidocaine, benzocaine, chirocaine*** or ***pramocaine*** ointment are used prior to opening the bowels if an anal fissure is present. As these can be absorbed through the rectal mucosa, excessive application should be avoided. They should only be used for a few days as they may cause sensitization of the anal skin.

Some preparations are combined with steroids for short-term use (e.g. ***Anusol-HC***).

Other treatments are available from specialists (e.g. injection sclerotherapy) using phenol in oil.

Section 7

Endocrine system

Section Outline

7.1 ENDOCRINE PANCREAS AND DIABETES MELLITUS

This section includes not only drugs used to treat diabetes mellitus and other endocrine disorders but also sex hormones and contraception, as well as pregnancy.

The pancreas produces two hormones that regulate blood glucose levels. *Insulin* is produced by the beta cells in the islets of Langerhans and is secreted when blood glucose levels rise. The overall impact is increased utilization of glucose and a reduction in the level of glucose in the blood. *Glucagon* is produced by the alpha cells in the islets when blood glucose levels are low and stimulates the conversion of glycogen stored in the liver to glucose, thus raising the level of glucose in the blood and preventing hypoglycaemia. In health the normal range for blood glucose is 4.0−7.0 mmol/L.

Diabetes mellitus

Diabetes mellitus is a syndrome characterized by a persistently raised blood glucose level and associated with a deficiency of or resistance to insulin. More than 4.7 million people in the United Kingdom have diabetes, and this is expected to reach 5.5 million by 2030 (Diabetes UK, 2020). Someone is diagnosed with diabetes every 2 minutes! Worldwide more than 422 million people have diabetes and diabetes was the seventh leading cause of death in 2016 (WHO, 2018).

Type 1 diabetes is an **autoimmune disease** where the beta cells that produce insulin are destroyed. Eventually no insulin at all is secreted. **Type 2 diabetes** is a different disease. The patient still produces some insulin, but this is either low in quantity or the cells are resistant to its action (insulin resistance). There are a great many more people with type 2 diabetes (more than

90% of all those with diabetes) than type 1 (approximately 8%). The remaining 2% have rarer forms of diabetes. The incidence of type 2 diabetes is increasing in this country and is linked to obesity, hypertension and heart disease. Simple lifestyle measures can delay or prevent the onset of type 2 diabetes.

Action of insulin

- Insulin secretion is dependent upon the level of glucose in the blood.
- A low basal level of insulin is secreted throughout the day and night, but after a meal when glucose levels rise, more insulin is secreted. There is a 7–10-fold difference in insulin concentrations between meals and following a meal. Secretion in health is approximately 30–40 units daily.
- Insulin is necessary to allow glucose to enter most body cells and so be used for energy. If there is excess glucose, insulin encourages its storage as glycogen in the liver and muscles and as fat in adipose tissue.
- If there is insufficient insulin, the body cannot utilize its glucose, which will then accumulate in the blood (hyperglycaemia) and spill over into the urine.

Effect of insulin on target cells

- Insulin causes the rapid uptake, storage and use of glucose by almost all tissues in the body but especially by the muscles, liver and adipose tissue.
- Binds with a specific membrane receptor protein on the surface of the target cell, which becomes activated and triggers the cell's response.
- Within seconds of binding, approximately 80% of all body cells become highly permeable to glucose. This allows the rapid entry of glucose into the cells by specific carriers.

Glucose uptake by the brain is not dependent on insulin secretion.

Type 1 diabetes mellitus

- Used to be called insulin-dependent diabetes mellitus (IDDM).
- No insulin is produced, and without insulin injections the patient would eventually die.
- Autoimmune disorder, the causes of which are not entirely understood. The beta cells in the pancreas are attacked by antibodies and eventually totally destroyed.

- Certain individuals have a genetic predisposition towards the disease, but an environmental trigger factor is needed. This may be a virus.
- The onset of the disease has its highest incidence around 11−12 years of age, and although it can occur at any age, it is uncommon older than the age of approximately 40 years.
  - Onset is reasonably acute over a period of weeks or months with polyuria (passing lots of urine), thirst, polydipsia (drinking lots), weight loss and lack of energy.
  - Without treatment the body has to utilize fat for energy and in doing so produces ketones. These are acidic and accumulate in the blood, being eliminated in the urine. If the person does not receive insulin therapy, a ketoacidotic coma may result. This is a medical emergency, and the patient is dehydrated, suffering from electrolyte imbalance and acidosis.

Type 2 diabetes mellitus

- This is due to insulin resistance or deficiency. There is some insulin available, but the body may not be able to utilize this adequately.
- The majority of people with diabetes have type 2 diabetes, and the numbers are increasing worldwide.
- The disease is associated with obesity, and although it used to be considered a disease of middle or old age, there are now cases occurring in children.
- Onset is insidious, and the person may have type 2 for years and not know about it.
- It is possible to prevent or delay the onset of type 2 diabetes by eating a healthy diet, keeping slim and exercising sufficiently.
- Type 2 can usually be controlled by diet alone or tablets, but some patients may eventually need insulin injections.
- There is no cure for diabetes at present, and the aim of treatment is to control the blood glucose levels and prevent long-term complications.

Long-term complications of diabetes

Uncontrolled diabetes may affect large blood vessels such as the aorta and coronary, carotid and femoral arteries. Atheroma is deposited more readily, and this results in a higher risk of cardiovascular disease. People with diabetes are more than twice as likely to have ischaemic heart disease or a stroke.

Small capillaries are affected by the raised glucose levels, and this may result in eye disease (retinopathy), kidney disease (neuropathy) or nerve conduction problems (peripheral neuropathy).

To prevent complications, blood glucose needs to be kept in as normal a range as possible. Blood pressure also needs to be tightly controlled and cardiovascular risk factors managed.

The diet in diabetes

- Although the patient with type 1 diabetes will need to have insulin injections, diet is still important.
- The patient will always see a dietician who will advise him or her and the family on the types of foods that may need to be avoided.
- The diet should be a balanced diet that is low in animal fats to reduce atheroma deposition. It is the sort of healthy diet that we should all be eating.
- Carbohydrate should be 'starchy' and long lasting such as that found in bread, rice and potatoes. Less should be eaten in the form of foods containing 'fast' sugar.
- At least five (preferably seven) portions of fruit and vegetables should be eaten daily, but it must be remembered that fruit does contain fructose, which is a fast sugar and so cannot be eaten freely.
- The use of foods labelled 'diabetic' is not encouraged, because these are unnecessary and expensive.
- The patient with type 2 diabetes usually needs to lose weight and will need advice on how this may be achieved.

Exercise

It is now realized that regular exercise should be encouraged for everyone, when possible. Half an hour of moderate exercise at least five times a week is recommended. It makes people feel good and helps with weight loss as well as increasing fitness.

Insulin therapy

Insulin was first isolated from the pancreas in 1922, and immediately the outlook for the patient with type 1 diabetes changed from rapid decline and death to practically that of a healthy person.

- The normal production of insulin by the pancreas has to be mimicked as closely as possible by the administration of insulin by injection. Insulin requirements in the body change from minute to minute and so this is a difficult task.
- Insulin cannot be given orally because it is a protein and so inactivated by enzymes in the gut. It is usually given subcutaneously, and the injection site is rotated on a systematic basis, using the thighs and the abdominal wall. Some patients also use the upper arms or buttocks.
- Injections may be up to four or even five times daily, and for some, this is the worst aspect of their illness. Very fine insulin needles have now made the process practically painless.

- Short-acting insulin may also be given by a continuous subcutaneous portable infusion pump. This delivers a continuous basal insulin infusion with patient-activated bolus doses at meal times.
- Insulin is a small protein, and its basic structure is common to all mammalian species which allowed patients to be treated with animal insulins until genetic engineering allowed the manufacture of recombinant human insulin analogues. Bovine insulin differs from human insulin by three amino acids, and porcine differs from human by only one. Currently, animal forms are not initiated in new cases of diabetes and are used nowadays only rarely, in those already established on this type of insulin.

Insulin as therapy in diabetes is indicated in:

- type I diabetes
- all patients presenting with ketoacidosis, regardless of age
- any type of diabetes where oral therapy has failed
- intercurrent illness (e.g. myocardial infarction)
- pregnancy
- surgery.

Aims of insulin therapy

- Abolition of symptoms.
- Maintenance of ideal body weight.
- Optimization of glucose control – without making the patient obsessional.
- Prevention of complications or delay in progress.
- Reduction in associated risk factors for coronary heart disease.

Close cooperation between the patient and the healthcare team is needed, and the patient should be involved in decision making about their treatment. The dose of insulin needs adjustment on an individual basis.

Healthy nondiabetic fasting glucose should be maintained very close to 4.3 mmol/L. After a meal it should not rise to greater than 7.0 mmol/L.

In diabetes the aim is to maintain blood glucose levels as close as possible to normal physiological levels without inducing hypoglycaemia.

Self-monitoring of blood glucose levels

- This is essential to maintain good control of blood glucose levels in type 1 diabetes.
- The aim is to keep the fasting blood glucose between 5 and 7 mmol/L on waking.
- A blood glucose concentration between 4 and 7 mmol/L before meals and at other times during the day.

- Target levels of <7.8 mmol/L 2 hours postprandial (after food) in type 1. In type 2 may accept up to 9 mmol/L.
- A blood glucose of at least 5 mmol/L when driving.
- The person with diabetes usually gives their own insulin injections and monitors their glucose levels.
- Self-monitoring of blood glucose levels (SMGLs) requires the use of **blood glucose testing strips** and meters or the **newer flash glucose devices**. The latter are usually used if the patient is requiring intensive insulin therapy or has difficulty in reaching his or her treatment targets and is having episodes of hypoglycaemia or hyperglycaemia.
- Using finger prick glucose, measurements are taken at least four times daily, and insulin doses and physical activity may be adjusted according to these levels. This may be extended to 10 times daily when control is poor or there are problems such as frequent hypoglycaemia.
- Flash monitoring is done by a small device that is inserted under the skin and monitors levels throughout the day and night. It does not measure blood glucose levels but the level of glucose in the interstitial fluid around the body cells. This means there is a small time delay in readings compared with those produced by finger prick monitoring. People using flash glucose devices will still have to do occasional monitoring using fingerprick when they are having problems such as hypoglycaemia.
- The levels should be checked when using the flash monitor at least eight times a day, and it should be worn at least 70% of the time (Diabetes UK, 2020). The patient has a reader that he or she swipes over the sensor to get the levels and also the trend of his or her levels. It can also be scanned using the patient's phone and gives the levels for the past 8 hours. Sensors can be worn for approximately 14 days, then they have to be changed. Box 7.1 looks at the advantages of flash glucose monitoring.
- Ketone testing strips are available to be used if the blood glucose level is very high or the patient is unwell.

HbA$_{1c}$ levels

This is another means of assessing control of blood glucose. It is a measure of the percentage of haemoglobin (Hb) in the blood that is carrying glucose — glycated Hb. It is slower to change than blood glucose and monitors glucose control over a period of 2—3 months. In a person without diabetes, the normal percentage is less than 6.5%.

Diabetes UK recommends that most people with diabetes should ideally aim for levels of 6.5% or less.

Types of insulin available

The half-life of insulin from the pancreas is 5—6 minutes — it is rapidly destroyed by the liver. This is ideal in the body where it is released as needed

---

BOX 7.1 Advantages and disadvantages of flash glucose monitoring

Fewer finger prick tests	Cannot set an alarm for high and low glucose levels and so will not help patient to recognize a hypoglycaemic attack (hypo)
Trends can be seen so the patient can see when levels are starting to drop or rise	Data overload may confuse some patients or worry them
Can increase confidence in diabetes management as decisions are made with more data available	Patient still needs to do some finger prick tests
Easier to stain target range for sugar levels as can see when they are likely to rise and fall	Some may find the sensor irritating to wear or may not like the look of it
You can see what your levels are like during the night by asking someone else to scan the sensor	

Adapted from information provided by Diabetes UK, 2017. https://www.diabetes.org.uk/guide-to-diabetes/ managing-your-diabetes/testing/flash-glucose-monitoring.

---

but not ideal for an injection given for replacement therapy. Sustained-release formulations have been developed to try and overcome this. To prolong the action of insulin it is bound to zinc or proteins.

The main types of insulin are:

- rapid-acting or short-acting insulins with short duration — analogues such as *aspart* and soluble insulin
- intermediate-acting insulin (e.g. isophane insulin)
- long-acting (e.g. insulin zinc suspension [IZS]) and analogues (e.g. *glargine*).

Types of insulin and their actions are summarized in Table 7.1.

The action profile of insulin is also affected by:

- dose
- injection site
- injection technique
- exercise
- temperature.

TABLE 7.1 The different action of various types of insulin.

Types of insulin	Brand names	Following subcutaneous administration			Description
		Onset	Peak	Duration	
Recombinant human insulin analogues	Insulin Lispro (*Humalog*) Insulin Aspart (*NovoRapid*) Insulin Glulisine (*Apidra*)	*5–20 min*	*30–60 min*	*2–5 h* *2–4 h*	Amino acid structure slightly altered to make action faster and of shorter duration
Soluble insulin (insulin injection; neutral insulin)	Human sequence insulins: *Actrapid, Humulin S* Highly purified animal insulins: *Hypurin Bovine Neutral, Hypurin Porcine Neutral*	*30–60 min*	*2–4 h*	*4–8 h*	Structure as in the human body. Porcine 1 AA different to human
Intermediate-acting					
Isophane insulin (isophane protamine, isophane NPH)	*Insulatard, Humulin I, Insuman Basal, Porcine and Bovine Isophane, Pork Insulatard*	*1–2 h*	*5–8 h*	*12–18 h*	Soluble insulin and the protein protamine in equal amounts
Long-acting					
Insulin zinc suspension Protamine zinc insulin	*Hypurin Bovine Lente Hypurin Bovine Protamins Zinc*	*1–2 h*	*6–20 h*	*Up to 36 h*	Combined with zinc for longer action
Basal insulin analogue	Glargine Detemir Degludec	*90 min*	*Flat profile*	*24 h*	Amino acid structure changed – long action for basal level

continued

TABLE 7.1 The different action of various types of insulin.—cont'd.

| Types of insulin | Brand names | Following subcutaneous administration | | | Description |
		Onset	Peak	Duration	
Biphasic insulins					
Biphasic isophane	*Humulin M3, Insuman Comb 15, 25, 50. Pork Mixtard 30, Hypurin porcine 30/70 mix*				Mixture of fast-acting soluble and intermediate-acting isophane Mixtard 30 is 30% soluble, 70% isophane. Reduces the number of injections. Often twice daily
Biphasic insulin lispro	*Humalog Mix 25* *Humalog Mix 50*				25% lispro and 75% insulin lispro protamine 50% of each
Biphasic aspart	*NovoMix 30*				30% aspart and 70% aspart protamine

NPH, Neutral protamine Hagedorn.

Short-acting insulins

- Soluble insulin was the original form of insulin.
- Clear solution. Additive such as phenol prevents growth of microorganisms.
- Injected subcutaneously 15–30 minutes before food.
- Can be given intravenously and intramuscularly as well as by continuous subcutaneous infusion and is used in medical emergencies (e.g. diabetic ketoacidosis [DKA]) and also in surgery.
- Given intravenously has half-life of only 5 minutes and duration of action only 30 minutes.

Subcutaneous administration results in onset of action at approximately 30 minutes to 1 hour; peak action 2–4 hours; duration of action 4–8 hours.

Medicinal forms include *Actrapid, Humulin S, Hypurin Bovine Neutral, Hypurin Porcine Neutral, Insuman Infusat, Insuman Rapid.*

Recombinant human insulin analogues

Rapid-acting insulin, such as insulin lispro (Humalog), insulin aspart (NovoRapid) and insulin glulisine (Apidra), has a faster onset of action than soluble insulin.

Insulin aspart is a modified soluble insulin where two amino acids have changed places.

- Faster onset and shorter duration of action than soluble.
- This results in higher preprandial glucose levels and lower postprandial levels.
- Hypoglycaemia occurs less frequently.
- Convenient as the injection is given just before eating or while eating.
- Can also be given intravenously and is an alternative in diabetic emergencies or surgery.
- May be given by continuous subcutaneous infusion as a basal dose with injectable bolus doses.

Subcutaneous administration results in onset of action in 10–20 minutes; time to peak 1 hour; duration of action 3–4 hours.

Intermediate-acting insulins

These have a slower onset and act for varying periods depending on what the insulin is combined with to increase its length of action.

Isophane insulin injection (human – Insulatard, Humulin I, Insuman Basal. Animal – Hypurin, porcine isophane)

Equal amounts of soluble insulin and protamine (a protein) that join together to form a bonded pair. They are always in equal amounts. The insulin has to detach itself from the protamine before it can act on the body.

- Onset 1–2 hours; time to peak 4–8 hours; duration 8–12 hours.
- Neutral protamine Hagedorn (NPH) peaks 3–5 hours; duration 14 ± 3 hours.

Long-acting insulins

IZS (mixed; e.g. Hypurin), Bovine Lente, Protamine Zinc Insulin Hypurin, bovine protamine zinc.

There is more zinc than insulin. It is crystallized and the duration of action varies by varying the size of the crystal. A smaller crystal has a proportionately larger surface area and so a faster onset of action.

Must not be mixed with soluble because there is excess zinc and this will combine with the soluble to make it longer acting.

- Onset 2—4 hours; time to peak 6—20 hours; duration up to 36 hours.

Long-acting analogue insulins

Insulin detemir (Levemir), insulin glargine (Abasagla, Lantus, Toujeo), insulin degludec (Tresiba)

- Long-acting basal insulins usually given once daily at bedtime.
- Human insulins produced by recombinant DNA technology.
- Clear insulin. Must not be mixed with other types.
- When injected form a microprecipitate in the subcutaneous tissue that delays absorption and extends action.
- Allows a fairly constant basal insulin supply and smoothes out unwanted peak effects that are seen with other intermediate- and long-acting insulins.
- Low, flat profile of systemic insulin exposure over 24 hours.

Biphasic insulins

These are premixed set ratios of short-acting and isophane insulin that have been prepared in the pen/vial by the manufacturer.

The soluble or analogue component acts quickly and the isophane component last longer. This allows twice-daily administration before breakfast and evening meal.

Biphasic isophane insulin

(Humulin M3, Insuman Comb 15, 25, 50. Pork Mixtard 30, Hypurin porcine 30/70 mix)

The figures give the percentage of soluble insulin in the combination (e.g. **Humulin M3** is 30% soluble insulin and 70% isophane insulin).

All the range of mixtures that are needed is covered so there is no need to mix.

This improves patient compliance. Available from 10% soluble, 90% isophane to 50% soluble, 50% isophane.

The most common formulation is 30% short acting, 70% isophane.

Biphasic insulin lispro

(Humalog Mix 25, Mix 50)
  25% or 50% *lispro* and 75% or 50% *lispro protamine*.

Biphasic insulin aspart
  (Novomix 30)
  30% aspart and 70% aspart protamine.
  Different types of insulin are summarized in Table 7.1.

Duration of insulin action varies in individuals, and each patient needs his or her own individual assessment.

Administration of insulin
  The standard strength of insulin in the United Kingdom is 100 international units per mL.
  The word units should not be abbreviated, to avoid confusion.
  Small amounts can be measured accurately using special insulin syringes.

- Absorption after subcutaneous injection is variable and influenced by many factors, such as site, angle and depth of injection, time of day, environmental temperature, phase of menstrual cycle, insulin species and formulation used.
- Absorption is slowest from the thigh, but physical activity will affect this.
- There is no difference in potency between human and animal insulins. Human insulin is absorbed from subcutaneous tissue slightly more rapidly than animal insulins, and it has a slightly shorter duration of action. The chief reason for using human insulin is not difference in biological activity but reduced immunogenicity.
- Some sources report that there may be less warning of a hypoglycaemic attack after human than animal insulin.
- The rate of absorption may be affected by smoking, alcohol intake (vasodilation) and drugs such as *propranolol* (peripheral vasoconstriction) and *nifedipine* (vasodilation).
- It has been said that the problem in type I diabetes is not the insulin deficiency but the insulin therapy. This is because getting the correct type of insulin and the regimen right can be difficult.

Insulin regimens
The number of available insulins, injection devices and pumps produce a daunting array of choices.

Insulin is often administered using pen devices which are much more convenient for some patients, especially children.

The overall aim is to produce as near a normal glycaemic profile as is achievable in the individual.

In the young person with type 1 diabetes we need to emulate the body's secretion patterns, where there is a sharp rise in available insulin following meals and snacks with a rapid return to the low basal rate between meals and at night.

To acquire a similar profile with injected insulin would need continuous blood glucose monitoring, together with minute-by-minute insulin regulation.

Insulin devices

Subcutaneous insulin is often injected via a pen device that is either disposable or contains a cartridge refill. Pens are easy to use and always display the number of units to be administered. Many pens have an audible click that can be heard when the dose has been fully administered.

The insulin pump is a small piece of equipment that holds rapid acting insulin in a reservoir. The pump delivers programmed small doses of insulin automatically to keep the blood glucose stable overnight and between meals. The programmed rate can be different from hour to hour if this is necessary and is delivered via a canula inserted subcutaneously. The patient can then administer bolus doses of insulin at mealtimes, at the touch of a button, by using carbohydrate counting.

Common insulin regimens

Because there is absent or near-absent beta cell function in type 1 diabetes, it is essential that insulin is given with an aim to maintaining as near normal blood glucose levels as possible without hypoglycaemia occurring. Evidence accumulated over the past 30 years has shown that multiple daily injections or continuous subcutaneous infusion together with blood glucose monitoring are the most effective forms of treatment. Insulin regimens can be quite complex and need to be targeted to each individual so only examples are given here. Insulin should always be prescribed by brand rather than by generic name because not all brands of insulin are directly interchangeable.

1 Twice-daily short-acting mixed with intermediate-acting insulins
Usually premixed nowadays in a vial or penfill (biphasic insulins) but can be mixed by the patient.

- Advantage — only two injections daily.
- Disadvantage — lack of flexibility. Lunch must be eaten on time to avoid the risk of hypoglycaemia.

Commonest split is 30% soluble and 70% isophane.

Injections should be no closer than 8 hours apart and preferably more than 10.

If postprandial hyperglycaemia is a problem, the percentage of soluble insulin in the mixture can be increased.

Not usually recommended for newly diagnosed adults where a basal-bolus regime offers better control.

2 Twice-daily isophane

Provides good control with minimum risk of hypoglycaemia.

- Particularly effective in older people with type 2, changing to insulin from oral hypoglycaemic agents.
- Some patients with type 2 diabetes may receive just once-daily insulin before breakfast or at bedtime.

3 Basal/bolus regimen This is usually the regimen of choice for those with acute-onset diabetes.

Rapid-acting insulin (soluble insulin or insulin analogue such as *aspart*) is given before meals, three times daily and isophane or a long-acting insulin analogue (e.g. *detemir, glargine*) at bedtime to provide a 24-hour basal level.

NICE recommends using insulin *detemir* (Levemir) as the basal insulin of choice. It was found to be the most clinically and financially effective (NICE, 2019g).

This regimen emulates the body's basal insulin secretion with mealtime boluses.

- Advantages — flexibility of lifestyle, mealtimes, meal sizes and when exercising.
- Disadvantage — need four injections daily.

Basal insulin is usually best given in the late evening. This reduces overlap with the action of the evening soluble.

- Most people need more soluble with breakfast than other meals.
- Most people need less soluble with lunch.
- May vary according to individual lifestyles.
- May not necessarily achieve better control than twice-daily insulin.

Sometimes fast-acting analogue insulins may be given before eating up to five times daily with long-acting insulin at night.

4 Continuous subcutaneous insulin infusion pump

Continuous supply of preprogrammed basal insulin with addition of boluses whenever food is taken. A small pump is attached to the abdomen via a cannula.

This is approved by NICE and usually provides the best control. Not all can manage this system, but it is best when control is difficult to achieve and in pregnancy when good control is vital.

Advantages:

- Most closely matches normal functioning.
- Flexibility of lifestyle.
- Can make adjustments for exercise more easily.

Disadvantages:

- Cost of equipment and disposables.
- Inconvenience of wearing pump.
- Can cause problems on abdominal site.

Side effects of insulin therapy

Hypoglycaemia

This is the main immediate side effect that can occur following the administration of insulin. It is a low blood glucose level that can result in loss of consciousness and can quickly lead to death. It occurs if an insulin injection is not followed by eating. It requires immediate treatment by the administration of quick-acting carbohydrate (e.g. Lucozade or glucose tablets).

The risk of hypoglycaemia is highest before meals and during the night.

Causes include too high a dose of insulin, irregular eating habits, unusual levels of exercise or excessive alcohol intake (Table 7.2).

It is important not to let glucose levels fall less than 4 mmol/L. The saying is 'four is the floor'.

TABLE 7.2 Changes in insulin requirements.

Increased insulin requirements	Decreased insulin requirements
Stress	Renal or hepatic impairment
Accidental or surgical trauma	Some endocrine disorders (e.g. Addison's
Puberty	disease, hypopituitarism)
Second and third trimesters of pregnancy	Coeliac disease

Signs and symptoms of hypoglycaemia
The brain is totally reliant on the blood glucose for its energy and so is the first organ to suffer when glucose levels are low.

- At first there may be just a headache, but as the glucose levels fall, thinking processes are disrupted. Confusion follows and the person may behave strangely, often becoming aggressive.
- Some symptoms of hypoglycaemia are due to adrenaline (epinephrine) release, and these include tremor, pallor and sweating.
- The blood pressure will be normal or even raised slightly.
- If the condition is not corrected, consciousness will be lost.
- Warning signs of hypoglycaemia may be less in those who have had diabetes for many years.

Treatment of hypoglycaemia
Oral glucose or sugar in any form may be given if the patient is fully conscious and cooperative. The person with diabetes should always carry some form of glucose with them in case they feel hypoglycaemic. At first 10–20 g of glucose should be given; 10 g of glucose is found in approximately 3 sugar cubes or 2 teaspoons of sugar. Nondiet forms of Lucozade, Coca-cola, Ribena (take care to check the label because the carbohydrate content of drinks is subject to change) or sparkling glucose drink may be used. If necessary, this can be repeated every 10–15 minutes and should be followed by a snack providing longer lasting carbohydrate such as a sandwich or the next meal, if due.

Glucose is available as a gel for buccal administration in the form of **Glucogel**. This is available on prescription for patients to keep at hand if needed.

Hypoglycaemia causing unconsciousness is an emergency. It may be treated by the administration of **glucagon**, 1 mg, intramuscularly. If it is not effective within 10 minutes, intravenous glucose should be administered. Glucagon is the hormone produced by the alpha cells in the islets of Langerhans. Its action is the reverse of insulin, and glucagon is secreted when glucose levels are low. It stimulates the conversion of glycogen stores in the liver to glucose and so raises blood glucose levels. As soon as possible the patient should be given some longer-lasting carbohydrate (e.g. toast) to restore the liver's levels of glycogen.

Intravenous glucose may be used to treat hypoglycaemia when the patient is unconscious – 50 mL of 20% glucose is given into a large peripheral vein. Glucose is irritant, especially if the needle comes out of the vein and enters the tissues. Glucose 50% is not recommended because of this. Glucose 10% may be used as an alternative, but larger quantities are required.

Lipohypertrophy

Changes in the fat deposits beneath the skin may occur at injection sites after they have been used repeatedly. The fat becomes lumpy and may be unsightly but is otherwise harmless. The site should not be used further as absorption may be erratic.

Drug interactions with insulin

The most important interactions are those that result in a rise or fall in blood glucose levels.

Drugs that may increase the action of insulin

- **Beta blockers** may increase the hypoglycaemic effects of insulin and may also mask the symptoms of hypoglycaemia (e.g. tremor). Recovery from hypoglycaemia is slower. Normally we release adrenaline (epinephrine) in hypoglycaemia, and this increases blood glucose. Beta blockers block the adrenergic receptor and so interfere with this. There is greatest risk with nonselective drugs such as ***propranolol*** and less risk with cardioselective agents such as ***atenolol***.
- **Angiotensin-converting enzyme (ACE) inhibitors** may increase sensitivity in some patients. Three times the incidence of hypoglycaemia has been reported in one trial.
- **Alcohol** gives enhanced hypoglycaemic effect.
- **Some antidepressants** – monoamine oxidase inhibitors (MAOIs) – enhance hypoglycaemic effect. ***Moclobemide*** appears not to do this (see Section 4.5).
- **Anabolic steroids (e.g. *nandrolone* and *testosterone*)** may possibly enhance blood glucose–lowering effects of insulin in some patients. An average reduction of insulin dose of one-third is needed in approximately one-third of patients (Stockley, 2005). The reason is uncertain.
- ***Quinine*** given as an antimalarial or sometimes when used for cramp has been associated with hypoglycaemia in patients without diabetes and thus not receiving insulin. The effect in diabetes has not been studied.
- ***Aspirin*** in large doses can lower blood sugar levels.

Drugs that antagonize the action of insulin or impair glucose tolerance

- Corticosteroids (e.g. ***prednisolone***) can raise blood sugar levels and induce diabetes.
- ***Levothyroxine***.
- ***Furosemide*** may occasionally raise blood glucose levels. Thiazide diuretics (e.g. ***bendroflumethiazide***) do raise blood glucose and can impair the control of diabetes.

- Oral contraceptives and hormone replacement therapy (HRT) may occasionally require adjustment of insulin.
- Calcium channel blockers (e.g. *nifedipine*) – occasional reports only. No precautions appear necessary but just to monitor the effects on glucose control.
- *Lithium* may occasionally impair glucose tolerance.
- Antipsychotics such as *chlorpromazine, clozapine, risperidone* and *olanzapine* are associated with an increased risk of glucose intolerance.
- Studies have shown that those who smoke require more insulin. This may be due to reduced absorption of insulin due to peripheral vasoconstriction and a rise in hormones that oppose the action of insulin.

Oral antidiabetic drugs

These are used in type 2 diabetes that is not controlled by diet alone. Dietary and lifestyle changes will be tried for at least 3 months. If there is no/little response, tablets may be needed in addition to weight loss and regular exercise.

There are several groups of drugs:

- Biguanides (e.g. *metformin*).
- Sulfonylureas (e.g. *gliclazide*).
- Glitazones (e.g. *rosiglitazone*).
- Prandial glucose regulators, the meglitinides (e.g. *nateglinide*).
- Enzyme inhibitors (e.g. *acarbose*).
- Gliptins (dipeptidylpeptidasa-4 inhibitors) (e.g. *alogliptin*).
- Sodium-glucose cotransporter 2 (SGLC2) inhibitors (e.g. *dapagliflozin*).
- Glucagon-like peptide-1 receptor antagonists (e.g. *liraglutide*).

Those with type 2 diabetes should initially be treated with a single oral antidiabetic drug (usually *metformin*), but some patients may be taking more than one type of antidiabetic drug.

- Target HbA$_{1c}$ of 6.5% (48 mmol/L) is recommended when type 2 is treated by diet and lifestyle management alone or a single antidiabetic drug not associated with hypoglycaemia (e.g. metformin).
- When a drug such as a sulfonylurea which can cause hypoglycaemia is used, or the patient is taking two or more antidiabetic drugs, a target level of 7% (53 mmol/L) is aimed for.
- If the HbA$_{1c}$ is poorly controlled on one drug and is 7.5% (58 mmol/L) or more, the drug treatment can be intensified together with reinforcement of the dietary advice and lifestyle measures. Always check that the patient is taking their drugs as prescribed.

Initial treatment

Metformin is recommended as the first drug for the initial treatment of all patients. The majority of patients with type 2 diabetes are overweight, and the main problem is insulin resistance. *Metformin* increases the body's sensitivity to insulin. Other advantages include a reduced risk of hypoglycaemia and additional long-term cardiovascular benefits. If it is contraindicated or the patient cannot tolerate it, then alternatives are offered.

First intensification of treatment

When metformin does not control the HbA_{1c} to less than the agreed level, then it is combined with one of the following:

- A sulfonylurea (e.g. *gliclazide, glipizide*)
- Pioglitazone
- Gliptins (dipeptidylpeptidasa-4 inhibitors) (e.g. *alogliptin*)
- Sodium glucose co-transporter 2 inhibitors (e.g. *dapagliflozin*) but only when sulfonylureas are contraindicated or not tolerated or there is a high risk of hypoglycaemia.

Second intensification of treatment

If still unsuccessful then a triple therapy regimen may be prescribed. One example is *metformin*, a sulfonylurea and a gliptin. Others are found in the British National Formulary (BNF), diabetes section.

Alternatively, it may be appropriate to start insulin-based treatment.

Insulin sensitizers

These act directly against insulin resistance.

Biguanides – metformin

Originated from a plant remedy, French lilac, in the 1950s.

Metformin is the only drug available at the moment. *Phenformin* was discontinued in the 1970s due to high incidence of lactic acidosis.

Metformin is the most extensively used oral agent for type 2 diabetes worldwide.

Mechanism of action

Decreases the endogenous/exogenous insulin requirement. Has a variety of metabolic effects, being antihyperglycaemic rather than hypoglycaemic.

- Does not alter insulin production or release. Increases insulin sensitivity and requires the presence of insulin to work.
- Reduces blood glucose by increasing the body's ability to use it.
- Reduces the production of glucose by the liver mainly by increasing sensitivity to insulin.
- Increases the uptake of glucose by the cells as long as there is some insulin available.
- May interfere with the absorption of glucose.
- Decreases fatty acid oxidation and reduces triglyceride levels.
- Increases intestinal use of glucose with the production of lactate.
- Especially useful in the obese when dietary management has failed.
- May be used on its own or in combination with other antidiabetic drugs or insulin.
- Equally effective in normal weight patients and is now used extensively as monotherapy in all patients with type 2 diabetes inadequately controlled by diet.
- Decreases basal and postprandial glucose measurements after 2−6 weeks of treatment.
- Decreases HbA$_{1c}$, plasma insulin, total cholesterol, low-density lipoprotein (LDL) and triglyceride levels. Slightly increases high-density lipoprotein (HDL) after 3−4 months of treatment.
- Reduces the risks of thromboembolism by making platelets less sticky and increasing clot breakdown.
- Intensive management with *metformin* has been found to significantly reduce diabetes-related complications and mortality (UK Prospective Diabetes Study Group 1998).

Pharmacokinetics
- Quickly absorbed and quickly eliminated unchanged in the urine.
- Time to peak plasma concentration is 1−2 hours, half-life is 2−5 hours. Effect lasts approximately 5 hours.
- Not metabolized and is eliminated unchanged in the urine (90% in 12 hours).
- Gastrointestinal absorption is complete within 6 hours of ingestion.

Contraindications
Need sufficient renal function to avoid accumulation of the drug. Tubular secretion is more important than glomerular filtration.

Lactic acidosis may occur with other chronic conditions and metformin is contraindicated in renal failure or impairment, hepatic impairment, cardiac or respiratory insufficiency and alcohol dependence.

Adverse/side effects

- Side effects are less troublesome if small doses are used at first.
- 5% of patients are not able to tolerate the drug due to gastrointestinal side effects.
- 20% have transient gastrointestinal disturbances − anorexia, epigastric discomfort/pain, nausea, vomiting, wind, diarrhoea.
- Unpleasant metallic taste.
- Lactic acidosis is a very rare but potentially fatal complication. The risks are greatly reduced if metformin is avoided in the presence of hepatic, renal, chest or cardiac disease. Most cases are due to bad prescribing.
- On its own is extremely unlikely to cause hypoglycaemia.
- Does not result in weight gain. Useful in the obese patient.
- With long-term use it may interfere with the absorption of vitamin B_{12} and folic acid.

Efficacy

- Long-term blood glucose−lowering effects are similar to sulfonylureas, although mechanism of action is different.
- Reduces fasting plasma glucose (FPG) by approximately 2−4 mmol/L and HbA_{1c} by 1%−2%.
- Action is dependent on presence of insulin but is independent of weight, age and duration of diabetes.
- Has been shown to delay the onset of type 2 in those with impaired glucose tolerance.
- If used alongside insulin in type 2 diabetes, it decreases the amount of insulin the patient needs (Box 7.2).

BOX 7.2 Advantages of monotherapy with metformin

Unlikely to cause hypoglycaemia
Improves insulin sensitivity
Reduction or stabilization of body weight
Improved blood lipid profile
Reduced risk of myocardial infarction of 39% (UK Prospective Diabetes Study Group 1998) after 10 years
Increased fibrinolysis and reduced clotting tendency.

Thiazolidinediones (glitazones)

Pioglitazone

These drugs were introduced in the late 1990s and reduce insulin resistance. They are known as insulin sensitizers and require the presence of insulin to work. They are used less frequently and carefully monitored due to long-term risks, especially in cardiovascular disease, bladder cancer and eye disease.

Mechanism of action

- Combine with a receptor inside the cell nucleus — peroxisome proliferators-activated receptor-gamma (PPARγ). Known as PPARγ agonists. They may take several weeks for their effect to be seen on blood glucose levels because the drugs act by increasing gene transcription in the nucleus. Full expression of the drug may not occur for 2–3 months after first administration.
- They enhance the response of the tissues to insulin and so target insulin resistance. They aid insulin action by promoting glucose utilization in the tissues and decrease hepatic glucose production and overall cause a decrease in circulating insulin and triglycerides in type 2 diabetes. They reduce insulin resistance and preserve beta cell function when added to metformin or sulfonylureas.
- Lower incidence of hypoglycaemia than sulfonylureas but give an additional decrease in HbA$_{1c}$ of approximately 1%–1.2% that is sustained for at least 2 years.

Cardiovascular safety

Patients with diabetes are at an increased risk of heart disease. The use of these drugs may be associated with weight gain and fluid retention that may make some heart conditions worse. They are contraindicated in heart failure and their use is carefully monitored. They are not advised in the elderly due to the risk of heart failure and have been shown to be associated an increased risk of bladder cancer.

Adverse reactions

- Liver function tests should be done as a precautionary measure before commencement of treatment. Liver function monitored every 2 months for 12 months and then occasionally while still taking the drug.
- Increased risk of fracture mainly of the foot and arm in women.
- Worsening of macular oedema in some patients with decreased vision.
- Increased risk of bladder cancer.
- May cause ovulation to resume and so may be a risk of pregnancy.

Secretagogues

These drugs stimulate the release of preformed insulin from the pancreas.

There are two classes:

- Sulfonylureas.
- Prandial regulators.

Sulfonylureas

The oldest class of antidiabetic drugs that are derived from sulfonamide antibiotics originally.

- Stimulate insulin secretion to lower blood glucose concentration, therefore do require some residual beta cell function to work.
- They can cause weight gain so caution here.
- *Tolbutamide* was introduced in 1956 and *chlorpropamide* in 1957. These are known as first-generation sulfonylureas.
- Second-generation drugs have been developed and display greater potency (e.g. *glibenclamide, gliclazide, glipizide*).
- There is now a third-generation drug that acts on a different part of the sulfonylurea receptor, *glimepiride*.
- May be given as monotherapy or in combination with any differently acting oral antidiabetic agent.

Mechanism of action

- Stimulate insulin secretion by binding to a receptor on the beta cell in the pancreas and allowing an influx of calcium into the cell. This stimulates the release of preformed insulin and results in a fall in plasma glucose levels.
- They are of no use in type 1 diabetes where the beta cells are largely destroyed.
- The drugs have different potencies according to their ability to bind to receptors on the beta cells and stimulate insulin release.
- Usually reduce FPG by 2−4 mmol/L.
- Associated with a fall in HbA_{1c} of 1%−2%.
- Action dependent on adequate beta cell function but independent of age and body weight.
- As the disease progresses, there is a deterioration in beta cell function and insulin may then be required. Insulin resistance remains essentially unchanged.
- There appears to be a lower secondary failure rate with *gliclazide,* and this is the most commonly prescribed drug in this group.

Pharmacokinetics

The drugs are well absorbed orally and reach their peak plasma concentration after 2−4 hours.

Should be taken at least half an hour before food. This is because they are not absorbed until they reach the duodenum.

Their duration of action varies, and this determines the number of doses needed daily.

Sulfonylureas are mostly excreted in the urine and so action is increased in the elderly (whose renal function is impaired) and in those with renal disease.

Cross the placenta and so may cause hypoglycaemia in the newborn.

Adverse/side effects

Hypoglycaemia

Because these drugs increase the release of insulin, hypoglycaemia may occur with their use. The incidence is related to the potency of the drug and its duration of action.

- More likely on the longer-acting preparations and in those with irregular eating habits. Also more likely in patients with good control.
- The hypoglycaemia may be prolonged because the drug will still be exerting its action for some time.
- *Glucagon* should not be used in this hypoglycaemia because it may induce endogenous insulin release.
- Greatest risk in the elderly, when the shorter-acting drugs (e.g. *gliclazide*) should be used.
- Drugs that compete for plasma binding (e.g. *aspirin* and *trimethoprim*) have caused hypoglycaemia.

Severe sulfonylurea-induced hypoglycaemia, although rare, has a high fatality rate. Long-acting sulfonylureas (e.g. glibenclamide) should be avoided in the elderly.

Weight gain

- No glucose is being lost in the urine now and a reduction in calorie intake is needed to prevent weight gain.
- Weight gain is typically approximately 1–4 kg and stabilizes after approximately 6 months.
- The appetite may be stimulated due to lowering of blood glucose.
- Anabolic effects of extra insulin.

Other side effects

- Usually well tolerated.
- Gastrointestinal upset (3%), headache, allergic skin rashes can occur.
- Bone marrow depression and jaundice are extremely rare reactions.
- Sulfonylureas are not recommended in severe hepatic impairment.

Drug interactions

- All bind strongly to plasma albumin and so are involved with interactions with some other drugs (e.g. nonsteroidal anti-inflammatory drugs [NSAIDs], *warfarin, fibrates* and *sulphonamides*) that also bind to albumin.
- Increased action with *aspirin, alcohol, fibrates* and *MAOIs*.
- Decreased action with *thiazides, corticosteroids, furosemide*, oral contraceptives.

Gliclazide

- Taken once or twice daily, half an hour before meals.
- Excreted in the bile and can therefore be used in impaired renal function.
- Less prone to cause hypoglycaemia in the elderly.
- Now available in modified-release preparation — reproducible and predictable progressive release of the drug over 24 hours. No reported incidents of nocturnal hypoglycaemia.

Prandial insulin releasers (meglitinides)

Repaglinide, nateglinide

- Plasma insulin rise during digestion of a meal is lost early in type 2 diabetes.
- These drugs stimulate insulin release. They have a rapid onset and short duration of action.
- Taken immediately before each meal, according to patient's normal pattern of eating.
- Stimulatory effect on beta cell is short lived and so the risk of hypoglycaemia is less.
- May be associated with less weight gain than sulfonylureas.

Adverse/side effects

Despite short duration of action, hypoglycaemia remains the main adverse effect. Incidence much lower than sulfonylureas. Sensitivity reactions (usually transient) have been reported. Caution with erythromycin and antifungals (reduce rate of metabolism).

Other blood glucose lowering drugs

Alpha-glucosidase inhibitors

Acarbose (Glucobay), miglitol

Slows the rate at which glucose enters the circulation after a meal and reduces the rise in postprandial hyperglycaemia.

Inhibit the enzyme alpha-glucosidase in the brush border of the intestine and so delay the splitting down of complex sugars to monosaccharides. This delays the absorption of glucose and reduces the post rise in blood glucose levels, having a smoothing effect on the glucose profile.

- Antihyperglycaemic rather than hypoglycaemic.
- Good safety profile – not usually associated with hypoglycaemic events.
- Does not cause weight gain.
- Not well tolerated.
- Start low – go slow is the motto as acarbose can cause gastrointestinal upset, bloating, flatulence and diarrhoea.
- Cannot lead to hypoglycaemia when given alone but can in combination with a sulfonylurea.

Sodium-glucose cotransporter 2 inhibitors
Canagliflozin, dapagliflozin, empagliflozin

- Reversibly inhibits the SGLT2 transporter in the renal proximal tubule which then reduces the reabsorption of glucose and increases its excretion in the urine.
- Usually combined with other antidiabetic drugs if control poor but may be used alone if the patient is intolerant of metformin.
- Increase the risk of urinary tract infections and rashes in the genital area. Not recommended in kidney disease.
- There may be an increased incidence of DKA, and this may occur atypically when the blood glucose is only moderately raised. Patients should be taught the signs and symptoms of DKA and the SGLT2 inhibitor discontinued if DKA suspected.

Canagliflozin may increase the risk of lower limb amputation, mainly the toes. The Medicines and Healthcare products Regulatory Agency (MHRA) has issued advice while further clinical trials are ongoing. The advice includes careful monitoring of patients with peripheral vascular disease and stopping the drug if any lower limb complications such as skin ulcers occur.

Glucagon-like peptide-1 receptor antagonists
Dulaglutide, exenatide, liraglutide, lixisenatide

- An incretin mimetic that binds to and activates the GLP-1 receptor which increases insulin secretion, suppresses glucagon secretion and slows gastric emptying.
- They have to be given by subcutaneous injection and may be used in combination with metformin or a sulfonylurea, or both, in patients who have not achieved adequate glycaemic control with these drugs alone or in combination.

- They may cause hypoglycaemia.
- *Liraglutide* may be used alongside dietary measures and increased physical activity to manage weight loss.
- Contraindicated in gastrointestinal disease.
- May cause loss of appetite.

Dipeptidylpeptidase-4 inhibitors (gliptins)

Alogliptin, linagliptin, saxagliptin, sitagliptin vildagliptin

Inhibit the enzyme dipeptidylpeptidase-4 (DPP-4). This enzyme normally destroys the hormone incretin which increases insulin secretion and lowers glucagon secretion.

Incretins are produced throughout the day, and levels increase after meals. They increase the levels of insulin when it is needed and reduce glucagon. They usually stay in the bloodstream only a short time before they are broken down.

They are all taken orally.

Associated with less risk of hypoglycaemia and less weight gain than some other antidiabetic drugs.

Prolong the action of insulin and reduce glucagon secretion without appearing to promote weight gain. Research shows that they may improve and preserve beta cell function.

Pancreatitis is a possible side effect, and patients should be warned of the symptoms.

The different groups of oral antidiabetic drugs are shown in Table 7.3.

Insulin in type 2 diabetes

The ability to secret insulin may decline with time, and many patients with type 2 diabetes eventually are given insulin by injection. Sometimes this may be just once daily and may be alongside metformin.

In type 2, insulin should be considered if blood glucose is not controlled by metformin and another oral antidiabetic drug. There should be caution if the patient is obese, because insulin may cause further weight gain with little improvement in blood glucose levels in this instance. Personal preference and fear of needles should also be taken into account. Physical and mental health is important too, and the risk of hypoglycaemia should be taken into account (NICE, 2016).

Obesity management

NICE has produced guidance on the management of obesity because this is a growing problem in the United Kingdom.

TABLE 7.3 Oral hypoglycaemic agents and their action.

Type of drug	Name	Mode of action	Special features	Side effects
Sulfonylureas	Gliclazide Glibenclamide Glimepiride Glipizide Tolbutamide	Augment insulin secretion Need residual pancreatic activity	May rarely cause hypoglycaemia – especially in elderly – may last many hours – treat in hospital Can encourage weight gain	Usually mild and infrequent Gastrointestinal (e.g. nausea, diarrhoea, constipation)
Biguanides	Metformin	Decreases gluconeogenesis Increases peripheral utilization of glucose	Drug of choice in type 2 Do not gain weight Very little danger of hypoglycaemia Reduced risk of cardiovascular disease	Anorexia, nausea, diarrhoea, metallic taste, lactic acidosis
Glitazones	Pioglitazone	Reduce peripheral insulin resistance	Used with other oral hypoglycaemics Not with insulin	Check liver function tests Higher incidence of fractures in females
Meglitinides	Repaglinide Nateglinide	Stimulate insulin release	Rapid onset, short duration of action	Hypoglycaemia Rashes
Glucosidase inhibitor	Acarbose	Enzyme inhibitor – delays digestion of starch and sucrose	May be used in combination with oral drugs or insulin	Flatulence, soft stools, diarrhoea

continued

TABLE 7.3 Oral hypoglycaemic agents and their action.—cont'd.

Type of drug	Name	Mode of action	Special features	Side effects
DPP-4 inhibitor	Alogliptin Linagliptin Saxagliptin Sitagliptin Vildagliptin	Inhibits enzyme DPP-4 Slows inactivation of incretin hormones	May be used in combination with sulfonylurea or metformin Not with insulin	Allergic reactions, runny nose, sore throat, headache
GLP-1 (Glucagon-like peptide-1) receptor antagonists	Exenatide Dulaglutide Liraglutide Lixisenatide	Stimulates insulin secretion when glucose levels raised	In combination with metformin/ sulfonylureas if not controlled on max doses	Nausea, vomiting Hypoglycaemia can lead to pancreatitis
SGLT2 (Sodium glucose cotransporter 2) inhibitors	Canagliflozin Dapagliflozin Empagliflozin	Reversibly inhibit sodium-glucose cotransporter in the renal tubule to reduce glucose reabsorption and increase urinary glucose excretion	Can be used as monotherapy or combined with insulin or other antidiabetic drugs	MHRA (2017) – increased incidence of lower limb amputation – mainly toes. Warning of increased incidence of DKA with dapagliflozin and empagliflozin

DKA, Diabetic ketoacidosis; *DPP-4*, dipeptidylpeptidase-4; *MRHA*, Medicines and Healthcare products Regulatory Agency.

Obesity is a risk factor for type 2 diabetes, heart disease, gallstones and osteoarthritis, and the government has targeted obesity via the media.

Possible underlying causes should be ruled out (e.g. hypothyroidism) and current medication reviewed in case any is likely to cause weight gain (e.g. atypical antipsychotics, insulin, sulfonylureas, lithium or tricyclic antidepressants).

A healthy diet and increased exercise should lead to weight loss. Some may need psychological support, and organizations such as Weight Watchers may help here.

Patients should be monitored for changes in weight as well as changes in blood lipids and blood pressure.

Body mass index

This is calculated by dividing your weight measured in kilograms by your height in metres squared (multiplied by itself). Body mass index (BMI) is expressed in kg/m^2:

$$BMI = \frac{weight\ (kg)}{height \times height\ (m^2)}$$

BMI is used as a measure to classify weight as healthy, overweight or obese (Table 7.4).

Realistic maximum targets for weight loss are 0.5–1 kg weekly with the aim of losing 5%–10% of the person's original weight.

Antiobesity drugs

Over the years there have been many attempts to find suitable drugs to aid in weight loss. Amfetamines were developed as appetite suppressants, as was *fenfluramine,* but there are currently only two drugs on the market to aid weight loss. *Orlistat* acts on the gastrointestinal tract, and *sibutramine* is an appetite suppressant.

Drug treatment should never be used as the only treatment and should be part of an overall weight loss plan which includes diet and exercise.

TABLE 7.4 Classifying overweight and obesity.

Classification	Body mass index (kg/m^2)
Healthy weight	18.5–24.9
Overweight	25–29.9
Obesity I	30–34.9
Obesity II	35–39.9
Obesity III	40 or more

An antiobesity drug should be considered only when the BMI is 30 kg/m^2 or greater and following at least 3 months of supervised diet and exercise failing to achieve a satisfactory reduction in weight. If other risk factors for heart disease or diabetes are present, the drugs may be prescribed with a BMI of 28 kg/m^2. They should be used alongside a reduced calorie diet as an aid to weight loss.

NICE recommends that treatment should not be continued beyond 3 months unless 5% of the original body weight has been lost. If type 2 diabetes is present, the rules may be less strictly applied. Treatment should not be continued beyond 1 year, and two different antiobesity drugs should not be prescribed at the same time.

Drugs that produce a feeling of satiety (e.g. methylcellulose) have been tried in the past to control appetite but have had little success.

Orlistat

Mechanism of action

Orlistat reduces the absorption of fat in the diet by irreversibly inhibiting lipase enzymes in the pancreas and alimentary tract that are needed for the digestion of fats. This prevents the breakdown of dietary fat to fatty acids and glycerol, and there is a dose-related decrease in fat absorption that peaks at approximately 30% of fat eaten. The fat is now lost in the stools making them offensive.

There is no increase in energy expenditure.

Adverse/side effects

These are due to an inability to absorb fat in the diet. There is urgency associated with the need to defaecate, and sometimes this is sufficient to stop the patient taking the drug. May also get an oily leakage from the rectum and some faecal incontinence. Flatulence, abdominal pain and distension, liquid and oily stools and fatigue may also occur. These are lessened if the amount of fat in the diet is reduced.

Liraglutide used in type 2 diabetes (see earlier) may be used as an adjunct in weight management along with the usual measures of increased physical activity.

Appetite suppressants

e.g. Sibutramine

These drugs work centrally and inhibit the reuptake of noradrenaline (norepinephrine) and serotonin in areas within the hypothalamus that regulate food intake. Food intake is reduced, and there is dose-dependent weight loss. There does appear to be an increased rate of energy expenditure that may be related to an adrenergic increase in thermogenesis. Currently, they have been withdrawn or are no longer recommended because of their addictive potential.

Bariatric surgery may be considered with a BMI greater than 40 kg/m² or slightly less if there is a disease that may benefit from weight loss (e.g. hypertension, type 2 diabetes).

7.2 PITUITARY GLAND AND ADRENAL CORTEX

Important hormones that affect the workings of virtually all cells in the body are synthesized and released from these glands. The pituitary gland secretes hormones that control many other endocrine glands but is actually controlled itself by hormones secreted by the hypothalamus. These hormones are shown in Table 7.5.

Anterior pituitary gland

Hormones secreted by the hypothalamus, anterior pituitary and associated glands are controlled by negative feedback systems, and it is beyond the scope of this small text to discuss this. The reader is referred to a physiology text in the further reading list.

TABLE 7.5 Hormones secreted by the hypothalamus and anterior pituitary gland.

Hypothalamic hormone	Anterior pituitary hormone	Effect of anterior pituitary hormone
Corticotropic releasing factor	Adrenocorticotropic hormone	Stimulates secretion of hormones from the adrenal cortex, mainly cortisol
Thyrotropin releasing hormone	Thyroid-stimulating hormone (thyrotropin)	Stimulates secretion of thyroid hormones from thyroid gland
Growth hormone (GH) releasing factor GH inhibitory factor	GH (somatotropin)	Regulates growth Increases lipolysis and protein synthesis Increases blood glucose
Gonadotropin-releasing hormone	Follicle-stimulating hormone Luteinizing hormone	Stimulates growth of ovum Stimulates ovulation Regulates testosterone secretion
Prolactin releasing factor Prolactin inhibitory factor	Prolactin	Development of breast tissue during pregnancy and promotion of milk secretion
Melanocyte-stimulating hormone (MSH) release factor MSH inhibitory factor	MSH	Promotes formation of melanin Also anti-inflammatory and regulates appetite

Growth hormone (somatotropin)

Natural secretion is high in the newborn baby and decreases at approximately 4 years to an intermediate level that is maintained until after puberty, when there is a further decline. Deficiency in growth hormone (GH) results in very slow growth and small stature with normal body proportions are maintained.

- **Synthetic GH (somatotropin)** is used to treat a GH deficiency in children and adults. **Somatotropin** is produced by recombinant DNA technology and is given by subcutaneous injection daily.
- NICE guidance recommends the use of somatotropin in children for proven GH deficiency. Progress is carefully monitored by a paediatrician.
- It is also used in Prader–Willi syndrome, Turner syndrome and chronic renal insufficiency.
- Occasionally the drug is given to adults with severe deficiency.

GH receptor antagonists

Pegvisomant is a synthetic analogue of GH that is a highly selective antagonist at the GH receptor and is used in severe cases of acromegaly.

Adrenocorticotrophic hormone (corticotropin)

Controls the release of glucocorticoids (mainly cortisol) from the adrenal cortex. Used to be used in therapy for inflammatory and autoimmune disorders but has currently been replaced by corticosteroids with a more predictable action.

Posterior pituitary gland

Peptides manufactured in the nervous tissue of the hypothalamus are passed down nerve fibres to the posterior pituitary, where they are stored and secreted as needed.

The two main hormones are antidiuretic hormone (ADH) and oxytocin.

Antidiuretic hormone (Vasopressin)

Released when there is an increase in the concentration of the plasma (as in dehydration or heavy salt intake). Decreases urine output.

ADH is used clinically in diabetes insipidus where there is a deficiency of ADH and large volumes of dilute urine are passed. It is given as **vasopressin** (ADH) or its analogue **desmopressin**. **Vasopressin (Pitressin)** has a vasoconstrictor effect and is used for this action in bleeding **oesophageal varices**. It is given by injection or infusion.

Desmopressin may be given orally or intranasally for maintenance therapy but is also available by injection. It is more potent than vasopressin with a longer effect and does not promote vasoconstriction. **Desmopressin** is used to treat diabetes insipidus and also in primary nocturnal enuresis (bed wetting).

The adrenal cortex

The adrenal glands are situated above the kidneys, and each gland has an outer cortex and an inner medulla. The medulla secretes the hormones adrenaline (epinephrine) and noradrenaline (norepinephrine) and the cortex secretes glucocorticoids (cortisol), mineralocorticoids (aldosterone) and some sex steroids (mainly androgens).

The adrenal gland is essential to life. A deficiency in production of hormones from the adrenal cortex is called **Addison's disease** and is characterized by low blood pressure, muscular weakness, weight loss, depression and hypoglycaemia. Sometimes this occurs as a result of an autoimmune process, but it may follow destruction of the gland by chronic disease such as tuberculosis.

Oversecretion of cortisol by the adrenal cortex results in **Cushing's syndrome**. This is shown in Fig. 7.1. Cushing's may also be secondary to prolonged steroid therapy.

Oversecretion of mineralocorticoids results in a rare hyperaldosteronism called **Conn's syndrome** that is one cause of hypertension.

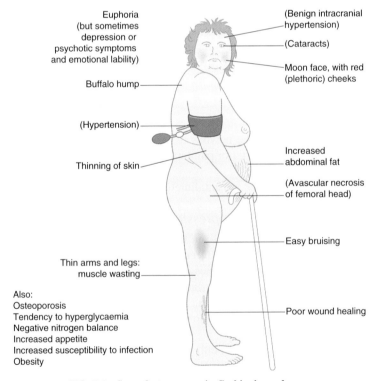

Euphoria
(but sometimes
depression or
psychotic symptoms
and emotional lability)

Buffalo hump

(Hypertension)

Thinning of skin

Thin arms and legs:
muscle wasting

Also:
Osteoporosis
Tendency to hyperglycaemia
Negative nitrogen balance
Increased appetite
Increased susceptibility to infection
Obesity

(Benign intracranial
hypertension)

(Cataracts)

Moon face, with red
(plethoric) cheeks

Increased
abdominal fat

(Avascular necrosis
of femoral head)

Easy bruising

Poor wound healing

FIG. 7.1   **Some features seen in Cushing's syndrome.**

Glucocorticoids

These are synthesized from cholesterol and released as required. In health there is a circadian rhythm of secretion whereby circulation is highest in the morning, reaching a low point in the evening or night time.

- Essential to life and are secreted more in stress.
- It is not known exactly why they are so vital to life.
- Cortisol is the main hormone.
- There are a number of synthetic compounds with similar action, and these are known as corticosteroids. Synthetic steroids include ***prednisolone, methylprednisolone, betamethasone*** and ***dexamethasone***.
- Glucocorticoids have an anti-inflammatory and immunosuppressive action, and it is for these actions that they are used therapeutically. All their other actions then become unwanted side effects.

Mechanism of action

- Bind to specific receptors in the cytoplasm of the cell and then pass into the nucleus of the cell. Receptors are found in nearly all tissues.
- Steroid receptor complex binds to DNA and directs the synthesis of specific proteins by regulating gene expression.
- This means there is a delay of several hours before some beneficial effects become manifest.
- Studies are showing that some effects are immediate and mediated by membrane-bound receptors.
- Some genes are negatively regulated by corticosteroids — those coding for some cytokines (regulatory molecules in immune and inflammatory response) and those for collagenase, an enzyme that plays a role in destruction of joints in rheumatoid arthritis.

Clinical effects

These are the actions when steroids are administered for therapeutic purposes. Unwanted effects occur with large doses or prolonged administration and these are as seen in Cushing's syndrome shown in Fig. 7.1.

Metabolic actions

Mainly affect carbohydrate, lipid and protein metabolism.

- Facilitate the production of glucose in the body (gluconeogenesis).
- Protect glucose-dependent tissues such as the brain and heart from starvation.
- Decrease in uptake and utilization of glucose results in a tendency to hyperglycaemia.

- Decrease sensitivity to insulin. Prolonged treatment may precipitate diabetes mellitus.
- Decrease protein synthesis and increase protein breakdown, particularly in muscle, can lead to muscle wastage.
- Activate lypolysis (fat breakdown) to make glycerol available for gluconeogenesis.
- Produce a negative calcium balance − decrease calcium absorption in the gastrointestinal tract and increase calcium excretion in the kidney. This can result in osteoporosis with long-term steroid use.
- In nonphysiological concentrations have some mineralocorticoid effects and cause retention of sodium and water in the body and loss of potassium. This is not so powerful as aldosterone, but this may lead to hypokalaemic alkalosis, hypertension, oedema and heart failure in some patients.
- Fat redistribution occurs from the extremities to the trunk, neck and face. This leads to the development of a 'moon face' and a 'buffalo hump'. The abdomen tends to be large and striae (stretch marks) may be present.

Anti-inflammatory and immunosuppressive effects

- All inflammatory responses are suppressed including generalized ones such as pyrexia and malaise. May be dangerous in infections as the body no longer responds to the bacteria which can then reproduce freely.
- Decreased production of many cytokines that are inflammatory mediators and a reduced production of prostaglandins (PGs) and leukotrienes that are also involved in the inflammatory response.
- Get decreased production of white blood cells and decreased levels of antibodies.
- Steroids are therefore antiallergic and suppress the allergic response.
- Circulating polymorphs and macrophages are prevented from reaching inflamed tissue.
- Production of inflammatory mediators is suppressed by inhibition of phospholipase A_2 that normally facilitates the breakdown of phospholipids in the cell membrane to arachidonic acid (AA). AA is the precursor of inflammatory mediators, including PGs.
- This may reduce the patient's resistance to infection and may also reduce the clinical features until the infection is advanced.

Overall there is a reduction in chronic inflammation and autoimmune reactions but also decreased healing and a diminished protective inflammatory response.

The MHRA has given advice (2017) that there is a rare risk of central serous chorioretinopathy with local as well as systemic administration of corticosteroids.

Psychological effects
- Steroids tend to cause euphoria mostly. Occasionally, however, severe psychoses can occur.

Some other effects
- Cause growth of body hair in women, including facial hair, and may promote acne.
- Resistance to stomach acid is decreased and prolonged administration may lead to peptic ulceration. Not such a great risk as was believed in the past.
- The skin also will atrophy and become thinner due to decreased collagen production. The capillaries become more fragile and increased bruising may result.
- Inhibition of growth in children is not likely unless continued for more than 6 months.
- There is a small increased risk of cataract formation that is greater in children but is rare.
- Negative feedback results in adrenal suppression and a decrease in production of glucocorticoids.
- Prolonged administration may lead to atrophy of the adrenal gland and an inability to produce cortisol in an emergency. The gland remains atrophic for many months after treatment has stopped.
- Abrupt withdrawal leaves the patient in a state of adrenocortical insufficiency that may be life threatening and leads to a shock-like syndrome.
- In any trauma, those on steroids need more hydrocortisone and should always carry a card to say they are on these drugs.
- Recovery of function of the adrenals takes approximately 2 months but may take up to 18 months in some patients.

If supplementary hydrocortisone is not given perioperatively, these patients are at risk of hypotension and possible cardiovascular collapse.

Mineralocorticoid side effects include hypertension, sodium and water retention and potassium loss. This is most marked with ***fludrocortisone*** but also occurs with ***hydrocortisone***.

Kinetics

Steroids may be administered via many routes, including intravenously, orally, rectally, by inhalation, as nasal spray or eye drops and as cream or ointment for skin conditions.

- ***Prednisolone*** is readily absorbed from the stomach. Plasma concentration peaks in approximately 15 minutes; therefore there is little point in intravenous administration.

- The maximum biological effect occurs after 2—8 hours.
- *Prednisolone* and *dexamethasone* are synthetic drugs with more anti-inflammatory action than hydrocortisone and less salt-retaining properties.

Therapeutic uses

- Replacement therapy. Small doses only are needed here.
- In acute adrenocortical insufficiency hydrocortisone is given intravenously in an infusion of saline.
- Suppression of disease processes. Anti-inflammatory actions in many disorders such as systemic lupus, polyarteritis nodosa, rheumatoid arthritis, ulcerative colitis and Crohn's disease. In inflammation that is due to bacterial infection, steroids can be life-threatening.
- Antiallergic actions. Useful in asthma (see Section 6.1), hay fever and eczema.
- Suppress immune response after organ transplants and also in certain autoimmune diseases such as rheumatoid arthritis, systemic lupus erythematosus (SLE) idiopathic thrombocytopenic purpura and haemolytic anaemias.
- Antitumour properties.
- Antilymphocyte properties and so are given in leukaemia and lymphomas, where steroids may help to delay the progress of the disease.
- In cerebral oedema, *dexamethasone* is used to reduce raised intracranial pressure, especially in cerebral tumours and encephalitis. It is probably an anti-inflammatory effect which reduces vascular permeability.
- *Dexamethasone* is also used in croup to suppress inflammation.
- In anaphylaxis as an adjunct to treatment with adrenaline.

Dosage

- Dosage varies widely in different diseases and in different patients, but the dose given is the smallest needed to produce the required response. This is to try and minimize the side effects.
- The suppressive action on cortisol secretion is least when the steroid is given as one dose in the morning.
- Large doses may be needed in life-threatening disease processes (e.g. acute leukaemia).
- When possible, local administration should be used (e.g. cream in eczema, inhalation is asthma and nasal spray in hay fever). Box 7.3 provides a checklist for patients taking steroids.
- Although inhalation gives fewer systemic effects than oral use, cases of adrenal suppression have occurred. Use of two routes of administration increases this risk.

BOX 7.3 Checklist for patients on systemic steroid therapy.

Patients on systemic steroid therapy must always:
- carry a card giving details of therapy and simple instructions
- be aware of the importance of taking their medication as prescribed
- know what to do if they develop an intercurrent illness or other severe stress – double their dose and tell their doctor
- take an omitted dose as soon as possible so that the daily intake is maintained.

Treatment of intercurrent illness

- When a disease intervenes during the course of another disease, e.g. infection, the normal adrenal response to the stress is to secrete more than 300 mg of cortisol daily. In an intercurrent infection the dose of steroid needs to be doubled and gradually reduced as the patient improves.
- Effective therapy in bacterial infections is important.
- Viral infections can be overwhelming because the immune response may be largely suppressed.

  Table 7.6 shows the relative potencies of some steroids to hydrocortisone.

Thyroid hormones

The thyroid gland is situated in the neck and secretes three main hormones. These are:

- thyroxine (T_4)
- triiodothyronine (T_3)
- calcitonin.

  T_3 and T_4 are important for normal growth and development and also in energy metabolism. Calcitonin is involved in the control of plasma calcium and is discussed later.

  To manufacture its hormones, the thyroid gland requires iodine which is actively taken up from the plasma.

TABLE 7.6 Relative potencies of some steroids to hydrocortisone.

Drug	Relative anti-inflammatory potency	Equivalent anti-inflammatory potency (mg)
Hydrocortisone	1	100
Prednisolone	4	25
Dexamethasone	25	4

Thyroid hormone manufacture and secretion are governed by the anterior pituitary and the hypothalamus (see Table 7.5).

Actions of thyroid hormones

- Increase the metabolism of carbohydrates, fats and proteins, leading to an increase in oxygen consumption, heat generation and basal metabolic rate. Important in a cold environment.
- Excess thyroid hormone leads to tachycardia and possible arrhythmias such as atrial fibrillation.
- Thyroid hormones are also important in normal growth and maturation of the nervous system.

Thyroid disorders

- Hyperthyroidism (thyrotoxicosis) is an overactivity of the gland resulting in an increased metabolic rate, weight loss, tachycardia, increased temperature and sweating and sensitivity to heat.
- Hypothyroidism is decreased activity of the thyroid (used to be known as myxoedema). It is autoimmune in origin and results in bradycardia, slow metabolic rate, weight gain, slow speech, deep voice, sensitivity to the cold and slow thinking.

Drugs used in treatment of thyroid disease

Hyperthyroidism is sometimes treated by surgery, or, more commonly, radioactive iodine is given orally. This is taken up by the thyroid, damaging cells. If underactivity results it is treated by thyroid replacement with T_4.

Carbimazole is a drug that interferes with the production of thyroid hormones and is used to reduce thyroid activity before partial thyroidectomy or for long-term treatment of hyperthyroidism.

Thyroid activity is usually reduced to normal levels in approximately 4 weeks. For long-term therapy the dose is reduced for maintenance therapy for a further 12–18 months.

A rare but dangerous adverse reaction is **bone marrow suppression and agranulocytosis**. Patients should report any sore throat to their doctor.

Propylthiouracil is an alternative to carbimazole that very rarely causes agranulocytosis.

Propranolol (a beta blocker) is sometimes used for rapid relief of symptoms of hyperthyroidism and may be useful alongside other antithyroid drugs.

Hypothyroidism is treated by replacement therapy with thyroid hormones. *Levothyroxine sodium* (thyroxine sodium) is usually used and is given in a daily dose of 100–200 micrograms as maintenance.

7.3 DISORDERS OF BONE AND BONE METABOLISM

Bone is the hardest and most enduring tissue in the human body, and, although it appears inert, its composition is constantly changing. Bone remodelling is due to the activity of two main types of bone cells. Osteoblasts secrete new bone matrix, and osteoclasts break it down. The main hormones involved in bone remodelling are parathyroid hormone (PTH), the vitamin D family (calcitriol), oestrogens and calcitonin.

The mechanical strength of bone is due to deposition of calcium phosphate within its matrix. More than 98% of the calcium in the body is found in bone. Calcium has many other functions in the body and is needed for muscle contraction, glandular secretion, transmission of nerve impulses and blood clotting, to mention a few.

Regulation of calcium metabolism

Calcium absorption in the intestine involves a Ca^{2+}-binding protein, whose synthesis is regulated by calcitriol (the active form of vitamin D). Absorption probably regulates the overall level of calcium in the body.

One form of vitamin D (ergocalciferol) is obtained from plants in the diet. The other form (cholecalciferol) is generated from the skin by the action of ultraviolet (UV) radiation (sunlight). From these, calcitriol (vitamin D) is made in the kidney.

The level of calcium circulating in the plasma is controlled by PTH, calcitriol and calcitonin (from the thyroid gland).

Reduced levels of calcium ions in the plasma stimulate the secretion of PTH. Its secretion is inhibited when calcium levels rise.

- PTH stimulates the formation of the hormone calcitriol from vitamin D in the kidney. This increases calcium absorption from the gut and the mobilization of calcium from bone.
- PTH increases reabsorption of calcium in the kidney tubules and increases phosphate elimination in the urine.
- PTH mobilizes calcium and phosphate from bone and stimulates bone cells (osteoblasts) to secrete new bone matrix.

Calcitonin inhibits bone resorption by inhibiting osteoclasts. In the kidney it decreases the reabsorption of Ca^{2+} and phosphate in the proximal tubule.

Before the menopause in women, oestrogens oppose bone resorbing and calcium mobilization by PTH. Loss of oestrogen after the menopause can lead to osteoporosis.

High therapeutic levels of glucocorticoids inhibit bone formation and may stimulate osteoclasts leading to osteoporosis. This can also happen in over-secretion by the adrenal cortex (see Section 7.2).

Phosphate metabolism

Phosphates play an important role in bone structure but also in the structure and function of all body cells. They are necessary for enzyme action and help to regulate acid–base balance in the body.

Calcitriol regulates active absorption of phosphate in the intestine and PTH increases its elimination in the urine.

Disorders of bone

Osteoporosis is the commonest bone disorder in the United Kingdom. It is a reduction in bone mass that mostly affects women after the menopause. Osteomalacia and its juvenile form, rickets, are due to vitamin D deficiency leading to poor mineralization of bone or Paget's disease, where bone resorption and remodelling are distorted.

Osteoporosis

This is a reduction in bone mass. A reduction in mineral content is osteopenia. In osteoporosis bones fracture easily and this is the reason why so many elderly people fall and fracture the neck of the femur.

Risk factors for osteoporosis

As the population is living longer, osteoporotic fractures are increasingly common.

Osteoporosis occurs most commonly in **postmenopausal women** and those on long-term oral **steroid therapy**.

There are other risk factors and these include:

- smoking
- low body weight
- excess alcohol intake
- lack of physical activity
- early menopause
- family history of osteoporosis.

Women of Afro-Caribbean origin appear less at risk of osteoporosis than those who are white or of Asian origin.

Elderly people who are housebound or in residential homes have an increased risk of deficiency and so may be given supplements of calcium and vitamin D. Supplements are only necessary if dietary intake is inadequate.

NICE has produced guidance (2017) for drug use in postmenopausal osteoporosis available on its website (www.nice.org.uk). *Bisphosphonates* are recommended in osteoporosis to prevent fractures. Only if these are not tolerated, or fractures continue to occur with treatment, are other products recommended.

A combination of lifestyle changes and drug treatment are used to try and prevent bone fractures in those with osteoporosis.

Drugs used to prevent and treat osteoporosis

Bisphosphonates

Alendronic acid, disodium etidronate, ibandronic acid, pamidronate disodium, risedronate sodium, zoledronic acid

Inhibit bone resorption and turnover by action on the osteoclasts. They bind to minerals in bone after administration and are ingested by the osteoclasts when they resorb bone thus exposing them to a high concentration of the drug.

Have been shown to decrease the rate of both vertebral fractures and nonvertebral and hip fractures.

Usually given orally but may be given intravenously in malignancy.

They must be taken on an empty stomach, at least 30 minutes before food, because their absorption is impaired by food, especially milk.

Uses

- Treatment and secondary prevention of osteoporotic fractures.
- Paget's disease.
- Hypercalcaemia in malignancy.
- Bone metastases in breast cancer.

Adverse effects are mainly gastrointestinal but may be severe. Occasionally bone pain may occur.

MHRA advise that atypical femoral fractures have been reported rarely with bisphosphonate treatment, usually when long term for osteoporosis (2011). Patients should be advised to report any thigh, hip or groin pain. Osteonecrosis of the jaw was reported in 2009, and the incidence is greater when receiving intravenous bisphosphonates for the treatment of cancer. All patients should have a dental check before commencing therapy, should maintain good oral hygiene and report any pain or swelling.

Alendronic acid may cause oesophagitis, ulcers and erosions of the oesophagus. The tablets must be swallowed whole with plenty of water while sitting or standing.

Zoledronic acid is given once only by intravenous infusion and is used in hypercalcaemia of malignancy. Renal function and serum electrolytes must be checked prior to its use.

Calcitonin

- This is synthetic salmon calcitonin (*salcatonin*).
- It is considered only in osteoporosis if at high risk and cannot take bisphosphonates.
- May also be used to prevent acute bone loss due to sudden immobility, Paget's disease and hypercalcaemia in malignancy.
- Is given by subcutaneous or intravenous injection.

Adverse/side effects

Include nausea, vomiting, abdominal pain, diarrhoea, flushing, dizziness, headaches and taste disturbances.

Teriparatide

- A recombinant PTH fragment that is used in the treatment of postmenopausal osteoporosis. It increases bone mass and strength by increasing the number of osteoblasts.
- Given by subcutaneous injection once daily.
- NICE recommends its use only in those older than 65 years of age who have suffered two or more fractures with a very low bone density.

Hormone replacement therapy

This is an option (see Section 7.4), but the Committee on Safety of Medicines (CSM) has advised that it should not be used as first line therapy for long-term prevention in women older than 50 years of age. It is of most use when started early in the menopause and continued for up to 5 years. When the HRT is stopped, bone loss resumes, and this may be at an increased rate.

Selective oestrogen receptor modulators

- New nonoestrogen compounds have been developed.
- They are agonists on some tissues and antagonists on others.
- *Raloxifene (Evista)* is a selective oestrogen receptor modulator (SERM) that is licensed for the treatment and prophylaxis of vertebral fractures in postmenopausal women.
- It is an agonist in bone and cardiovascular tissue and an antagonist on breast tissue and the uterus.
- Dose-dependent increase in osteoblast activity and decrease in osteoclast activity.
- It is used when bisphosphonates cannot be tolerated or when bone density continues to decline while taking a bisphosphonate.
- Unwanted effects include hot flushes and leg cramps. It may be associated with an increased risk of thromboembolism.

Vitamin D preparations These are used in vitamin D deficiency and rickets, hypoparathyroidism and bone problems occurring in renal failure.

Vitamin D is taken as *ergocalciferol* to prevent deficiency. Sometimes it is taken combined with calcium.

7.4 SEX HORMONES

In this section, the secretion of both male and female hormones is considered, as are drugs that alter these secretions such as oral contraceptive agents, HRT and drugs used to treat certain forms of malignancy such as prostate cancer.

The events of the menstrual cycle will be briefly explained prior to a description of individual hormones and contraception.

The menstrual cycle

This is a regular cycle of approximately 28 days in women of child-bearing age. Its purpose is to release an ovum from the ovaries each month that could be fertilized by a spermatozoa and to prepare the uterine lining to receive the fertilized egg. Throughout the 28 days of the cycle, hormone levels are closely regulated and constantly changing. Hormones involved are:

- gonadotropin-releasing hormone (GnRH) produced in the hypothalamus
- follicle-stimulating hormone (FSH) and luteinizing hormone (LH) produced in the anterior pituitary
- oestrogen and progesterone produced in the ovary.

Hormonal control is through feedback mechanisms that involve the hypothalamus and the pituitary as well as the ovaries themselves.

There are three phases within the menstrual cycle – the proliferative phase, the luteal phase and menstruation. This is shown in Fig. 7.2.

The proliferative phase

GnRH acts on cells in the anterior pituitary, and FSH is released into the circulation.

FSH promotes the growth of ovarian follicles, one of which develops to become the Graafian follicle and synthesizes oestrogens. The release of oestrogens into the circulation prepares the uterus for ovulation by regenerating the endometrium and increasing the number of progestogen receptors in the endometrium, pituitary and hypothalamus.

Ovulation occurs approximately halfway through the 28-day cycle and is due to a massive surge of LH from the pituitary gland causing swelling and rupture of the follicle.

The luteal phase

The ruptured follicle becomes the corpus luteum and produces progesterone. This thickens the endometrium further, suppresses the release of LH and

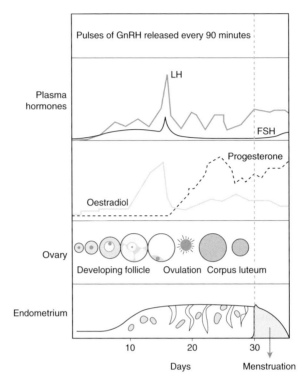

FIG. 7.2 Events in the menstrual cycle. *FSH*, Follicle-stimulating hormone; *GnRH*, gonadotropin-releasing hormone; *LH*, luteinizing hormone. *Reproduced with permission from Greenstein, B., 2004. Trounce's Clinical Pharmacology for Nurses, seventeenth ed. Churchill Livingstone, Edinburgh.*

makes cervical mucus thicker to create a hostile environment for sperm. Progesterone does cause some salt and water retention and increases body temperature by approximately 0.5°C.

If implantation does not occur progesterone secretion stops and menstruation follows. If pregnancy occurs the corpus luteum continues to produce progesterone until this function is taken over by the placenta.

Drugs effecting female reproduction function

Oestrogens

These are steroid hormones secreted by the ovary and placenta and in small amounts by the testes and adrenal cortex.

- All steroid hormones are synthesized from cholesterol. Bind to a nuclear receptor and affect gene transcription and protein manufacture in the nucleus.

- Three main oestrogens are secreted − *oestradiol* (the most potent), *oestrone* and *oestriol.*
- At the menopause, oestrogen replacement therapy prevents menopause symptoms and bone loss.
- Available as oral, transdermal, intramuscular, implantable and topical preparations.
- Well absorbed from the gastrointestinal tract and subject to enterohepatic recycling.
- May be given topically in the vagina as creams or pessaries for local effect.

Uses

- Replacement therapy in ovarian failure (e.g. Turner syndrome).
- At the menopause to control hot flushes, reduce vaginal dryness and preserve bone mass.
- As part of the oral contraceptive pill.
- As treatment in prostate and breast cancer. Now largely replaced by other treatments.

Unwanted effects

- Breast tenderness.
- Nausea, vomiting, anorexia.
- Salt and water retention and oedema.
- Increased risk of thromboembolism.
- Feminization in males.

Breast cancer

This is the most common form of malignancy in women.

Noninvasive breast cancer or ductal carcinoma in situ is restricted to the ducts, where it remains localized. Often though, the cancer is invasive at diagnosis, and this may mean that metastases are present already.

Surgery and radiotherapy may be used to remove the tumour and reduce the risk of its return. When the breast cancer is advanced, it is not curable, but the aim is remission and to have a period of disease-free life or to improve the quality of life by treating or relieving symptoms.

If operable then surgery may be followed by adjuvant therapy to try and eradicate any micrometastases.

How the cancer is treated depends on many factors, including tumour size and grade and spread, the aggressiveness of the cancer and the involvement of any lymph nodes.

A high-dose anthracycline-based chemotherapy regimen is usually preferred to a low-dose one or a non−anthracycline-based regimen (BNF, 2019).

Adjuvant anthracycline-taxane combination chemotherapy is used where this is likely to be beneficial.

Following surgery, *tamoxifen* alone or combined with chemotherapy can be given in premenopausal women if the tumour is oestrogen receptor positive. It is not recommended for ductal carcinoma in situ early breast cancer.

In postmenopausal women with oestrogen receptor–positive early invasive breast cancer, an aromatase inhibitor (e.g. *anastrozole* or *letrozole*) is first line therapy. *Tamoxifen* is an alternative if these are not tolerated.

Adjuvant bisphosphonate therapy has been shown to possible prevent recurrence in bones and improve survival in postmenopausal women with early breast cancer. Intravenous **zoledronic acid** is used.

Useful resource here is NICE (https://bnf.nice.org.uk/drug/zoledronic-acid.html).

Selective oestrogen receptor modulators

Raloxifene is a SERM, that does not affect oestrogen receptors in the breast and uterus but has effects on bone, lipid metabolism and blood coagulation. It can be used for the prevention and treatment of postmenopausal osteoporosis and reduces the incidence of oestrogen-dependent breast cancer with fewer side effects than **tamoxifen**.

Antioestrogens

These drugs compete with natural oestrogens at oestrogen receptors. In contrast to SERMs, which are partial antagonists in some tissues and antagonists in others, antioestrogens are pure oestrogen receptor antagonists.

Tamoxifen

Oestrogen antagonist in breast tissue and so used to treat hormone-sensitive breast cancers. It does give some menopausal side effects such as hot flushes.

Clomifene

Inhibits oestrogen binding in the anterior pituitary, and this causes increased secretion of GnRH with an increase in ovarian size and oestrogen secretion, inducing ovulation. It is used in the treatment of infertility caused by lack of ovulation. There is a risk of twins.

Progestogens

Progesterone is the natural hormone secreted by the corpus luteum and placenta. Small amounts are secreted by the testes and the adrenal cortex.

Acts on nuclear receptors. The density of receptors is controlled by oestrogen.

Progesterone is nearly inactive orally due to metabolism in the liver so other preparations are available.

Some progestogens are testosterone derivatives and so have some andro-genic activity (e.g. **_norethisterone_** and **_norgestrel_**).

Newer progestogens such as **_desogestrel_** and **_gestodene_** are not androgenic and have fewer adverse effects on lipids. They are used if others cause side effects such as depression and acne but have been associated with an increased risk of thromboembolism.

The pharmaceutical actions of the progestogens are the same as its phys-iological action of progesterone.

Uses

- Contraception – with oestrogen as combined pill, alone as progestogen-only pill, implants or injectable progestogen-only contraception, as part of intrauterine device for contraception.
- Combined with oestrogen in HRT.
- Endometriosis.
- In endometrial cancer.

Unwanted effects

- Acne.
- Fluid retention.
- Weight increase.
- Depression.
- Breast discomfort.
- Breakthrough bleeding.

Antiprogestogens

Mifepristone is a partial agonist at the progesterone receptor and sensitizes the uterus to PGs. It is used combined with a PG (e.g. **_gemeprost_**) to terminate pregnancy (see Section 7.5).

Oral contraception

Oral contraceptives ('the pill') are the most reliable and commonly used form of contraception. They may be either a combined pill containing both a syn-thetic oestrogen and a progestogen or they may be a progestogen alone.

Mechanism of action

Raised levels of oestrogen and progestogen do not allow the precise pattern of hormonally controlled events in the menstrual cycle to be maintained.

- In the combined pill, ovulation is prevented.

- The oestrogen inhibits the release of FSH and thus the development of the ovarian follicle.
- The progestogen inhibits LH release and ovulation.
- Oestrogen and progestogen work together to prevent implantation in the uterus.
- Oestrogen and progestogen in appropriate doses and taken perfectly give near-complete reliability with good cycle control unless there is intercurrent illness or drugs that interact are prescribed.
- Oestrogens alone can prevent ovulation but are not completely reliable and increase the risk of thromboembolism and endometrial cancer.
- In the progestogen-only pill, approximately 75% of women still ovulate but the uterine lining is less receptive to implantation and the cervical mucus is thicker and more hostile to sperm penetration.

The combined pill

Ethinyloestradiol is used almost exclusively as the oestrogen content of the combined pill. Occasionally ***mestranol*** is used, and this is metabolized in the liver to ***ethinyloestradiol***.

The oestrogen content of the pill has been reduced over the years since its introduction in 1960. Early oral contraceptives with high oestrogen content are called first generation, and those with lower oestrogen content are second generation.

- The progestogen content may be in the form of ***levonorgestrel*** or ***norethisterone,*** and these compounds do have some androgenic activity.
- There are third-generation pills with less androgenic activity. These contain modified progestogens such as ***desogestrel*** with a highly selective binding affinity for the progestogen receptor and not the androgen receptor. They do not reduce the levels of HDL in the blood which the earlier types do. It is undesirable to reduce HDL levels because this may promote atherosclerosis formation. These newer progestogens give a slightly higher risk of thromboembolism.
- Usually an oestrogen and a progestogen are given throughout the course. These are monophasic pills, and there are many preparations available.
- Oestrogen is given at as low a dose as possible because the risk of thromboembolism is related to the oestrogen content.
- The pill is started on the first day of bleeding in the menstrual cycle.
- It is taken for 21 days then stopped for 7 days. During this period, bleeding occurs. The cycle is then repeated.
- If a pill is missed or taken more than 12 hours late, alternative contraceptive measures must be taken for 7 days.

There are other formulations available, and these are listed fully in the BNF (2019). There are biphasic and triphasic pills with varying composition through the month, but these are less frequently used. They were developed to try and reduce side effects.

Beneficial effects

- Reliable and reversible contraception and avoidance of unwanted pregnancy.
- Reduction in menstrual symptoms such as irregular periods and inter-menstrual bleeding.
- Reduced incidence of benign breast disease, fibroids and ovarian cysts.
- Less premenstrual tension.
- Less benign breast disease.
- Small reduced risk of endometrial and ovarian cancer.
- Reduced risk of pelvic inflammatory disease.
- Less anaemia.

Possible unwanted effects

- Weight gain due to fluid retention and anabolic effects.
- Mild nausea, flushing, dizziness, depression or irritability.
- Acne or increased skin pigmentation.
- Temporary amenorrhoea when the pill is stopped.
- Some women develop hypertension linked to an increase in angiotensi-nogen just after starting the pill. This is reversed when the pill is withdrawn. Blood pressure should be monitored when oral contraceptives are started.
- Small increased risk of thromboembolism. This is increased in smokers, those with hypertension and long-term users, especially those older than 35 years. The incidence in users of the second-generation combined pill is approximately 15 per 100,000 users per year compared with 5 per 100,000 in nonusers per year. The incidence in pregnancy is 60 per 100,000 pregnancies.
- May be a small duration-related increased risk of breast cancer.
- Incidence of cervical cancer is slightly raised in pill users, but there are many variables here. It is advised that women have a smear every 3 years in the United Kingdom.

Drug interactions

Due to lowest effective doses being given, there is little latitude between success and failure if absorption or metabolism is affected.

Some drugs are potent inducers of hepatic drug-metabolizing enzymes.

This leads to enhanced metabolism of the pill and possible failure.

Rifampicin (an antibiotic) is an example. If given for 2 days, it increases metabolism for 4 weeks. *Phenytoin* and *carbamazepine* (antiepileptic drugs) also induce enzymes. Doctors have been sued effectively when epileptic treatment has been started when the woman is on the pill and pregnancy has ensued.

All drugs that induce hepatic enzymes, including alcohol, are a potential risk to efficacy.

Antibiotics and oestrogen

Antibiotics do not interfere with progestogen-only pills, unless enzyme inducers.

Bacteria in the large bowel split the metabolites of oestrogen that have been created in the liver and allow reabsorption of the active oestrogen which is then active again (enterohepatic circulation). The low dose of oestrogen used in oral contraception can be given only because this reabsorption occurs. Broad-spectrum antibiotics kill the bacteria that do this in the colon, and reabsorption of activated oestrogen is reduced. This means contraception will be less effective and pregnancy is possible.

Ampicillin, amoxicillin and related antibiotics as well as *tetracyclines* and *cephalosporins* may all be guilty.

The progestogen-only pill

Less reliable than the combined pill but may be preferred in older women where there is an increased risk of thromboembolism with oestrogen use or in those who cannot take oestrogen because of hypertension.

The pill is taken daily with no interruptions. Failure to take a pill may result in pregnancy.

It alters cervical mucous to prevent sperm penetration and may prevent ovulation in some women.

Disturbances in menstruation are common and include amenorrhoea and spotting of blood between periods.

Long-acting progestogen-only contraception

Medroxyprogesterone can be given intramuscularly as a contraceptive. It is safe and effective, but irregularities of menstruation are common and there can be infertility for many months after the treatment is stopped.

Levonorgestrel is implanted subcutaneously in the form of capsules that are nonbiodegradable. The release of progestogen is over 5 years slowly. Side effects include irregular bleeding and headaches.

Intrauterine devices are also impregnated with *levonorgestrel* and have contraceptive action for 3—5 years.

Emergency contraception

Intended only for occasional use to prevent pregnancy after unprotected intercourse. It is not a form of regular contraception.

Oral administration of *levonorgestrel* is effective and should be taken within 12 hours of unprotected intercourse if possible, and definitely within 72 hours.

- Sold over the counter in pharmacies.
- The next period may be early or late.
- There is an increased risk of ectopic pregnancy, and if lower abdominal pain develops the patient should seek medical advice.

Insertion of an intrauterine device is more effective than hormonal measures and may be inserted up to 5 days after unprotected intercourse or the earliest calculated ovulation date.

Postmenopausal hormone replacement therapy

- Ovarian function decreases after the menopause and oestrogen levels fall.
- Some women develop menopausal symptoms, and HRT may be appropriate to reduce these.
- It is given as oestrogen-only therapy or preferably combined with progestogen and will alleviate symptoms such as hot flushes, sweats and vaginal atrophy, although topical application of oestrogen is preferable for vaginal atrophy.
- HRT will protect against postmenopausal osteoporosis.
- There has been ongoing debate as to the safety of long-term HRT, and the CSM currently recommends the minimum effective dose for the shortest duration.
- Treatment should be reviewed annually and alternatives offered for osteoporosis (see Section 7.3).

Risks with prolonged therapy

- Increased risk of venous thromboembolism, stroke, breast cancer, ovarian cancer and, if oestrogen is given alone, endometrial cancer.
- HRT does not protect against coronary heart disease and does not improve cognitive functioning and so should not be prescribed for these purposes.
- HRT is given in cases of early menopause until the age of 50. This is because of an increased risk of osteoporosis.
- HRT does not provide contraception. A woman should be regarded as fertile for 2 years after her last menstrual period if younger than 50 and for 1 year if older than 50 years.
- The minimum effective dose should be given for the shortest possible duration.

Raloxifene is a bone resorption inhibitor and is licensed for the treatment and prevention of postmenopausal osteoporosis but does not reduce menopausal symptoms. It is not recommended by NICE (https://www.nice.org.uk/guidance/ta160) for the primary prevention of osteoporotic fragility fractures but is an alternative for the secondary prevention in women who are intolerant of other options such as *alendronate.*

Male sex hormones and antagonists

Androgens

Testosterone is the main natural male hormone and is a steroid synthesized from cholesterol. It is made by the interstitial cells in the testis and in small amounts in the ovaries and adrenal cortex.

Androgens are used in replacement therapy in castrated males or those with pituitary or testicular disease who have underactivity of the gonads.

- Treatment should only be given by specialists.
- Androgens are not normally of use in impotence or infertility due to any other cause.
- Intramuscular injections of testosterone esters are used for replacement. **Sustanon** is a longer acting compound and is given by injection monthly.
- Testosterone implants may be used and replaced every 4–5 months, but transdermal patches are currently available.
- Lower doses restore normal testosterone levels and improve sexual function in women following removal of ovaries and without ill effects.

Anabolic steroids

These are drugs with testosterone-like effects. The testosterone has been modified to have less masculinizing effects but still build up protein in bone and muscle. One example is **nandrolone**.

Their use in debilitating disease has been disappointing, but they are used in aplastic anaemia. They are abused by some athletes to increase muscle bulk, and approximately 50 of these preparations are on the prohibited list.

Actions

These depend on the age and sex of the recipient.

- If administered to boys at puberty lead to rapid development of secondary sex characteristics, maturation of reproductive organs and marked increase in muscular strength. There is a gradual increase in height.
- May be accompanied by salt and water retention.
- Skin thickens and may darken.
- Sebaceous glands more active and this may result in acne.
- Growth of facial hair and hair on pubic and axillary regions.
- Vocal cords thicken, and this leads to development of a deeper voice.
- May give a feeling of well-being, increased physical vigour and may increase libido.
- If given to males before puberty, they do not reach their full height due to closure of the epiphyses of long bones.
- Administration of male doses to women results in masculinization.

Adverse/side effects

- Eventual decrease of GnRH from pituitary with infertility following.
- Salt and water retention and oedema.
- Adenocarcinoma of the liver has been reported.
- Impair growth in children, cause acne and lead to masculinization in girls.

High doses of anabolic steroids may in addition cause:

- jaundice and liver tumours
- raised blood pressure
- harmful changes in cholesterol levels (increased LDL and decreased HDL)
- increased risk of coronary heart disease
- left ventricular hypertrophy
- acne.

Antiandrogens

Oestrogens and progestogens have antiandrogen activity. They inhibit GnRH and compete with androgens in target organs.

Cyproterone acetate is an antiandrogen that is a derivative of progesterone. It inhibits sperm manufacture and produces reversible infertility. It is not a contraceptive as it results in the production of abnormal sperm.

Uses

- Prostatic cancer.
- Masculinization and acne in women.
- Precocious puberty in males.
- Severe hypersexuality and deviation in males.

Enzyme inhibitors

Finasteride and **dutasteride** inhibit the enzyme that metabolizes testosterone into its more active form, dihydrotestosterone.

This leads to a reduction in size of the prostate gland, and the drugs are used in benign prostatic hyperplasia. More usually, alpha antagonists such as **terazosin** are used. These relax smooth muscle in the prostate.

GnRH agonists and antagonists

GnRH from the pituitary is inhibited by oestrogens, progesterone and testosterone. Only progestogens are used as inhibitors because they produce fewer unwanted hormonal effects.

Danazol is a synthetic steroid that inhibits GnRH and thus FSH, LH, oestrogen and progesterone secretion. It is used in conditions where it is necessary to reduce hormones such as endometriosis, breast dysplasia and gynaecomastia. It does have androgenic activity but reduces the manufacture of androgens and spermatogenesis in men.

Clomifene is an oestrogen antagonist that stimulates GnRH and is used to treat infertility. It is a stimulant of ovulation.

Gonadorelin

This is synthetic GnRH, and analogues have been made that are agonists initially and then, with continued administration, act as antagonists and reduce release of GnRH.

- *Buserelin, goserelin, leuprorelin, nafarelin* and *triptorelin* are available. They are given by subcutaneous injection, but some may be taken intranasally.
- Used mainly in the treatment of prostate cancer, advanced breast cancer and endometriosis.

Male erectile dysfunction (impotence)

This is the persistent inability to maintain an erection that would permit satisfactory sexual performance. It is a common disorder and may be secondary to ageing, vascular disease or autonomic neuropathy in diabetes. It may also be a side effect of alcohol use or certain drugs (e.g. antihypertensives [especially thiazides], antidepressants and neuroleptics).

Erection depends on both physiological and psychological factors. Relaxation of the smooth muscle in the penis and its arteries is followed by engorgement with blood. This involves the autonomic nervous system and nitric oxide as a vasodilator and smooth muscle relaxant.

The treatment recommended is a combination of lifestyle measures and drug treatment.

Regular exercise is important as well as weight loss if necessary, stopping smoking and reducing alcohol consumption.

Phosphodiesterase type V inhibitors

Sildenafil (Viagra) was the first drug of this type. *Avanafil* and *vardenafil* are also available. *Tadalafil* is longer acting and can be taken as a regular low dose when spontaneity is needed.

- Do not cause erection independent of sexual desire but enhance erectile response to sexual stimulation.
- Nitric oxide activates guanylate cyclase increasing cyclic guanosine monophosphate (cGMP), and this mediates vasodilation. This increases the blood flow to the penis.
- Phosphodiesterase (PDE) inactivates cGMP, and thus, if this enzyme is inhibited, the cGMP is not inactivated and its action is potentiated.

- Peak plasma concentration is reached in 30—120 minutes. This is delayed by eating.
- Given as a single dose as needed.
- Sildenafil is also used for pulmonary arterial hypertension.

Side effects

Mostly due to vasodilation and include flushing, hypotension, headache, dizziness and vomiting. Visual disturbances have also been reported.

If a prolonged erection of greater than 4 hours occurs, medical help should be sought.

The drug may be dangerous if taken with nitrates. Nitrates increase cGMP, and hypotension may be severe if *sildenafil* is also taken.

7.5 PREGNANCY

This section looks at the adverse effects drugs may have in pregnancy as well as drugs commonly used in pregnancy and labour.

Most women are exposed to drugs of one sort or another in pregnancy, so it is important to know which drugs are most likely to cause harm. A single exposure to a drug can affect the fetus when it is rapidly developing, and the recommendation in the BNF is that all drugs should be avoided in the first trimester if at all possible.

Drugs are sometimes given for their therapeutic effects on the fetus itself. Examples would be *dexamethasone* or other steroids when there is a risk of preterm birth. Steroids help to speed up the development of the baby's lungs and so lessen the chance of respiratory problems in babies born prematurely.

Nurses need to have a good working knowledge of the drugs in pregnancy so that women can be correctly informed and advised regarding the potential benefits and risks involved.

Folic acid, one of the vitamin B group and needed for successful cell division, is necessary in early pregnancy. Taking folic acid preconceptually and in early pregnancy is thought to lessen the risk of neural tube defects such as spina bifida.

Drug absorption and distribution

- Most drugs administered find their way to the bloodstream — this is necessary for a systemic action.

- Drugs will pass across the placenta or into breast milk in greater or less quantity depending on certain characteristics of the drugs themselves. Some will not pass at all; others will pass freely. Factors that affect absorption and diffusion across membranes are discussed in Section 1.5. Drugs that are fat soluble cross membranes most readily.

Influence of pregnancy on drug dosage

Pregnancy does cause some changes in pharmacokinetics.

- Transit time in the gut is prolonged.
- Circulating plasma volume is increased — this means a decrease in plasma concentration.
- Increased blood flow to the kidneys may mean more rapid elimination of the drug.
- Total body water and fat are increased.
- Some metabolic pathways in the liver are increased, speeding up metabolism.
- Changes in the level of plasma proteins may affect the amount of drug that is bound.

Most of the time these changes are not important, but where the blood level of the drug is critical (e.g. anticonvulsants), changes of dosage may be necessary.

Adverse effects of drugs in pregnancy

Drugs can have a harmful effect on the fetus at any time during pregnancy.

- Implantation (5–15 days). Abortion usually results from toxicity at this stage.
- First trimester — may be teratogenic (produce developmental abnormalities in the fetus). *Thalidomide* is the best known example.
- Second and third trimesters may affect the growth and functional development or may have a toxic effect on fetal tissues.
- Drugs given at term or during labour may have adverse effects on the neonate after delivery.

Very little information is often available so it can be difficult to give advice.

- Cannot perform the usual randomized clinical trials.
- Safety information is often accumulated through inadvertent use or unlicensed use. Many drugs that are in common use in pregnancy are not licensed for use in pregnant women.
- Drug companies are reluctant to license drugs for use in pregnancy since the thalidomide crisis and there is a fear of litigation.

- Few drugs have actually been proven to cause fetal malformation, but no drug is safe beyond all doubt.
- Drugs that have been available the longest and for which information has been gathered are most frequently used.
- New agents should be avoided if possible.

Drugs can be divided into those known to produce fetal abnormalities, those suspected and those probably not causing harm.

Teratogenesis

A teratogen is a substance that leads to the birth of a malformed baby. Table 7.7 shows some known teratogens and their effects.

- Organogenesis occurs between 18 and 55 days postconception (4–10 weeks).
- The woman may not be aware that she is pregnant or may not have attended a clinic for advice, and exposure to the teratogen may have occurred before the woman has had pregnancy confirmed.
- Identifying teratogens is not easy. Animal studies cannot confirm that a drug is not teratogenic in humans.
- Before **thalidomide** was identified as a teratogen, 10,000 incidences of limb abnormality were caused. It was not teratogenic in the rabbits used for testing the drug.
- Case reports and case studies are used to identify teratogens, but these are unreliable — just because a drug has been taken does not mean it is the definite cause of a malformation.
- There is a background rate of fetal abnormality of approximately 2%–3%.
- Larger cohort studies of several women exposed to the same drug are more reliable.

TABLE 7.7 Some known teratogens and their effects.

Drug	Effects
Lithium	Cardiac defects
Warfarin	Facial and CNS anomalies
Retinoic acid derivatives (vitamin A)	Craniofacial, cardiac and CNS anomalies
Thalidomide	Phocomelia (short or absent long bones)
Some anticonvulsants	Craniofacial anomalies
Phenytoin	Neural tube defects
Sodium valproate	Craniofacial anomalies
Carbamazepine	Neural tube defects

CNS, central nervous system.

Information on drugs and pregnancy is available from the National Teratology Information Service (Tel. 0344 892 0909). Useful website: www.uktis.org.

Other drug effects on pregnancy

- Any other process that occurs during the development of the fetus can be affected.
- Beta blockers can affect fetal growth rate.
- ACE inhibitors can cause renal failure.
- Iodine-containing medicines can affect fetal thyroid function.
- Drugs may be safe at one stage but not at another; for example, *trimethoprim* interferes with folate metabolism so should not be given in the first 3 months but is safe after that.

Where possible, ALL drugs should be avoided in the first trimester of pregnancy.

A risk assessment has to be done, and some drugs may need to be continued (e.g. anticonvulsants).

Prepregnancy counselling is needed when possible in such cases.

Women should be warned about the potential risks of any medication.

When exposed to a teratogen in the first trimester, a woman should be offered ultrasound for prenatal diagnosis.

Some common drug therapy problems in pregnancy

Antiemetics

If vomiting is significant, then you may see these prescribed by the doctor rather than risk dehydration.

Antibiotics

Diverse group with different indications and risks.

You may see penicillins, cephalosporins, erythromycin and trimethoprim used after the first trimester.

Analgesics

Paracetamol has a long and safe history when taken at the correct dosage and should be the first line analgesic agent in pregnancy. It is, of course, dangerous in overdosage because it can cause liver failure.

NSAIDs (e.g. *ibuprofen*) appear relatively safe in the first trimester but can cause problems in later pregnancy. These include fetal renal dysfunction, necrotizing enterocolitis, early closure of patent ductus and intracerebral bleeding.

Aspirin in analgesic doses has been shown to increase the risk of maternal, fetal and neonatal bleeding because it is an antiplatelet agent. In analgesic doses − 600 mg up to four times daily − it is **NOT recommended** in pregnancy. It is used in small doses of 75 mg daily to treat women with recurrent miscarriages and inherited risk of thromboembolism. It is used to prevent preeclampsia and intrauterine growth restriction.

Opiates (e.g. *pethidine, morphine* and *diamorphine*). In analgesic doses there is no evidence of teratogenesis, but with long-term use there is a risk of neonatal withdrawal. Large doses in labour run a risk of respiratory depression.

Anticoagulants

May be needed in those with an acute event or history of previous thromboembolic problems.

Warfarin crosses the placenta and is a teratogen. The critical time of exposure is 6−9 weeks, and the risk of fetal warfarin syndrome is approximately 10%, but there is also a risk of central nervous system abnormalities.

Characteristics of fetal warfarin syndrome include nasal hypoplasia, epiphyseal abnormality, eye defects, shortening of extremities, deafness, developmental retardation, congenital heart disease and scoliosis.

In the second and third trimester there is a danger of fetal intracerebral haemorrhage.

Women on warfarin long term should be converted to heparin as soon as they become pregnant.

Heparin does not cross the placenta or pass into breast milk.

Anticonvulsants

Treatment of epilepsy in pregnancy is problematic because most anticonvulsants are associated with an increased risk of fetal abnormality.

The incidence of congenital abnormality in women taking anticonvulsants is 6%.

Fetal anticonvulsant syndrome (craniofacial abnormalities, growth retardation and intellectual underfunctioning) may occur with *phenytoin, sodium valproate, phenobarbital* and *carbamazepine*.

Carbamazepine and *sodium valproate* are also associated with an increase in neural tube defects.

Risks from the newer drugs such as *lamotrigine* and *gabapentin* are not known. They do not appear to be teratogenic in animal studies.

Corticosteroids

- May be administered for preexisting maternal disease. No evidence of adverse effects on the fetus, but if the mother takes steroids throughout the pregnancy there is a danger of adrenal suppression and extra hydrocortisone may be needed in labour.
- Oral steroids only cross the placenta in very small amounts.
- Used in actual or threatened preterm delivery for lung maturation. ***Dexamethasone*** is used as this crosses the placenta more easily. Given in divided doses over 24–48 hours. Use is associated with decrease in respiratory distress syndrome. Most significant if 48 hours have elapsed between administration and delivery. Significant reduction in perinatal mortality and intraventricular haemorrhage.

Some common medical problems in pregnancy

Diabetes mellitus

- Careful management of preexisting diabetes is essential in pregnancy to avoid complications.
- Oral hypoglycaemic agents hold a risk of teratogenesis and should be stopped. There is also a risk of prolonged hypoglycaemia in the newborn following their use.
- Insulin should be used in all cases of diabetes in pregnancy.
- **Gestational diabetes** is diabetes that is diagnosed for the first time in pregnancy. It usually needs treatment with insulin during the pregnancy, but the blood glucose usually returns to normal following the birth. The woman is at an increased risk of developing type 2 diabetes later in life.

Hypertension in pregnancy

The development of albuminuria in conjunction with hypertension in the second half of pregnancy implies a diagnosis of preeclampsia. Delivery of the baby presents a cure, but the raised blood pressure needs to be treated until this time.

Antihypertensive drugs may be prescribed in pregnancy for preexisting hypertension, pregnancy-induced hypertension or preeclampsia.

Antihypertensive medication in pregnancy

1. **ACE inhibitors** are contraindicated in pregnancy. They have been associated with congenital abnormalities, growth retardation, intrauterine death and fetal anuria.
2. **Beta blockers** – information is currently available that ***atenolol, bisoprolol*** and some other beta blockers may be associated with reduced fetal

blood supply and smaller babies if commenced before 28 weeks' gestation. Better used in the third trimester of pregnancy. The combined beta and alpha blocker *labetalol hydrochloride* has been used extensively and does not appear to be associated with any growth retardation.

- Beta blockers should not be used in those with asthma − they can induce an attack.
- Do cross the placenta and may reduce fetal heart rate.

3. *Methyldopa* is the first line of choice in asthmatic mothers. *Methyldopa* has long been used in pregnancy to lower blood pressure because there is extensive experience with its use in pregnancy and no evidence of adverse effects on the fetus or newborn infant.

- It has recently moved out of favour because it can cause sedation and lethargy and may possibly be implicated in postnatal depression. These side effects may be dose dependent.
- Onset of action is slow so not suitable when rapid control is needed.
- Caution when withdrawing after several weeks, because insomnia and anxiety may occur. The drug should be stopped gradually.

4. **Diuretics** are not used to treat hypertension in pregnancy. This is because they may cause a reduction in circulating blood volume and an impairment in uteroplacental blood flow.

5. The emergency management of hypertension in mothers with **eclampsia** may require intravenous and intramuscular drugs such as *labetalol* or *hydralazine.* Anticonvulsants may be needed too. *Magnesium sulphate* has been shown to have a major role in eclampsia for the prevention of recurrent seizures.

- Given by intravenous infusion and usually continued for 24 hours after the last convulsion.
- Probably exerts its effect by being a cerebral vasodilator and relieving vasospasm. It thus increases cerebral blood flow.
- Care taken to avoid overdosage − signs include loss of patellar reflexes, weakness, nausea, sensation of warmth, flushing, drowsiness and slurred speech. *Calcium gluconate* by injection is used for magnesium toxicity.

Asthma

Drugs used in asthma − *salbutamol, steroid* inhalers − are considered safe in pregnancy and risks are less than the risks of an acute asthma attack to the fetus.

Drugs affecting uterine contractions

Uterine muscle (myometrium) contracts rhythmically with the contractions originating in the muscle itself. Myometrial cells in the fundus act as pacemakers and give rise to action potentials. The activity of these pacemaker cells is regulated by the action of sex hormones.

- The nonpregnant uterus shows weak spontaneous contractions during the first part of the menstrual cycle and stronger, more coordinated contractions during the latter part and in menstruation.
- In early pregnancy the contractions are depressed but return towards the end, increasing in force.
- During pregnancy a condition of relative inexcitability is produced by progesterone release.

Innervation of the uterus

Includes both excitatory and inhibitory sympathetic nerve fibres.

- **Adrenaline**, acting on the **beta adrenoreceptors** inhibits uterine contraction.
- **Noradrenaline**, acting on the **alpha adrenoreceptors**, stimulates uterine contraction.

Myometrial relaxants – tocolytics

There is no perfect agent for abolishing uterine activity in those in preterm labour.

Tocolytics are sometimes beneficial for short-term use to allow transfer to a centre or to allow 48 hours of steroid to be given. There is no evidence that delaying delivery longer than this is of benefit and so these drugs are usually only used short term to allow steroids to be given and to have action.

Atosiban

This is an oxytocin receptor antagonist that may be used between 24 and 33 weeks' gestation to inhibit premature labour. Other drugs occasionally used are *nifedipine*, a calcium channel blocker, and *salbutamol* and *terbutaline*, beta$_2$ agonists.

Contraindications

Abruption placenta, antepartum haemorrhage (requiring immediate delivery), eclampsia, intrauterine fetal death, intrauterine infection, intrauterine growth restriction with abnormal fetal heart rate, placenta praevia, premature rupture of membranes after 30 week's gestation, severe preeclampsia.

Adverse/side effects

- Common or very common – dizziness, headache, hot flushes, hyperglycaemia, hypotension, injection site reaction, nausea, tachycardia, vomiting.
- Uncommon – fever, insomnia, pruritus, rash.

NSAIDs (e.g. indomethacin)

Used in the past because they also delay the onset of labour by preventing the formation of PGs. They may produce unwanted effects on the baby such as impaired renal function.

Drugs that stimulate the uterus

PGs and oxytocics (drugs that induce the uterus to contract) are used to induce abortion or induce or aid labour and to minimize blood loss from the placental site. They include:

- oxytocin and carbetocin
- ergometrine
- PGs E and F (PGE and PGF).

All induce uterine contractions with varying degrees of pain according to the strength of the contractions induced.

Oxytocin

A hormone released from the posterior pituitary gland. Acts on smooth muscle to cause contraction. Receptors are found in the myometrium. It is prepared synthetically for clinical use.

Actions on the uterus

- Contracts the uterus.
- Given by slow intravenous infusion *(Syntocinon)* at term, causes regular coordinated contractions which travel from the fundus to the cervix.
- The strength and frequency of contraction are related to the dose.
- The uterus relaxes completely between contractions.
- Very high doses cause sustained contractions, which interfere with the blood flow through the placenta and lead to fetal distress or even death.

Other actions

Causes contraction of cells in the mammary gland − leads to 'milk let-down' − the expression of milk from the alveoli and ducts.

Given intravenously has a vasodilator effect.

Weak antidiuretic action − can result in water retention which occurs if large doses are infused − may cause a problem if there is a history of eclampsia, cardiac or renal problems.

Uses

- Used to induce or aid labour when the uterine muscle is not functioning adequately.

Can also be used to treat postpartum haemorrhage (bleeding following childbirth).

Unwanted effects

- Large doses can cause transient but serious hypotension with associated tachycardia.
- If given by rapid intravenous injection, electrocardiogram abnormalities can occur.
- Water retention in both mother and fetus can occur with large doses.
- Hyponatraemia (low sodium level in the blood).
- Uterine spasm or hyperstimulation. Uterine activity must be monitored carefully.

A PG, *dinoprostone*, is also available as vaginal tablets, pessaries and vaginal gels for the induction of labour.

Ergometrine

Isolated in 1935 and recognized as the principal oxytocic component in ergot — a fungus that infects rye.

Actions

- Rapid stimulant effect on the uterus following delivery of the baby.
- It is a vasoconstrictor as well.
- Very rapid onset of action — within 5 minutes.

A preparation containing both oxytocin and ergometrine is available for the management of the third stage of labour *(Syntometrine)*.

Unwanted effects

- Can induce vomiting.
- Vasoconstriction can cause a rise in blood pressure with nausea, blurred vision and headache. Vasospasm of the coronary arteries can occur and also angina.

Prostaglandins

- These are **locally acting chemicals** derived from fatty acids within cells.
- They are not preformed but generated as needed by the cells. AA is acted upon by cyclooxygenase (COX) enzymes to form PGs.
- They actually play a part in controlling many physiological processes and are among the most important mediators of the inflammatory process.
- PGs cause contraction of the pregnant and nonpregnant uterus.

- Sensitivity of the uterine muscle to PGs increases during gestation.
- They play a role in dysmenorrhoea and menorrhagia.
- Do have confusing names, but **PGE** and **PGF** families are important in obstetrics.
- **PGE**$_2$ and **PGF**$_2$ have a potent contractile effect on the human uterus and ripen and soften the cervix. Promote a series of coordinated contractions of the uterine body and relax the cervix. **PGE**$_2$ has been most effective in induction.

Gemeprost is a PG given vaginally in a pessary form and suitable for the medical induction of late therapeutic abortion. It is also used before surgical abortion, to ripen the cervix.

Dinoprostone

A synthetic **PGF**$_2$ which is available as vaginal tablets, pessaries and vaginal gels for the induction of labour. The uterus is sensitive to its action at all stages − oxytocin is reliable only in the later stages of pregnancy. It produces frequent, low-intensity contraction of the uterus. May not be felt by all women and wear off after 3−4 hours. Labour will result in 30%−50% of cases.

Side effects

Include nausea and vomiting, diarrhoea, uterine pain, flushing, headache, hypotension, fever and, very rarely, a ruptured uterus.

Carbetocin is used to prevent **uterine atony** (lack of contraction) in patients after a caesarean section. This is to prevent postpartum haemorrhage.

Carboprost is used in postpartum haemorrhage due to uterine atony if patients are unresponsive to ergometrine and oxytocin.

Breastfeeding

Most drugs will pass into the breast milk to some degree, but this is usually in amounts too small to affect the health of the baby. However, the same guidelines need to be applied as in pregnancy, and drugs should be prescribed only when the benefits to the mother outweigh the risk to the baby. Insufficient information is available to produce guidelines, and most drugs cannot be regarded as safe. There is a section at the beginning of the BNF that provides advice on the effects of drugs while breastfeeding. Some useful information:

- Some drugs do not pass into breast milk in significant amounts (e.g. digoxin).
- Other drugs such as lithium do enter into the milk in significant amounts.
- Many sedative drugs do pass into breast milk and may make the baby drowsy and less willing to feed.
- The baby may also develop hypersensitivity to drugs in breast milk (e.g. penicillin).

- Small amounts of alcohol have not been reported to harm the baby, but excessive amounts can produce effects in the baby.
- The concentration of caffeine in breast milk is approximately 1% that in maternal blood, so moderate use of coffee and tea appears safe.
- Opioids do pass into breast milk and may be sufficient to make the baby dependent if the mother is a regular drug user.

Section 8

Chemotherapy, antimicrobials and the immune system

Section Outline

8.1 CANCER CHEMOTHERAPY

This is a very complex area of pharmacology and is the realm of the specialist in oncology. The drugs have anticancer activity but may also damage our normal body cells and so can have severe side effects.

Chemotherapy is a term that was first used to describe treatment by chemical agents that are selectively toxic to micro-organisms, but came to include agents that targeted cancer cells and is now more strongly associated with drugs used in the treatment of cancer. The aim is to manufacture a drug that kills the micro-organism or the cancer cell without affecting normal body cells.

In cancer there is uncontrolled multiplication of body cells that invade and destroy adjacent structures and spread to distant sites (metastasize). It can occur in most cell types and is named according to the tissue of origin — for example, cancer occurring in epithelial cells is carcinoma and in blood-producing cells is leukaemia. It does occur in most plants as well as animals.

Sometimes cancer is referred to as a malignant tumour or neoplasm, and these terms have the same meaning.

- The rate of growth of malignant tumours varies, as does their speed of spread around the body. Some cancers grow very slowly and others extremely quickly. Their response to treatment is also variable.
- Cancer cells are no longer within the body's control and fail to respond to the regulation of cell division.
- They are also invasive and spread to other parts of the body by local invasion, the lymphatic system or the circulatory system. Cancers grow by progressive infiltration, invasion, destruction and penetration of surrounding tissue.

A Nurse's Survival Guide to Drugs in Practice. https://doi.org/10.1016/B978-0-7020-7658-9.00008-1

- Normally if a cell spreads outside its normal tissue it would die, but cancer cells do not. They can continue to grow in another organ — so, for example, a breast cancer may spread to the brain and produce a secondary tumour there.
- Cancer occurs in 1 in 3 of the population in their lifetime, and approximately 25% of people in the UK die from cancer.
- Treatment may be by surgical removal, chemotherapy, radiotherapy or sometimes all of these.
- Systemic therapy where anticancer drugs are introduced into the bloodstream, and thus the whole body, is often used alongside local therapies such as surgery and radiotherapy.

Cell division and cytotoxic drugs

The majority of cells consist of a nucleus surrounded by cytoplasm and a cell membrane. The nucleus contains the genetic material in the form of deoxyribonucleic acid (DNA), and this replicates in cell division. Also within the nucleus is ribonucleic acid (RNA), which determines the type of proteins manufactured by the cell. Most anticancer drugs are intracellular poisons that inhibit mitosis. They are cytotoxic, but susceptibility varies widely between different cancer types. The drug damages and stresses the cell, which then may initiate apoptosis (self-destruction).

- Many cytotoxic drugs target DNA or RNA but cannot do this just in the cancer cells. This means that normal body cells are also affected, giving rise to side effects such as myelosuppression and alopecia. The drugs may be used to actually treat some autoimmune diseases — for example, rheumatoid arthritis and multiple sclerosis, because of their impact on immune cells in an overactive immune system.
- Rapidly dividing cells are usually most sensitive to cytotoxic drugs. They are killed more readily, as they are constantly reproducing their DNA.

Sensitivity to chemotherapy

Twenty-eight per cent of tumours diagnosed in England are treated by curative or palliative chemotherapy, as part of the primary treatment (NCRAS, 2017). This may be chemotherapy alone or as part of a regimen with radiotherapy or tumour removal. The figure varies according to the type and stage of cancer at diagnosis.

Tumours can be divided according to their responsiveness to chemotherapy into those that are highly sensitive, moderately sensitive or resistant.

- **Chemosensitive tumours** may be eradicated by the use of drugs and are usually sensitive to several drugs. Combination chemotherapy is often used and has a greater success rate. Examples include acute lymphatic leukaemia, testicular cancer and Hodgkin lymphoma.

- **Moderately sensitive tumours** only have about 10% complete response to chemotherapy but have about 50% partial response rate. Chemotherapy is not used as first-line treatment but is often used alongside surgery and radiotherapy. Examples include breast cancer, prostate cancer and bladder cancer.
- **Resistant tumours** have a response rate of only about 20%, and it is rare to get a complete response, but chemotherapy may be used alongside other treatments and may be used to reduce symptoms. Examples include colorectal cancer, gliomas and pancreatic cancer.

The cell cycle

Some cells within the body have the ability to divide rapidly because they are constantly replaced as they wear out. Examples include the epidermis of the skin, the lining of the gastrointestinal tract and the blood-producing cells in the bone marrow. Other cells (e.g. liver) rarely divide but retain the ability to divide in organ damage, and cells such as neurones have little or no ability to divide when mature.

The cell cycle is the period from the beginning of one cell division to the beginning of the next. It is the orderly sequence of events by which a cell duplicates its contents and divides in two.

- Cell division replaces dead or injured cells and adds new ones for tissue growth.
- When a cell divides, each original cell becomes two daughter cells.
- Both will be genetically identical to the parent cell.

The cell cycle involves five phases. These are G_1, S, G_2, M and G_0 and are shown in Fig. 8.1. Interphase is the period from cell formation to cell division (G_1, S and G_2 phases), during which the DNA in the nucleus replicates.

G_1 phase

- Occurs immediately after a new cell has been produced.
- G stands for 'gap' or 'growth', and G_1 is the period between the end of cell division and DNA replication.
- It is a period of growth, RNA and protein synthesis.
- It is the most variable phase in terms of length. Cells with a rapid division time have a G_1 of minutes or hours in length. In those that divide slowly, it can last days or even years.

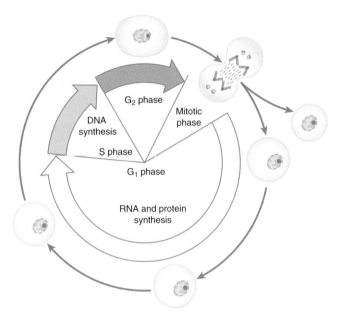

FIG. 8.1 **Phases in the cell cycle.** *DNA,* Deoxyribonucleic acid; *RNA,* ribonucleic acid. *Reproduced with permission from Greenstein, B., 2004. Trounce's Clinical Pharmacology for Nurses, seventeenth ed. Churchill Livingstone, Edinburgh.*

S phase

- S stands for 'synthesis'. It is in this phase that the DNA replicates precisely.
- It lasts about 6–8 hours but is variable.

G₂ phase

- This is the second gap phase and growth continues.
- It is very brief, about 4–6 hours.
- Synthesis of enzymes, RNA and other proteins needed for division is completed.
- Before mitosis can occur, the cell must approximately double its mass and contents.

M (mitotic) phase

Division of the cell that involves both division of the nucleus and of the cytoplasm.

The duration varies according to the type of cell; it is typically about 2 hours from start to finish.

G_0 phase

The cell is in a resting state. In adult tissue, not all cells divide at once and many are in this resting state.

Control of cell division

- Chemical signals released by other cells and the availability of space have an influence.
- Availability of nutrients and the presence or absence of growth factors are important.
- Normal cells stop dividing when they are touching. This is contact inhibition, and it is lost in cancer cells.
- Doubling time is the time a cancer cell takes to complete the cell cycle once.
- Cancer cells may not complete the cell cycle more rapidly than normal cells, and some take much longer.

Drugs used in cancer chemotherapy

The beginnings of cancer chemotherapy can be traced back to the drugs, such as nitrogen mustard gas, that were used in the Second World War and killed body cells. Anticancer drugs did not really come into use until the 1960s, and since then, the number available has been steadily increasing. As understanding of cellular biology, the immune system and cell death increases, new drugs with greater selectivity for the cancer cell are likely to be developed. The immune system is becoming the target for more therapies.

Mechanism of action

Most drugs target the rapidly dividing cancer cell, although they have a variety of mechanisms and act at different points in the process of DNA synthesis during the cell cycle.

- By targeting the rapidly dividing cell, the drugs affect our normal body cells less but will attack those cells that are still dividing regularly, such as the lining of the gastrointestinal tract. Because of this, many cancer drugs have the same side effects and are extremely toxic.
- Cells that are resting in the G_0 phase are resistant to many anticancer drugs.
- The sensitivity of the cancer depends on the number of its cells that are in the growth phase when the anticancer drug is given.
- We can sometimes target different points of the cell cycle with different drugs.

- **Burkitt's lymphoma** is an extremely fast-growing cancer, and nearly all the cells are in the growth phase. It is extremely responsive to even one dose of chemotherapy.
- In slow-growing tumours, such as most types of **colorectal cancer**, only about 5% of cells are in the growing phase, and this makes the tumour relatively insensitive to chemotherapy.
- Complete eradication of the cancer is needed or the growth can recur. This is not usually possible because of the side effects of the drugs.
- Drugs kill a certain percentage of cells each time they are given, and thus multiple treatments are needed.
- Sometimes clinical remission is induced in fast-growing tumours, such as **acute myeloid leukaemia** and **small-cell lung cancer**, but if all cells are not eradicated, the fast-growing cells can quickly produce a clinical relapse.

Resistance

Cancer cells may develop resistance to chemotherapy by several different mechanisms. They may:

- reduce drug uptake by a transporter as in ***methotrexate***
- use new biochemical pathways instead of those blocked by the drug as with ***asparaginase***
- inactivate the drug as with ***cisplatin***
- increase removal of the drug from the cancer cell by a glycoprotein pump, as occurs with multiple drug resistance (MDR) to unrelated compounds such as ***etoposide*** and ***taxanes***. The pump can be inactivated by unrelated drugs such as ***nifedipine, ciclosporin*** and ***tamoxifen.*** More effective inhibitors are being developed
- decrease the activation of a prodrug as with ***cytarabine***
- reduce sensitivity of the target of the anticancer drug as with anthracyclines

Cytotoxic drugs fall into a number of classes, each with their own anti-tumour activity, toxicity and sites of action. The drugs are dangerous and can be more toxic if not handled according to guidelines. Each trust will have its own policies, and here we provide the guidelines published in the British National Formulary (BNF, 2019). These guidelines include:

- Trained personnel should reconstitute cytotoxics.
- Reconstitution should be in designated pharmacy areas.
- Protective clothing (gloves, gowns and masks) should be worn.
- Pregnant staff should avoid exposure to cytotoxic drugs.
- The local procedures for spillage and safe disposal of waste material should be used.
- Staff exposure to cytotoxic drugs should be monitored.

There is special guidance for safe practice if the drugs are given intra-thecally, and this is available on the Department of Health website (www.dh.gov.uk).

Doses of cytotoxic drugs are calculated using a variety of different methods. These include body weight or body surface area, but other factors are increasingly taken into account as more is learned about genetic differences in the metabolism of these drugs. Ideally, each drug dose is calculated specif-ically for the patient who is to receive it.

Unwanted effects of drugs

Rapidly growing cells in normal body tissue are often affected by cytotoxic drugs. Many have a therapeutic index of 1, meaning that the dose needed to be effective is also the toxic dose. They are the most toxic group of drugs used in therapeutics, and courses have to be planned so that healthy cells such as those in the bone marrow can recover between doses of the drug. The cancer cells do not recover as fully and so more are eradicated with each dose of the drug.

Many side effects do not occur immediately but days or even weeks later. Patients need to know and understand this so that they can identify the symptoms and contact their team for advice.

The adverse effects listed here are common to many anticancer drugs.

Extravasation of intravenous cytotoxic drugs

Many cytotoxic drugs will cause local tissue necrosis if the needle comes out of the vein and into the tissues.

Extravasation of intravenous drugs can lead to severe local tissue necrosis, and drugs must only be administered by those trained in their use.

Sore mouth (oral mucositis)

This is a common complication, especially with *fluorouracil, methotrexate* and the *anthracyclines*.

- The aim is to prevent mucositis and ulceration by good mouth care. This includes rinsing the mouth frequently and brushing the teeth with a very soft toothbrush.
- Ice chips may be sucked during short infusions of fluorouracil.

- The sore mouth is difficult to treat when it has occurred, but saline mouthwashes may be used.
- Although there is no evidence for the benefits of anti-inflammatory or antiseptic mouthwashes, the patient may find these helpful.
- The danger is the entry of bacteria into the bloodstream if oral hygiene is poor.

Nausea and vomiting

This can be severe with high doses of certain drugs. It is worse with **cisplatin, cyclophosphamide** and **dacarbazine** and may limit the patient's tolerance of the drug.

- Patients vary in their susceptibility to nausea and vomiting, but it often increases with the number of treatments.
- The most effective antiemetics are the 5-HT$_3$ antagonists such as **ondansetron**, and in those at high risk of vomiting, this may be combined with other drugs such as the corticosteroid **dexamethasone** or the anxiolytic **lorazepam**.
- **Aprepitant** is a neurokinin 1 receptor antagonist licensed to control vomiting with **cisplatin**.
- **Nabilone** is a synthetic cannabinoid that may be used if patients are unresponsive to other antiemetics.
- The cytotoxic drug may be given at night so that the patient can be sedated, and sleep may reduce the nausea.
- Antiemetics are given 24 hours before starting the therapy and continuously to prevent symptoms.
- Delayed nausea and vomiting may occur more than 24 hours after treatment. This is best controlled using **dexamethasone** often combined with an antiemetic such as **ondansetron**.

Bone marrow suppression

All cytotoxic drugs except **vincristine** and **bleomycin** cause bone marrow suppression usually 7–10 days after they are given, but this may be longer in some cases. This leads to a fall in blood cells, especially white cells, and thus increased risk of infection by bacteria, viruses and candidiasis (thrush).

- All patients must have their white cell count (WCC) checked before each treatment.
- The treatment cannot be given if the WCC is too low because the bone marrow has not recovered from the last drug treatment.
- If the temperature is raised in those with a low WCC, it must be treated immediately with a broad-spectrum antibiotic, as sepsis may be fatal.

- Sometimes bone marrow growth factors may be given.
- Red cell transfusions are used to treat anaemia.

Gastrointestinal tract

Ulceration here may be associated with diarrhoea.

Alopecia

Reversible hair loss occurs with many drugs due to the effect on the hair follicle.

Reproductive function

Most of these drugs are teratogenic and so should not be administered in pregnancy, especially the first 3 months.

- Contraception should be used prior to, during and for a period following therapy.
- In women, menstrual irregularity or amenorrhoea may occur.
- Occasionally infertility may occur and is commoner with alkylating agents. This is more frequent in women over 35 and men. Sperm may be banked prior to therapy.
- Women may have a shortened reproductive life and an early menopause.

Tumour lysis syndrome

This is secondary to the breakdown of so many cells.

- Features include raised levels of potassium, uric acid and phosphates but low levels of calcium in the blood.
- It may lead to renal damage and cardiac arrhythmias.
- *Allopurinol* is used to prevent hyperuricaemia and is given prior to treatment in certain lymphomas and leukaemias where this is common.
- The patient should be well hydrated.

Thromboembolism

There is an increased risk in cancer, and this is raised when chemotherapy is used.

Growing tissues

- Cytotoxic drugs can impair growth in children.
- There is an increased risk of developing a second malignancy, often leukaemia.

The individual groups of drugs will now be listed and briefly described under the headings of their mechanism of action.

Specific cytotoxic agents

This is a very specialized area, and the reader should look up individual drugs in the BNF for a full description of their uses and side effects. A broad outline is given here.

Drugs affecting deoxyribonucleic acid synthesis and function

Alkylating drugs

Bendamustine, cyclophosphamide, chlorambucil, busulfan, carmustine, estramustine, lomustine, ifosfamide, melphalan, streptozocin, temozolomide, thiotepa, treosulfan

- They damage DNA and thus interfere with cell replication, preventing DNA and RNA synthesis.
- They are not cell cycle specific.
- Some may be given orally.
- Widely used group of drugs that contains some of the earliest to be licensed.
- First developed from nitrogen mustard gas used in the First World War as chemical warfare.

Unwanted effects
- Gametogenesis is severely affected giving impaired fertility.
- Long-term use is associated with an increased risk of acute myeloid leukaemia.
- Bone marrow depression and neutropenia.
- Pulmonary fibrosis with **busulfan, carmustine** and **treosulfan**.
- Skin pigmentation with **busulfan** and **treosulfan**.
- Haemorrhagic cystitis with **cyclophosphamide** and **ifosfamide**. This is prevented by treatment with **mesna** before therapy. There is an increased risk of bladder cancer years later.

Platinum compounds

Cisplatin, carboplatin, oxaliplatin These enter cells and break the DNA chain by crosslinking guanine units. This is a similar action to the alkylating drugs.

- Used in ovarian and testicular cancer. **Oxaliplatin** is used in advanced colorectal cancer.
- Not absorbed well orally and are given intravenously.

Unwanted effects

- Severe nausea and vomiting, especially with *cisplatin*.
- Nephrotoxicity with *cisplatin*, so renal function must be monitored. Good hydration reduces the risk.
- Peripheral neuropathy may also occur.
- These effects are less with *carboplatin*, but bone marrow suppression is greater.
- Ototoxicity that can result in tinnitus and deafness.

Topoisomerase I inhibitors

Irinotecan, topotecan Derived from an alkaloid in the Chinese tree *Camptotheca acuminata.*

- Topoisomerase I is important in DNA replication, and these drugs are active in the S phase of the cell cycle.
- Used in metastatic ovarian and colorectal cancer.
- Given by intravenous infusion.
- Side effects include bone marrow suppression that is dose related and diarrhoea that may be delayed.

Cytotoxic anthracycline antibiotics and related drugs

Anthracyclines are among the most effective anticancer drugs and are effective against many types of cancer. Their main side effects are cardiotoxicity and myelosuppression.

They act by intercalating with DNA and interfering with DNA metabolism and RNA production.

Anthracycline antibiotics – daunorubicin, doxorubicin, epirubicin, idarubicin.

Related drugs – bleomycin, mitomycin, mitoxantrone, pixantrone.

Some increase reactive chemicals (free radicals) and these cause DNA damage.

Some cause breaks in the strands of DNA while others interfere with cell membrane function.

- Widely used drugs but many of them are radiomimetics and should not be used alongside radiotherapy as this increases toxicity.
- Not usually cycle specific.
- Not well absorbed so given intravenously.

Unwanted effects

- *Doxorubicin*, epirubicin and mitoxantrone cause myocardial cell damage that is dose dependent.
- *Bleomycin* and *mitomycin* cause dose-related pulmonary fibrosis.

Antimetabolites

Azacitidine, capecitabine, cladribine, clofarabine, cytarabine, decitabine, fludarabine, fluorouracil, gemcitabine, mercaptopurine, methotrexate, tioguanine, trifluridine

Interfere with normal metabolism and prevent normal cellular division by either combining with enzymes needed or by being falsely incorporated into new DNA.

Methotrexate

Inhibits the enzyme *dihydrofolate reductase* and blocks the synthesis of purines and pyrimidines that are needed to make DNA, RNA and proteins.

- Active in the S phase of the cell cycle and slows G_1 to S phase.
- Used in acute lymphatic leukaemia and non-Hodgkin lymphoma.
- Is also used to treat nonmalignant conditions such as rheumatoid arthritis, severe Crohn's disease and psoriasis.

Unwanted effects Include bone marrow suppression and pulmonary fibrosis with chronic administration.

- Nonsteroidal anti-inflammatory drugs (NSAIDs) such as aspirin may reduce renal excretion and so increase blood levels into the toxic range.
- Folinic acid *(leucovorin)* is often administered after high doses to provide folate and rescue some of the normal body tissues, so reducing suppression of the bone marrow and inflammation of mucous membranes.

Base analogues

Capecitabine, cladribine, cytarabine, fludarabine, fluorouracil, gemcitabine, mercaptopurine, tegafur, tioguanine

- These drugs have been produced by modifying purine and pyrimidine bases and so interfering with DNA synthesis.
- Most are given by injection as absorption orally may be predictable.
- Suppression of the bone marrow is usually severe.

Capecitabine is metabolized to *fluorouracil*. It is given alone or with *oxaliplatin* in treatment of advanced colorectal cancer. It is also used in gastric cancer.

Cytarabine is used to produce a remission in acute myeloid leukaemia.

Gemcitabine is first-line treatment for pancreatic cancer where surgery is not possible.

Details of other drugs in this group can be found in the BNF.

Vinca alkaloids and etoposide

Vincristine, vinblastine, vindesinc, vinflunine, vinorelbine Isolated from the periwinkle plant *(Vinca rosea)*. ***Etoposide*** is a synthetic derivative of the mandrake root.

- Cycle specific and stop metaphase.
- Mostly used for leukaemias and lymphomas.
- Usually given intravenously.

Unwanted effects
- With ***vinblastine*** and ***vinorelbine*** suppression of the bone marrow limits the dose, but this does not usually occur with ***vincristine.***
- ***Vincristine*** is neurotoxic.
- Produce severe tissue damage if they come out of the vein.

Taxanes

Paclitaxel, cabazitaxel, docetaxel Extracted from the bark of the Pacific Yew tree *(Taxus brevifolia).* They interfere with microtubules in the cell similar to vinca alkaloids but attach to a different site. The microtubules are needed for many cell functions, including cell division, so these drugs inhibit mitosis.

Poor absorption orally and so are given intravenously.

National Institute for Health and Care Excellence (NICE) guidance is available for the use of taxanes in the treatment of breast cancer, ovarian cancer and prostate cancer.

Unwanted effects

Severe hypersensitivity reactions can occur with hypotension, bronchospasm and angioedema. To lessen this, ***dexamethasone*** may be given prior to administration.

Trastuzumab (Herceptin)

Licensed for the treatment of early breast cancer that overexpresses human epidermal growth factor receptor-2 (HER-2).

Also licensed in other sensitive metastatic breast cancers, and there is NICE guidance available for its use.

- Given by intravenous infusion. Resuscitation facilities must be available, and only a specialist can initiate treatment.

- Infusion side effects such as shivering, fever and hypersensitivity reactions may occur.
- Unwanted effects include cardiotoxicity, hypotension, chest pain, headache, gastrointestinal disturbances and peripheral neuropathy.

Tretinoin

This is a form of vitamin A that is licensed for some types of leukaemia. It is also used in the treatment of extremely severe acne under the care of a specialist.

It must be avoided in those who may become pregnant or are pregnant, as it may cause fetal deformities.

Bexarotene

This is an agonist at the retinoid X receptor which is involved with the regulation of cell proliferation and differentiation.

It is used in cutaneous T-cell lymphoma where it may cause a regression.

Other antineoplastic drugs

Amsacrine is used in acute leukaemia which is not responding to anthracycline chemotherapy. It intercalates into the DNA of tumour cells.

Asparaginase is an enzyme that disrupts protein synthesis in tumour cells. It is used in acute lymphoblastic leukaemia as part of a drug regimen.

Eribulin is a synthetic analogue of a substance found in marine sponges. It is a mitotic inhibitor and is used occasionally in metastatic breast cancer after treatment with other drugs.

Hydroxycarbamide is occasionally used in polycythaemia vera, thrombocytopaenia, sickle cell disease and chronic myeloid leukaemia.

Panobinostat is a histone deacetylase inhibitor and is important in the treatment of multiple myeloma.

Pegaspargase breaks down the amino acid asparagine and interferes with the growth of malignant cells which cannot synthesis this amino acid. It is used in acute lymphoblastic leukaemia.

Procarbazine is a monoamine oxidase inhibitor that is used in Hodgkin lymphoma.

Raltitrexed is a thymidylate synthase inhibitor that causes damage to DNA and is used in palliative care in advanced colorectal cancer when other regimens cannot be used.

Hormones and antagonists used in cancer therapy

Some malignant cells have steroid receptors and are hormone dependent. This means their growth can be inhibited by blocking the receptors or by giving hormones with an opposing action. This is not usually sufficient to cure but can be an important element in treatment, especially of sex hormone−dependent cancers.

Glucocorticoids − dexamethasone, prednisolone

- These are used in leukaemias and lymphomas because they suppress lymphocyte proliferation.
- Also useful in reducing raised intracranial pressure and oedema around a tumour.

Oestrogens

Diethylstilbestrol and *ethinylestradiol* are used in palliative care to suppress androgen-dependent prostate cancer cells and metastases.

Gonadotropin releasing hormone analogues − *goserelin, buserelin, leuprorelin* and *triptorelin* are used to treat advanced breast cancer and prostate cancer (see Section 7.4).

Oestrogen antagonists

- *Tamoxifen* is very effective in some types of breast cancer. This is given orally and binds to oestrogen receptors. Its effects on bone are oestrogenic, but its effects on breast tissue are antioestrogenic (Section 7.5). It has side effects similar to menopausal symptoms − for example, hot flushes.
- Synthesis of oestrogen from androgens is prevented by aromatase inhibitors that block the enzyme needed for this reaction − for example, *anastrozole*. These are used in some types of breast cancer.

Androgen antagonists

These suppress prostate cancer − for example, *flutamide, cyproterone* and *bicalutamide*.

Monoclonal antibodies

These are antibodies that react with proteins on cancer cells and so can be used to target the cancer cell.

Rituximab is used in certain lymphomas, and *alemtuzumab* is used in resistant chronic lymphocytic leukaemia.

Trastuzumab (Herceptin) binds to HER-2, which is a human growth factor receptor that is overexpressed in about a quarter of breast cancers, causing them to grow rapidly. Treatment with this monoclonal antibody is combined with other agents and has increased survival in a high percentage of patients with aggressive breast cancer of this type.

Treatment regimens

Often combinations of anticancer drugs are used to increase cytotoxicity without always increasing the side effects.

This decreases the chance of resistance to individual drugs developing.

Drugs are usually given in high doses with intervals of 2—3 weeks between courses to allow the bone marrow to recover. If the drugs were given in smaller doses constantly, the activity of the bone marrow would be depressed.

NICE guidance for the use of many of these drugs in certain cancers is available on their website: www.nice.org.uk.

8.2 ANTIMICROBIAL DRUGS

Micro-organisms are too small to be seen by the unaided eye. They include bacteria, viruses, protozoa and some fungi. Drug treatment used to destroy any parasite without destroying the host is termed chemotherapy and this includes antibiotics and antiviral agents. The term is now mostly used to describe anticancer drugs where the aim is to destroy the cancer cell without destroying the body's normal cells. Ehrlich invented the word, 'chemotherapy' in 1906 when he found he could selectively kill certain bacteria with aniline dyes used to stain them. Chemicals had been used before this to combat infection such as mercury to treat syphilis (16th century) and the use of certain ferns by the Ancient Greeks as anthelmintics that kill parasitic worms.

Sulphonamides were the first group of drugs to be used as effective antimicrobials. They were developed from dyes and are occasionally used today.

Antibiotics are substances produced by micro-organisms that are antagonistic to other micro-organisms. Their clinical use began with the discovery of penicillin in 1928 by Fleming and its use as an antibiotic in 1946. This revolutionized the treatment of bacterial infections and many other antibacterial drugs have followed. Drugs effective against viruses were much more difficult and discovered more recently.

Classification of antimicrobial drugs

These drugs may be classified according to the type of organism they are effective against:

- antibacterial drugs
- antiviral drugs
- antifungal drugs

- antiprotozoal drugs
- anthelminthic drugs.

Not all microbes cause disease. Those that do are referred to as ***pathogens***.

Mechanism of action of antimicrobial drugs

These drugs rely on selective toxicity so that the parasitic organism is killed but not the host cells. The differences between parasitic and human cells are targeted. This is easier in bacteria than viruses, as the virus lives inside the human cell.

Most infectious diseases are caused by bacteria, and it is unfortunate that bacteria have been able to develop resistance to some antibiotics. Almost as fast as new drugs are discovered so the microbes develop mutations that allow them to counteract the effects of the antibiotic.

Prokaryotic and eukaryotic cells

Cells with a nucleus are eukaryotic. Those with no nucleus are prokaryotic and include bacteria. There are similarities and differences between prokaryotes and eukaryotes, and some of these allow an attack to be made on microorganisms.

- DNA is the carrier of genetic material in most cases, although some viruses have only RNA.
- Bacteria have a cell wall, whereas animal cells do not. This keeps the shape of the bacterium and supports the underlying plasma membrane. It usually contains a chemical called peptidoglycan that is not found in animal cells and thus can be a target for antibiotics – for example, ***penicillins, cephalosporins***.
- There are no mitochondria in bacteria, and energy is produced by enzyme systems in the cytoplasmic membrane inside the cell wall. Drugs can interfere with this membrane and affect its permeability, thus causing leakage of the products within – for example, **polymyxins**.
- Protein synthesis may be attacked, as the ribosomes of bacteria are structurally different from ours – for example, ***erythromycin***.
- Bacteria have no nucleus, and the genetic material is a single thread in the cytoplasm with no nuclear membrane. Some drugs interfere with microbial DNA (e.g. ***quinolones*** and ***metronidazole***), or with RNA (e.g. ***rifampicin***).
- May block metabolic processes that are different in bacteria – for example, ***trimethoprim***.

Gram-positive and Gram-negative bacteria

There is an outer wall outside the cell wall, and it is this that allows bacteria to be classed as Gram negative or Gram positive according to whether this outer wall takes up the Gram stain. In Gram-negative bacteria, the outer wall is more difficult to penetrate and so they are more resistant to certain antibiotics. The majority of important bacteria can be classified as gram positive or negative, and this is useful in deciding which antibiotic should be prescribed. Examples of some of the important pathogenic bacteria in hospitals are given in Table 8.1.

Anaerobic bacteria

Bacteria that can live and replicate in an environment without free oxygen. An example is *Clostridium tetani.* Spores lie dormant in the soil and can gain entry into cuts to produce tetanus. Some anaerobes live in the gut and may cause severe sepsis following abdominal surgery.

Broad- and narrow-spectrum antibiotics

Some antibiotics are described as broad spectrum and have an extensive spectrum of activity. Others are narrow spectrum and only kill a limited number of types of micro-organism.

Some are mainly active against Gram-positive organisms — for example, *penicillins, erythromycin*. Others are mainly active against Gram-negative organisms — for example, *polymyxin*. Broad-spectrum antibiotics are active against both — for example, *ampicillin, cephalosporins*.

Bacteriostatic and bactericidal drugs

- Some antibiotics are bactericidal and kill the bacteria present — for example, *penicillin.*
- Some are bacteriostatic and stop the bacteria replicating but do not kill those already present. They rely on body defences to do this, and so in those with ineffective immune systems, bactericidal drugs must be used.
- Some are bactericidal at high doses and bacteriostatic at lower ones.

TABLE 8.1 Some important pathogenic Gram-positive and Gram-negative bacteria.

Gram-positive bacteria	Gram-negative bacteria
Staphylococcus aureus	*Neisseria meningitidis (meningococcus)*
Streptococcus pyogenes	*Escherichia coli*
Streptococcus pneumoniae (pneumococcus)	*Pseudomonas*

Antimicrobial resistance

Resistance is when a safe dose of the antibiotic is ineffective. Resistance to some antibiotics is already present in certain micro-organisms. Bacteria mutate and change their genetic structure more readily than higher organisms, enabling resistance to occur. The bacteria that acquire a characteristic that enables survival in the presence of an antibiotic will reproduce, producing genetically identical cells that are also resistant. This means that just one mutant bacterium can rapidly produce an identical colony of bacteria, all resistant to the antibiotic.

Bacteria may acquire resistance in several ways. They may:

- produce an enzyme that will inactivate the drug — for example, β-lactamase enzymes that attack penicillins and acetylating enzymes that inactivate aminoglycosides
- pump the drug out of their cell or adapt so that the drug can no longer enter their cell — for example, *Pseudomonas aeruginosa* prevents the penetration of *imipenem*
- change the structure of the molecule in their cell that the antibiotic targets — for example, change in the bacterial ribosome may prevent the binding of aminoglycosides
- produce a new biochemical pathway to bypass the one affected by the antibiotic — for example, some develop a new enzyme not inhibited by *trimethoprim*.

Opportunistic infection

The antibiotic will kill some of the normal bacterial flora of the patient, and the bacteria killed depends on the antibiotic used. This may allow drug-resistant organisms to multiply now that competition from other organisms has been removed.

- *Candida albicans* is an example presenting as thrush in the mouth or vagina.
- More serious is antibiotic-associated colitis, when a broad-spectrum antibiotic has been used, killing the normal flora in the bowel, leading to pseudomembranous colitis with bloody diarrhoea, abdominal pain and dehydration. This is most frequently caused by *Clostridium difficile* and may cause problems even when antibiotics have been discontinued. Some people do have the bacteria in their colon already, but in many cases it is acquired by cross infection in hospital. Treatment is with *metronidazole* and *vancomycin*.
- Some people are carriers of *C. difficile*, and it can spread in hospitals and care homes where patients with diarrhoea should be isolated, if possible.

In the young and healthy, the bacteria are not usually a problem, but in the elderly and ill or those on broad-spectrum antibiotics, the infection can be devastating. Thorough hand washing and hygiene are essential, and the use of gloves is needed. The diarrhoea of those with the infection contains many, many spores that can be transferred readily to others.

Selection of an antibiotic

This needs to take into account the causative organism but also the patient.

Factors in the patient to consider include any history of allergy, renal and hepatic function, whether immunocompromised, severity of the illness, age, ethnic origin, other medication, possible pregnancy, breast feeding and ability to tolerate a drug orally.

The causative organism alongside its sensitivity to antibacterials can then be used, alongside the patient factors, to select an antibiotic. Local policies may limit the antibacterials that may be used to try and prevent the development of resistant organisms and also for economic reasons.

Other considerations before starting therapy (in a non-emergency)

Antibacterial drugs do not eradicate viruses and should not be used in viral infections. However, they may be used to treat a secondary infection, such as bacterial pneumonia secondary to influenza.

- Samples should be taken for culture and sensitivity of the organism before an antibiotic is prescribed. Treatment may need to be changed when the bacteria has been cultured and its sensitivity is known. The diagnosis is made more difficult if antibiotics have been prescribed 'blind'.
- Narrow spectrum antibiotics are usually preferred unless there is a serious situation such as life-threatening sepsis, when broad spectrum may be preferred.
- The dose of an antibiotic should be decided according to the age of the patient, their weight, liver function, renal function and the severity of the infection. One dose for all is not appropriate and may be inadequate to treat the infection. Too small a dose may also increase the chance of bacterial resistance, but care is required as some antibiotics — for example, aminoglycosides — are toxic in too high a dose.
- The route of administration does depend on the severity of the infection, and intravenous administration is usually the choice in life-threatening infections. There are some antibiotics that are very well absorbed from the gastrointestinal (GI) tract and can be given orally, even in some severe infections.
- Parenteral administration is required if the patient is vomiting or cannot absorb well from the gut.

- Intramuscular administration is often painful and so should be avoided where possible, especially in children.
- The duration of therapy varies according to the actual infection and the response to the antibiotic. If administered over too long a period, this can encourage resistance. In some infections such as tuberculosis (TB), prolonged courses of antibiotics are required. At the other end of the spectrum, a single dose of antibiotic may cure an uncomplicated urinary tract infection (UTI).
- The prescription should state the period over which the antibiotic is to be administered and the date for review.

Sepsis

A broad-spectrum antibiotic at the maximum recommended dose should be commenced immediately (within 1 hour if possible) in all cases of suspected sepsis.

- Before the antibiotic is administered, blood cultures and microbiological samples should be taken and the prescription changed if necessary when the results are known.
- The patient will have a full clinical examination to try and identify the source of the infection, and if this is identified, it should also be treated locally with a recommended antibacterial agent.
- If there is no diagnosis, treatment with an intravenous antibiotic will be according to the local formulary and national guidelines.
- In severe cases, the patient may require oxygen, intravenous fluids, vaso-pressors and inotrope, dependent on their condition.

Details of the recommended antibiotics for specific infections are given in BNF (2019), Section 5, and the reader is referred to this (also available online at www.bnf.org).

Types of antimicrobial agent

Agents affecting the cell wall

β-Lactam antibiotics

All have the same β-lactam ring in their chemical structure. They include penicillins, cephalosporins, monobactams and carbapenems.

Some bacteria produce an enzyme, β-lactamase (penicillinase), that splits the β-lactam ring and renders the antibiotic ineffective. Some antibiotics in this group have been modified to include a β-lactamase inhibitor, so that they are resistant to this enzyme.

Penicillins
- Ampicillin.
- Amoxicillin.
- Azlocillin.
- Benzylpenicillin (penicillin G).
- Co-fluampicil.
- Co-amoxiclav.
- Flucloxacillin.
- Phenoxymethylpenicillin (penicillin V).
- Piperacillin.
- Pivampicillin.
- Pivmecillinam hydrochloride.
- Temocillin.
- Ticarcillin.

Penicillin was discovered by Fleming in 1928 when he noticed that a culture plate of staphylococci had been contaminated by the mould *Penicillium* and there was no bacterial growth around the mould. Only tested in humans in 1941 with a small amount of purified penicillin given intravenously and found to have a dramatic effect in a staphylococcal infection.

Mechanism of action
- Inhibit the synthesis of the peptidoglycan layer of the bacterial cell wall that surrounds some bacteria and is necessary for survival.
- Bactericidal.
- Penetrate body fluids well but cannot cross the blood–brain barrier (BBB) unless inflammation is present as in meningococcal meningitis when *benzylpenicillin* can still be used.
- Penicillins are still widely used and are very effective antibiotics but unfortunately can be destroyed by bacterial enzymes – β-lactamases (penicillinases) and amidases. This is the case with the staphylococcus.

Unwanted effects
- Very safe antibiotics with a high therapeutic index.
- Encephalopathy due to cerebral irritation is a rare side effect of penicillins and may be due to large doses with high concentrations in the cerebro-spinal fluid.

Benzylpenicillin is not given intrathecally for this reason. It may also occur in renal failure, as penicillin is eliminated unchanged in the urine. If the kidneys are not functioning adequately, it will accumulate.

Hypersensitivity
- Hypersensitivity is the biggest problem in up to 10% of those exposed to the drug.
- This may present with a rash but may result in anaphylaxis in 0.05% of people and can be fatal.

- Those with a history of allergies or hay fever, asthma or eczema are at greater risk.
- Penicillin should not be given again to anyone who has developed a rash following previous administration, as it could result in a severe anaphylactic response.
- If allergic to one penicillin, will be allergic to all, and this sensitivity may cross to cephalosporins or other β-lactam antibiotics as well.
- Gastrointestinal side effects are not an allergy. Patients may develop diarrhoea due to the balance of bacteria in the large bowel being changed.

Types of penicillin

Benzylpenicillin (penicillin G). The first penicillin to be used. It is destroyed by the acid in the stomach and so is only given by intramuscular or intravenous injection.

Effective against many streptococcal infections, such as the pneumococcus, meningococcus and gonococcus, although some now have decreased sensitivity.

Intravenous benzylpenicillin is the drug of choice in meningococcal meningitis and may be administered by paramedics if the rash of meningococcal septicaemia is present.

Phenoxymethylpenicillin (penicillin V) is a form of penicillin that is not destroyed by acid in the stomach and can be taken orally.

Penicillinase-resistant penicillins. Flucloxacillin is not inactivated by penicillinase and is effective in penicillin-resistant staphylococcal infections. This is the only time *flucloxacillin* is used, and it is especially important in hospitals. It can be given by mouth or by injection.

Temocillin is also stable in the presence of penicillinases and is reserved for infections by those bacteria where resistance to other β-lactam antibiotics is present. It is used in septicaemia due to UTIs and in lower respiratory tract infections caused by susceptible bacteria.

MRSA (methicillin-resistant *Staphylococcus aureus*)
This is infection by *S. aureus* that is resistant to **methicillin**, an antibiotic that has now been discontinued. It is resistant to other antibiotics such as **flucloxacillin** and is extremely difficult to treat.

Broad-spectrum penicillins. These are effective against a greater range of bacteria.

Ampicillin is an example but is inactivated by penicillinases, including those produced by the streptococcus and some gram-negative bacteria — for example, *Escherichia coli*. In hospital, it should not be used without checking the sensitivity of the organism first.

When given orally, less than half the dose is absorbed. This is even less if there is food in the stomach.

In patients with glandular fever, a maculopapular rash frequently occurs. This is not due to a penicillin allergy.

Amoxicillin is derived from ampicillin and is better absorbed orally and not affected by food in the stomach.

Co-amoxiclav (Augmentin) is amoxicillin with a β-lactamase inhibitor (clavulanic acid) added. This increases activity against some bacteria resistant to penicillin and should be reserved for those infections.

Antipseudomonal penicillins. Ticarcillin is reserved mostly for serious infections caused by *P. aeruginosa* or *proteus* and is combined with clavulanic acid *(Timentin)*. It is given by intravenous infusion.

Piperacillin is more active than ticarcillin against *Pseudomonas* and comes combined with tazobactam as *Tazocin*. It is given by intravenous infusion.

Given in hospital-acquired pneumonia, septicaemia, complicated infections of the urinary tract, skin or soft tissues.

Pivmecillinam is active against many gram-negative bacteria, including *E. coli*, but not against *P. aeruginosa*. It is given orally in cystitis and UTIs.

Cephalosporins

- First generation — cefadroxil, cefalexin, cefradine.
- Second generation — cefaclor, cefuroxime.
- Third generation — cefixime, cefotaxime, cefpodoxime, ceftazidime, ceftriaxone.

First isolated from *Cephalosporium* fungus and chemically related to penicillin. Semisynthetic broad-spectrum cephalosporins have been created by changing the chemical structure.

Cephalosporins vary in their susceptibility to β-lactamases.

About 10% of those allergic to penicillin will also be allergic to cephalosporins.

Mechanism of action

- Similar to penicillins and interfere with bacterial peptidoglycan synthesis, preventing manufacture of the bacterial cell wall.
- Broad-spectrum antibiotics used in the treatment of septicaemia, pneumonia, meningitis, peritonitis, biliary tract infections and UTIs.
- Succeeding generations have increased activity against gram-negative bacteria but less against gram positive, and third generation are less effective against *S. aureus* than *cefuroxime*, which is less susceptible to inactivation by β-lactamases.

- Gram-negative bacteria are able to develop resistance to cephalosporins more easily than to penicillins.
- First generation can be given orally, but most others are acid labile and are given by injection or infusion.
- Some — for example, *cefotaxime, cefuroxime* and *ceftriaxone* — cross the BBB; others do not penetrate the BBB unless it is inflamed.
- Mostly eliminated in the urine but about 40% in the bile.

Uses
- Depending on the sensitivity of the bacteria, used for septicaemia, pneumonia, meningitis, biliary tract infection, UTIs, peritonitis and sinusitis.

Unwanted effects
- Skin rashes and hypersensitivity.
- Antibiotic-associated colitis may occur with broad-spectrum drugs, especially those given orally.
- Nausea, vomiting, abdominal pain.

Other β-lactam antibiotics

Monobactams (aztreonam), carbapenems (imipenem, meropenem and ertapenem) These were developed to work against β-lactamase-producing Gram-negative bacteria that were resistant to penicillin. All work in a similar way to penicillins.

Aztreonam should not be prescribed alone 'blind', as it is not effective against Gram-positive organisms. Given by inhalation, intramuscular injection or intravenous infusion. Used in *Pseudomonas* and *Haemophilus influenzae*, as well as *Neisseria meningitis* and lung infections in cystic fibrosis.

The carbapenems are not effective against MRSA and *Enterococcus faecium.*

Imipenem with *cilastatin* is a very broad-spectrum antibiotic that was resistant to all β-lactamase-producing bacteria at first, but resistance has now developed in strains of MRSA and *P. aeruginosa*. It is given with *cilastatin*, an enzyme inhibitor, to decrease renal breakdown of the drug. It is used in hospital-acquired septicaemia and in infection is febrile patients with neutropaenia.

Full details of their use are found in the BNF (2019).

Drugs affecting bacterial protein synthesis

Tetracyclines

Tetracycline, oxytetracycline, demeclocycline, doxycycline, lymecycline, minocycline Although these are broad-spectrum antibiotics, their use has declined as bacteria have developed resistance.

They are bacteriostatic and used in infections caused by chlamydia, rickettsia, brucella and Lyme disease.

They may also be used for UTI, skin infections and bronchiectasis caused by MRSA. They do have a role in MRSA infections (BNF, 2019).

Other uses include respiratory tract infections, acne and exacerbations of chronic obstructive pulmonary disease (active against *H. influenzae*).

They are all similar in action, except minocycline, which has a broader spectrum but has the side effects of vertigo and dizziness and a greater risk of lupus-erythematosus-like syndrome.

Unwanted effects

- Commonest is gastrointestinal upset, as they are irritant to the mucosa. Also change the range of bacteria within the gut and occasionally produce suprainfection.
- Vitamin B deficiency may occur, so supplementation may be needed.
- Hypersensitivity.

Caution — tetracyclines bind to calcium (and other metal ions) and can be deposited in growing bones and teeth, causing staining. They should not be given to children under 12 years of age, in pregnancy or when breast feeding.

Should not be given with milk because this will also bind and reduce absorption as with various antacids or iron supplements.

Tigecycline is related to tetracyclines but is active against tetracycline-resistant bacteria and MRSA. It is only used for skin and soft tissue infections and abdominal infections caused by resistant organisms.

Chloramphenicol

Originally isolated from cultures of *Streptomyces* and inhibits protein synthesis in a similar way to erythromycin.

- Powerful broad-spectrum antibiotic that is bacteriostatic for most organisms.
- Associated with severe agranulocytosis that can be permanent and so only used in life-threatening infections with *H. influenzae* and typhoid fever.
- May also be given in meningitis if penicillin cannot be used.
- Available as eye drops or cream and the most frequent form of treatment for conjunctivitis. Also available as ear drops.

Aminoglycosides

Gentamicin, streptomycin, amikacin, tobramycin, neomycin

Gentamicin is the aminoglycoside most frequently used in the UK.

Aminoglycosides are bactericidal and inhibit bacterial protein synthesis.

- Require oxygen-dependent active transport to enter the bacteria, so have little action against anaerobic bacteria.
- Bacteriocidal and active against some Gram-positive organisms and many Gram-negative ones.
- *Streptomycin* is active against *Mycobacterium tuberculosis.*
- Bacterial resistance is now becoming a problem, and these antibiotics are inactivated by some microbial enzymes. *Amikacin* is less likely to be inactivated and is only used in gentamicin-resistant infections.
- Not absorbed from the gastrointestinal tract and have to be given by injections for systemic infections.
- Eliminated via the kidney, and accumulation reduces renal function. They should only be prescribed for 7 days. Blood levels must be monitored to prevent too high concentration.
- May produce dose-related deafness and damage the auditory nerve.
- *Neomycin* is too toxic for injection but is used orally prior to bowel surgery to reduce bacteria in the colon. It is also used topically for skin infections.
- *Gentamicin* is the aminoglycoside of choice in the UK and is used widely in the treatment of serious infections. Poor activity against *Haemolytic streptococci* and *pneumococci* and not active against anaerobes.
- If prescribed 'blind' in serious infections, gentamicin is usually combined with penicillin or metronidazole.
- Monitoring serum concentration by blood samples avoids both excessive or subtherapeutic concentrations of aminoglycosides.

Macrolides

Erythromycin, clarithromycin, azithromycin, spiramycin Inhibit bacterial protein synthesis by binding to the ribosome. May be bacteriostatic or bactericidal, depending on the dose and the bacteria.

Have an antibacterial spectrum that is similar (but not identical) to penicillin.

Erythromycin Used for more than 40 years but all other macrolides are more recent. Effective orally. Irritant to veins, so if intravenous injection is needed, it is given as an infusion.

Uses. Often used when there is penicillin sensitivity.

Also used in *Legionella* infection, whooping cough (pertussis), campylobacter enteritis, respiratory tract infections, skin infections and acne, prevention of recurrence of rheumatic fever.

Side effects. Irritant drug to the mucosa and may cause nausea, vomiting, abdominal discomfort and diarrhoea.

Clarithromycin is a derivative of erythromycin that has a slightly higher activity and greater tissue concentrations. It is used as part of a regimen in the elimination of *Helicobacter pylori*.

Spiramycin is used in the treatment of toxoplasmosis.

Azithromycin has less activity against gram-positive bacteria than erythromycin but better activity against some gram-negative bacteria, including *H. influenzae*.

Lincosamides

Clindamycin is active against Gram-positive cocci, including streptococci and penicillin-resistant staphylococci. It reaches bone and is used to treat staphylococcal infections of bones and joints as in osteomyelitis. It is also effective against some anaerobes and is similar in action to macrolides. It can be used for the treatment of dentoalveolar abscess when penicillin and metronidazole are not effective. Can also be used to treat MRSA in bronchiectasis.

Oxazolidinones

Linezolid Different mechanism of action on bacterial protein synthesis to all other antibiotics. Treatment can only be initiated by a specialist and in severe, resistant infections. Is effective orally or by intravenous infusion.

- Active against a wide range of Gram-positive organisms, including MRSA and glycopeptide-resistant enterococci.
- Can be used to treat pneumonia and septicaemia.
- Active against some anaerobes, including *C. difficile*.
- Not active against most Gram-negative bacteria.
- Resistance can occur with prolonged treatment or if the dose given is smaller than that recommended.
- Full blood count must be monitored weekly, as red cells, platelets and white cells may all fall in numbers. Close monitoring is needed if the patient is treated for more than 10−14 days.
- Damage to the optic nerve has occurred in some patients treated for longer than 28 days. Patients should be warned to report blurred vision or any other visual symptoms.
- Inhibits monoamine oxidase, and thus the patient has to avoid foods rich in tyramine (see Section 4.6).

Fusidic acid

Sodium fusidate (Fucidin) Narrow-spectrum antibiotic effective against Gram-positive bacteria. It inhibits bacterial protein synthesis.

- Should only be used in penicillin-resistant staphylococcal infections, especially osteomyelitis, as it concentrates well in bone. Used in combination with another antibiotic to reduce risk of resistance.

- Used for staphylococcal skin infections.
- Liver function should be monitored on high doses.

Quinolones

Ciprofloxacin, levofloxacin, ofloxacin, norfloxacin, moxifloxacin Inhibit topoisomerase, an enzyme needed by bacteria when DNA is replicated.

The MHRA has warned that quinolones may cause convulsions and that taking NSAIDs at the same time may also induce these.

Tendon damage, including rupture, has been reported rarely and within 48 hours of starting treatment.

Also a small increased risk of ruptured aortic aneurysm, especially in the elderly.

Ciprofloxacin Most commonly used of this group. It is active against Gram-positive but more effective against Gram-negative bacteria such as *salmonella, shigella, campylobacter, neisseria* and *pseudomonas*. Also active against chlamydia. Not active against most anaerobes.

Uses
- Fulminating Crohn's disease.
- Respiratory tract infections but not pneumococcal pneumonia.
- UTIs.
- Infections of the gastrointestinal tract.
- Bone and joint infections.
- Septicaemia if organism is sensitive.
- Anthrax, and may be used for 60 days following contact, as germination can be delayed.

Unwanted effects
- Nausea, vomiting, diarrhoea.
- Rash.
- Can induce seizures in epilepsy and in those with no history of convulsions sometimes.
- Photosensitivity, so avoid exposure to full sunlight.
- Tendon damage and rupture have rarely occurred within 48 hours of commencing quinolones. Should not be given if any history of tendon problems.

Glycopeptide antibiotics

Dalbavancin, teicoplanin, telavancin and vancomycin These are glycopeptide antibiotics that inhibit bacterial cell wall synthesis. They are bactericidal, including against various staphylococci. There are increased reports of resistance among enterococci and reduced susceptibility of some staphylococci.

Vancomycin is not absorbed orally and so is given by this route to treat *C. difficile* infection of the gastrointestinal tract (pseudomembranous colitis).

- It is given by intravenous infusion for other uses including MRSA.
- Long duration of action, so may be given every 12 hours.
- Reports of resistance in some MRSA strains and some enterococci.

Unwanted effects
- May be toxic to the kidneys and occasionally cause renal failure.
- Toxic to auditory nerve so discontinue if tinnitus occurs.
- Blood disorders.
- Rapid infusion should be avoided, as anaphylaxis may occur.

Daptomycin Lipopeptide with similar action to *vancomycin*. Reserved for skin and soft tissue infection by MRSA.

Polymyxins Colistimethate sodium (Colistin) is bactericidal and effective against Gram-negative organisms, including *P. aeruginosa* and *Klebsiella pneumoniae*.

- Not absorbed by mouth and has to be given intravenously.
- Used orally with *nystatin* to sterilize the bowel in patients with low WCCs.
- Given by inhalation in cystic fibrosis to manage chronic lung infection due to *P. aeruginosa*.

Sulfonamides

Sulfadiazine These were the very first drugs to be used to combat infection and were developed from the dye industry. The dye prontosil is an inactive prodrug that is metabolized to sulfanilamide, the active sulfonamide. Sulfadiazine is bacteriostatic against a broad spectrum of bacteria.

Many more drugs have been developed since its use in the 1930s, but the group has become less important as bacterial resistance has increased.

Mechanism of action
- Sulfanilamide is similar in structure to para-aminobenzoic acid (PABA), a chemical needed by bacteria to manufacture folic acid that is needed to make new cells. Bacteria cannot utilize dietary folic acid, as animals can and have to synthesize it. The sulfanilamide competes with PABA for an

enzyme. This means that if the concentration of PABA is increased, the effect of sulfanilamide will be reduced.

- Not effective if pus or products from cell breakdown are present, as these contain thymidine and purines, enabling the bacteria to make DNA without the use of folic acid.
- Bacteriostatic, not bactericidal.
- Resistance is common.
- May be used topically in burns to reduce infection.

Trimethoprim

Also a folate antagonist and is used on its own in UTIs and respiratory tract infections.

It is combined with a **sulfamethoxazole** as **co-trimoxazole** because of their synergistic activity (working together well). It is used in the prophylaxis and treatment of *Pneumocystis jiroveci (Pneumocystis carinii)* and toxoplasmosis but should only be considered for acute exacerbations of chronic bronchitis or UTIs where sensitivity of the bacteria causing the infection is known and there is a good reason to prefer it. This is because it can cause serious side effects, including bone marrow suppression and Stevens–Johnson syndrome.

Nitroimidazole derivatives

Metronidazole This drug is active against anaerobic bacteria and also against some protozoa. It is used in dental infections, against colonic anaerobes following gynaecological or bowel surgery and in pseudomembranous colitis.

It may be given orally, topically, rectally or intravenously. It interacts with alcohol, and the patient must not drink alcohol while on treatment.

Metronidazole can cause gastrointestinal tract side effects, a metallic taste, occasionally dizziness and headache. It is usually well tolerated.

Tinidazole has high activity against anaerobic bacteria and protozoa. It has a longer duration of action than metronidazole.

Antimycobacterials

Rifampicin Used in:

- treatment of brucellosis and Legionnaires disease in conjunction with other antibiotics
- treatment of TB (see below) and also in the prevention of TB in susceptible close contacts (alongside isoniazid)
- prevention of secondary cases of meningococcal meningitis and *H. influenzae*
- treatment of multibacillary leprosy alongside dapsone and clofazimine.

Aminosalicylic acid, bedaquiline, capreomycin, cycloserine, delamanid, ethambutol, isoniazid, pyrazinamide.

These drugs are used in TB and some in multiple drug-resistant TB, alongside other drugs.

Drugs used in the treatment of tuberculosis

This is a difficult disease to treat, as the bacteria can survive inside the macrophages following phagocytosis. TB was a major killer in this country until *rifampicin* and *ethambutol* were developed in the 1960s, when it became easily treatable. The problem now is that there are multi-resistant strains and TB is again a major threat in some countries.

NICE has produced guidance on the management of TB that is available on its website: www.nice.org.uk.

TB is treated in two stages. The **initial phase** uses four drugs for 2 months, and the **continuation phase** uses two drugs for a further 4 months. Specialist knowledge is required to treat this disease, and there are many resistant organisms.

The use of four drugs in the initial phase hopes to reduce the number of organisms rapidly and also prevent resistance developing.

There are two regimens recommended for the treatment of TB in the UK, but variations occur in other countries. There is an unsupervised regimen and a supervised regimen, which should not be used at the same time. Compliance is vital to have success in the treatment of TB.

Drugs usually given in the initial phase are *rifampicin, isoniazid, pyrazinamide* and *ethambutol* with *isoniazid* and *rifampicin* in the continuation phase.

Second-line drugs include *streptomycin, capreomycin* and *cycloserine*. They are used in resistance.

Drugs used to treat leprosy

Leprosy is an ancient disease that was documented in 600 BCE. The bacteria, like the tubercle bacillus, can survive following phagocytosis.

It is an extremely disfiguring disease, and those that had the disease were isolated in colonies, although it is not especially contagious.

Multidrug regimens are used, and the WHO is involved in the choices available.

Dapsone, rifampicin and *clofazimine* are used for at least 2 years in multibacillary leprosy.

Antiviral agents

Viruses are species specific, but virtually all species on Earth can be infected by some form of virus. Even bacteria can be infected by viruses called *bacteriophages*.

Most viral infections are dealt with by a healthy immune system and drugs are not needed − an example being the common cold. The main danger is when the immune system is not competent as in human immunodeficiency virus (HIV) or cancer chemotherapy treatment. A virus that is usually not problematic can now become virulent.

- Although viruses are extremely small, they have a very sophisticated structure and are not easy to kill.
- They live inside our cells so are not easily accessible.
- Viruses use the host's cells to replicate, so it is difficult to target the virus without damaging the host's cell.
- Much replication of the virus has already occurred before any symptoms are produced.
- Viruses mutate so rapidly that vaccine development can be extremely difficult. Influenza virus changes (mutates) from year to year, and new vaccines have to be produced annually.
- Effective vaccines include smallpox (now eradicated), mumps, rubella, measles and poliomyelitis.
- Most antiviral drugs have an effect against DNA or RNA synthesis and replication.
- Much more is now known about the structure and function of viruses, and this had led to the development of new drugs.
- There was pressure to develop drugs to help control the HIV, which is the cause of acquired immunodeficiency disease (AIDS). Much money has been put into this area of research with good effect.

Antiviral drugs are used specifically for viral infections, and they act by either killing or preventing the replication of the virus. Many antiviral drugs are used for one specific infection, although there are some broad-spectrum antivirals that work against a wide range of viruses.

The first antivirals were developed in the 1960s, mostly to combat the herpes virus. In the 1980s the full genetic sequence of viruses began to be revealed, and this made it easier to develop drugs to target these organisms.

Although the life cycles of different viruses vary, they have some common features, and these include:

- attachment to a host cell.
- release of viral genes and enzymes into the cell.
- replication of the viral components within the host cell, inducing it to replicate the viral genome.
- release of the newly created viruses from the host cell by various methods. The virus may wait for the cell to die before it is released. It is then able to infect more host cells.

There are many classes of antiviral drug that have been developed today, and the virus can be targeted at different stages of its life cycle.

- It could be targeted before it has entered the host cell by preventing the virus attaching to the receptor on the surface of the host cell.
- The synthesis of viral components can be targeted by, for example, inhibiting reverse transcriptase. *Lamivudine* for hepatitis B works this way. *Aciclovir* is a nucleoside analogue, as is AZT *(zidovudine)*, the first antiviral to treat HIV.
- Transcription and translation can be targeted as can protein processing. Some viruses contain an enzyme called a protease that cuts protein chains for final assembly. This can be targeted by protease inhibitors. *Rifampicin* acts at the assembly stage.
- Drugs have also been manufactured that prevent the release of the viral particles from the cell — for example, *zanamivir* for influenza.
- Another approach is to stimulate the body's own immune system to attack the viruses. These drugs often do not work on one specific virus. Interferons are an example.
- Antibodies are protein molecules that link up to target proteins on the pathogen and make it attractive for attack by the body's immune system. The synthesis of monoclonal antibodies that bind to the target on the pathogen is possible.

There are some specific antiviral treatments available for:

- herpes virus infections — herpes simplex virus and varicella zoster virus (chickenpox)
- HIV
- cytomegalovirus
- respiratory syncytial virus (RSV)
- hepatitis B and C
- influenza A and B viruses.

Antiviral resistance is when there is a decreased susceptibility of the virus to the drug. This is caused by changes to the viral genotype and is extremely problematic, as viruses constantly change their genetic makeup and mutate so quickly.

Recommendations about the use of antiviral preparations for flu are based on national and international surveillance of the effectiveness of the current flu antiviral drugs. Combination therapy is used, if available, when resistance to an antiviral has occurred.

Types of antiviral drug

Nucleoside analogues

These drugs contain a nucleic acid analogue and a sugar. They are used to prevent viral replication in cells that are infected.

Aciclovir (Zovirax)

This was the first antiviral drug, and it inhibits herpes virus DNA polymerase, thus blocking viral replication. It does not eradicate the virus.

- It can be used topically for herpes simplex eye infections.
- Used to treat genital herpes and cold sores but must be started early.
- Can be given orally as a liquid or tablets.
- Effective against shingles if started within 72 hours. It can reduce the severity and duration of pain. Usually continued for 7–10 days.
- Available intravenously for systemic infections and encephalitis.
- Similar drugs effective in herpes are *famciclovir* and *valaciclovir*.

Ganciclovir

- Related to *aciclovir* but more active against cytomegalovirus.
- Given by intravenous infusion for prevention of cytomegalovirus in those with drug-induced immunosuppression or in immunocompromised patients.
- It is much more toxic than acyclovir and so only prescribed when the benefits outweigh the risks.
- Other drugs active against cytomegalovirus include *valaciclovir, valganciclovir* and *foscarnet*.

Ribavirin

Inhibits a wide range of DNA and RNA viruses.

- Reduces replication of the virus by inhibiting viral RNA polymerase.
- Used by inhalation when treating infants and children with bronchiolitis caused by RSV.
- Has been used intravenously for Lassa fever.
- Used for chronic hepatitis C in combination with peginterferon α-2b.

Neuraminidase inhibitors

Oseltamivir (Tamiflu) and *zanamivir (Relenza)* reduce replication of influenza A and B viruses by inhibiting the viral enzyme neuraminidase. This prevents the release of the virus by budding from the host cell. The drugs are used for prophylaxis and treatment of influenza A and B, but vaccination is still the most effective way of preventing infection with influenza. There is NICE guidance for the treatment of influenza.

    Amantadine is an antiviral drug that is an antagonist of one of the surface proteins of the virus. It was active against influenza A but is no longer used because of the high levels of viral resistance.

While trialling this drug it was discovered to have anti-parkinsonian effects due to its antimuscarinic effects. Adverse effects include confusion, depression and insomnia.

Antiretroviral drugs active against human immunodeficiency virus infection

AIDS was first described in the early 1980s and the virus identified in 1984. HIV is a retrovirus that binds to lymphocytes via the CD4 receptor. There is a progressive fall in these cells, and this leads to a decrease in immunity. Eventually this leads to failure of the immune response and AIDS. Opportunist infections occur such as recurrent shingles or thrush. Other infections typical in AIDS include *P. carinii* pneumonia.

- Drugs can halt or slow progression of the disease but cannot cure it.
- Drugs increase life expectancy, but mortality and morbidity still remain slightly higher than in uninfected people.
- The drugs are toxic and prescription is by specialists.
- Treatment needs to be started as early as possible before the immune system has been permanently damaged.
- To prevent drug resistance, combinations of drugs are used, and these are carefully selected to work together without increasing toxicity.
- Sensitivity of the virus should be tested for before treatment.
- There has to be a strong commitment to treatment and willingness to stick to a regimen over many years
- The time for the initiation of treatment is dependent on the CD4 cell count. Other factors to take into account are the presence of symptoms and any other illnesses.
- There are national guidelines for the treatment of AIDS and these are regularly revised. The various regimens can be found in the British National Formulary.

Drugs attack important enzymes in the virus.

Nucleoside reverse transcriptase inhibitors

Zidovudine (AZT) was the first anti-HIV drug. Other drugs in this category include **abacavir, didanosine, emtricitabine, lamivudine, stavudine** and **tenofovir.**

Protease inhibitors

Atazanavir, darunavir, fosamprenavir, lopinavir, nelfinavir, ritonavir, saquinavir and tipranavir

- Block the active site on the enzyme in the virus.
- Usually two are given in combination to allow smaller doses and give less side effects.
- They are associated with lipodystrophy and some metabolic effects.

Other drugs used in human immunodeficiency virus

Enfuvirtide inhibits the fusion of HIV to the host cell and is licensed when the HIV has not responded to a regimen of other antiviral drugs. It is combined with other drugs. To treat HIV-1.

Maraviroc is an antagonist of the CCR5 receptor and is only given to those with tis specific type of HIV.

Dolutegravir, elvitegravir and **raltegravir** are inhibitors of the HIV enzyme integrase.

This is a very specialized and constantly evolving area, and new developments are constantly in the news.

Antifungal agents

Fungi were originally thought to be plants. They are simple organisms and include mushrooms, moulds and yeasts. Most are not problematic for man, but some cause superficial infections such as thrush (candidiasis) and athlete's foot (tinea pedis). Treatment is described in Section 9.4.

Systemic infections

These used to be extremely rare but have increased partly due to the use of broad-spectrum antibiotics that destroy our natural bacteria. The latter usually keep fungal infection down by offering competition for nutrients. Those with deficient immune systems as in HIV and cancer chemotherapy are also at risk of systemic fungal infections.

Antifungal agents are used for infections with such fungi as aspergillosis, candidiasis, cryptococcosis and histoplasmosis.

Echinocandin antifungals

Anidulafungin, caspofungin, micafungin

These are only active against *Aspergillus* spp. and *Candida* spp. They are not effective against fungal infections of the CNS.

Given by intravenous infusion.

Polyene antifungals

Include **amphotericin** and **nystatin**. They are not adsorbed orally. That means nystatin can be used locally for oral thrush.

Amphotericin

- Has a low therapeutic index and renal function must be monitored.
- Used for systemic candidiasis, cryptococcal meningitis and histoplasmosis.

- Given by intravenous infusion with a gradually increasing dose.
- Anaphylaxis may occur and a test dose should be given before infusion.
- Lipid formulations are available that are less toxic, especially in renal disease. The MHRA have warned that there have been tree fatal overdoses caused by a medication error when a non-lipid-based formulation of Amphotericin B was given instead of a lipid-based formulation. This means it is best to prescribe amphotericin via the complete generic name and the proprietary name each time.

Triazole antifungals

Fluconazole, isavuconazole, itraconazole, posaconazole, voriconazole

Have a role to play in the prevention and systemic treatment of fungal infections.

Fluconazole is well absorbed orally and penetrates the cerebrospinal fluid so it can treat fungal meningitis.

Itraconazole has been associated with liver damage.

Imidazole antifungals

These include *clotrimazole* and *econazole* used for treatment locally of vaginal candidiasis and intestinal infections. If *miconazole* gel is absorbed systemically, it can result in certain drug interactions.

Other antifungals

Include flucytosine, griseofulvin and terbinafine.

Some fungal infections

Aspergillosis

Usually affects the lungs, but if the patient is severely immunocompromised, then invasive forms can affect the skin, heart and brain.

Candidiasis (Thrush)

Superficial infections are treated locally, whereas widespread infection needs systemic treatment.

Vaginal thrush may be treated locally or with *fluconazole* by mouth.

Thrush in the mouth and throat is treated topically unless not responding or immunocompromised when systemic *fluconazole* may be used.

Cryptococcus

This is uncommon, but infection in HIV patients can be life-threatening, with cryptococcal meningitis being the most common form of fungal meningitis. *Amphotericin* is given by intravenous infusion, followed by *fluconazole* for 8 weeks.

Histoplasmosis

Can be life-threatening, especially in HIV-infected patients, but is rare in temperate climates. *Itraconazole* may be used or amphotericin IV for severe infections, followed by itraconazole orally.

Skin and nail infections

These include tinea corporis (ringworm), tinea pedis (athlete's foot) and tinea capitis. They usually respond to local therapy, but if this fails, systemic therapy can be used.

8.3 THE IMMUNE SYSTEM

Overview of the immune system

Immunology is the study of the way in which organisms fight off disease. It includes the study of how they differentiate between self and non-self.

The immune system is a defence system that will identify and destroy all substances — dead or alive — not recognized as self. The immune system has evolved to protect the organism against microbes and other parasites that may cause damage to the body. However, the immune system also contributes to wound healing and aids removal of cells dying through natural processes. The body relies heavily on two intrinsic defence systems that act both independently and co-operatively.

1. Innate immunity

These processes are the same no matter what the organism:

- surface barriers — skin and mucosae
- chemical defences — phagocytes, natural killer cells, inflammation
- antimicrobial proteins — complement, interferon
- increase in body temperature.

2. Specific immune responses

These are adaptive and display a number of characteristics:

- It is antigen specific — it recognizes and acts against particular antigens.
- It is systemic — not restricted to the initial infection site.

- Diverse – it will attempt to destroy any foreign matter that enters the body.
- It displays an immunological memory.
- Self/non-self-recognition.

Anything that stimulates a specific immune response is called an *immunogen:*

- bacteria
- viruses
- foreign cells
- proteins
- fungi
- parasites.

When an immune response is stimulated, it is a reaction to antigens, which are small molecules, found on the surface of immunogens and capable of inducing a specific immune response. These antigens are not normally present in the body, and as far as the body is concerned, they are identified as non-self.

The specialized cells of the immune system that recognize antigens are called lymphocytes, and originate from the bone marrow. Found in blood and lymphoid tissue. Two cell populations of lymphocytes are:

1. B cells – humoral or (antibody-mediated) immunity, returned to the bone marrow to mature.
2. T cells – cellular or (cell-mediated) immunity, matured in the thymus.

Both are able to specifically recognize parts of a virus or bacteria. These two populations of lymphocytes form a functional system that reacts to specific foreign substances and acts to immobilize, neutralize and destroy them.

Recognition of antigens

- Antigens are very large and complex and are not generally recognized in their entirety by lymphocytes.
- Both B and T lymphocytes recognize discrete sites on the antigen known as antigenic determinants or epitopes.
- Epitopes are immunologically active regions on a complex antigen, which bind to B-cell or T-cell receptors.
- The parts of an infectious agent that are usually recognized are usually either proteins or polysaccharides.
- Proteins function as the most potent immunogens and polysaccharides second.

Foreignness

- In order to elicit an immune response, a molecule must be recognized as non-self by the biological system.
- The external surfaces of all our cells are dotted with a huge variety of protein molecules.

- Among these cell surface proteins is a specific group of glycoproteins that mark a cell as self.
- These proteins called major histocompatibility complex (MHC) proteins are coded by genes of the MHC.
- There are two major groups of MHC proteins:
  - Class 1 MHC proteins are found in virtually all body cells.
  - Class II MHC proteins are displayed only by cells that act in the immune response.

B lymphocytes

Respond to antigens by secreting antibodies:

- The function of antibodies is to combine with an antigen.
- Can memorize specific antigens and this ensures a speedy response to the same stimulus when met again. This response is powerful and quickly made.
- It is thought that there are around 1 million antigens, and our immune system needs to be able to respond to all these.

Antibodies

Antibodies belong to a group of proteins called *immunoglobulins*, which act as receptors for antigens on the B cells. The lymphocytes respond to the antigen because they have these receptors on them. The functions of antibodies are to protect the host by:

- neutralizing viruses
- neutralizing bacterial toxins
- opsonizing bacteria
- activating components of the inflammatory response.

Protection always begins with antigen–antibody binding

Antigenic molecules are usually complex and bind to several antibodies. Secreted antibodies circulate in the blood and search out or eliminate antigens. Antibodies also function as antitoxins that neutralize bacterial toxins. The antibodies 'capture' toxin molecules by occupying their antigenic determinant sites. This prevents the toxins binding to the tissues and exerting their toxic effects. The complexes formed are then phagocytosed.

Immunoglobulins

Serum glycoproteins are secreted by plasma cells in response to a challenge by an antigen. When they develop antigen specificity, they are known as antibodies. They are antigen-binding proteins present on the B-cell membrane. Membrane-bound antibody confers antigen specificity to B cells. Antigen-specific proliferation of B cells depends on the interaction of membrane antibody and antigen. Immunoglobulins are found in all tissue fluid and secretions. There are five types of immunoglobulins (antibodies): IgG, IgE, IgM, IgD and IgA.

The primary immune response:

- When a B cell meets an antigen for the first time, it differentiates into either an antibody-secreting cell called a plasma cell or a memory cell, which may persist for many years. Plasma cells do not express membrane-bound antibodies. Instead, they produce antibodies in a form that can be secreted.
- Although the plasma cells only live for a few days, they secrete enormous amounts of antibodies. One plasma cell has been estimated to secrete more than 2000 molecules of antibody per second.
- Antibodies cannot destroy antigen-bearing invaders directly; they can inactivate them and tag them for destruction.
- The common event in all antibody-antigen interactions is formation of antigen-antibody (or immune) complexes. The defensive mechanisms used by antibodies are neutralization, agglutination, precipitation and complement fixation.
- Of these, complement fixation and neutralization are the most important.
- If memory cells are exposed to the same antigen again, they rapidly become activated and secrete more antibodies.

Active and passive humoral immunity

When B cells encounter antigens and produce antibodies against them, they are exhibiting active humoral immunity.

- Active humoral immunity may be naturally acquired during bacterial and viral infections. You may develop the symptoms of the disease and suffer a little or a lot.
- Artificially acquired active immunity is when a vaccine has been received. The response of the immune system is much the same, whether the antigen invades the body under its own power or is deliberately introduced in the form of a vaccine.

Passive humoral immunity is when instead of being made by your plasma cells, the antibodies are obtained from the serum of an immune human or animal donor. As a result:

- B cells are not challenged by antigens
- immunological memory does not occur
- the protection provided by the borrowed antibodies ends when they naturally degrade in the body.

There are a number of vaccines available (see Table 8.2).

TABLE 8.2 Vaccinations.

Vaccine	Type	Information
Anthrax	Made from antigens from *Bacillus anthracis*	Indicated for individuals who handle infected animals, exposed to imported infected animal products and laboratory staff who work with *B. anthracis.*
BCG	Bacillus Calmette-Guerin (diagnostic agents are available)	Recommended for nearly all age groups: www.gov.uk/phe.
Cholera	Contains inactivated strains of *Vibrio cholerae*	Oral cholera vaccine is licensed for travellers to endemic or epidemic areas (should be completed 1 week prior to travel).
Diphtheria	Prepared from the toxin of *Corynebacterium diphtheriae*	The vaccine stimulates the production of the protective antibody (not available as a single dose it is a combination product which includes other vaccines).
Haemophilus influence type B conjugate vaccine	Capsular polysaccharide conjugated with other proteins to increase immunogenicity	Included as part of childhood immunization.
Hepatitis A	Prepared from formaldehyde-inactivated hepatitis A virus grown in human diploid cells	Recommended for laboratory and healthcare staff; patients with haemophilia, liver failure; travellers to high-risk areas; drug users and those who partake in certain sexual risk behaviours.
Hepatitis B	Inactivated hepatitis B virus surface antigen (HBsAg)	Recommended for a wide variety of individuals, patients and healthcare personnel.
Human papillomavirus	Available in a variety of vaccine types	A two-dose schedule is recommended. Does not protect against all strains, routine cervical screening should continue.
Influenza	The influenza virus (A and C) constantly altering their structure	Recommended for persons at high-risk for those with chronic illness, immunosuppression, HIV infection, obesity
Japanese encephalitis		Indicated for travellers to Asia and the Far East (www.nathnac.org) and laboratory staff

Continued

TABLE 8.2 Vaccinations.—cont'd.

Vaccine	Type	Information
Measles, Mumps and Rubella (German measles)	Live combined vaccine	Every child should receive 2 doses by entry to primary school.
Meningococcal vaccines	Caused by *Neisseria meningitides* serogroups B and C	Separate vaccination is required.
Pertussis (whooping cough)	A cellular vaccine from components of *Bordetella pertussis*	Given in combination preparations with other vaccines. A 3-dose schedule is recommended with booster doses (BNF, 2019).
Pneumococcal	Protects against infection with *Streptococcus pneumoniae*	Recommended for patients with chronic disease, diabetes, immune deficiency, leakage of CSF and recurrent infection. A variety of vaccinations are available.
Poliomyelitis	Inactive virus for injection	Routine immunization and travel abroad (full 3-dose course recommended if travelling to areas of high incidence).
Rabies	Contains inactivated rabies virus	Can be used for both and pre and post exposure prophylaxis.
Rotavirus	A live oral vaccine used to protect against gastro-enteritis	Recommended course, see BNF (2019).
Smallpox		Limited supplies held for exclusive use of workers.
Tetanus	Contains purified toxin of *Clostridium tetani*	Three individual doses are required with an interval of 1 month between doses in children under 10; 2 booster doses at school entry and on leaving.
Typhoid	Drawn from *Salmonella typhi*, available in oral and injection forms	Recommended for travellers and laboratory personnel.
Varicella-zoster (chickenpox)	A live varicella-zoster vaccine	Usually recommended for sero-negative healthy children under 1 year, and healthcare workers.
Yellow fever	A live vaccine	Recommended for a wide variety of individuals, patients and healthcare personnel. The immunity usually lasts for 10 years.

CSF, cerebrospinal fluid.

T lymphocytes

Despite their immense versatility, antibodies provide only partial immunity. They are fairly useless against infections such as TB, and in these cases the second (cell-mediated) immunity comes into play. T cells are more complex. They contain pairs of cell differentiation glycoproteins displayed by mature T cells — for example, CD4 and CD8. In addition, there are also two major groups of T cells — for example, delayed hypersensitivity T cells (T_{DH}) and suppressor T cells (T_S).

CD4 cells (T4 cells) primarily helper T cells (T_H)

Play a central role in the immune response. Their major function is to chemically or directly stimulate proliferation of other T cells and of B cells that have already become bound to an antigen. Without the direct inclusion of T helper cells, there is no immune response. Their lymphokines furnish the chemical help needed to recruit other immune cells to fight off intruders.

CD8 cells (T8 cells) are cytotoxic T cells (T_C)

The only T cells that can directly attack and kill other cells. Activated cytotoxic T cells roam the body, circulating in and out of the blood and lymph and through lymphatic organs in search of body cells displaying antigens to which they are sensitized. Their main targets are:

- virus-infected cells
- intracellular bacteria (TB)
- parasites
- cancer cells
- foreign cells.

Suppressor T cells (T_S)

These are regulatory cells, as they release lymphokines that suppress the activity of both T and B cells. These cells are vital for winding down and finally stopping the immune response after an antigen has been successfully inactivated or destroyed. This helps prevent uncontrolled immune system activity.

Cytokines

As in the inflammatory response, chemical mediators enhance the immune response. Cytokines, the mediators involved in cellular immunity, include hormone-like lymphokines, released by T cells, and monokines, secreted by macrophages.

Some cytokines act as co-stimulators of T cells — for example, interleukins (ILs) 1 and 2. IL-1, released by macrophages, co-stimulates bound T cells to liberate IL-2 and also to synthesize more IL-2 that encourages activated T cells to divide even more rapidly. All activated T cells secrete one or more lymphokines that help amplify and regulate a variety of immune and nonspecific responses.

Each type of T cell has a unique role to play in the immune response, yet at the same time is heavily enmeshed in interactions with other immune cells:

- Cytotoxic T cells prevent infectious micro-organisms hidden from antibody surveillance within cells.
- Helper T cells co-stimulate both other T cells and B cells and recruit nonspecific defences.
- Suppressor T cells prevent runaway or undesirable immune reactions.

However, without helper T cells, **there is no immune response** because the helper cells direct and/or help complete the activation of *all* other immune cells. Their crucial role in immunity is painfully evident when they are destroyed, as in AIDS.

Immunosuppressants

This group of drugs is used to treat autoimmune diseases and prevent rejection of organ transplants. They impair the immune response; they decrease the response to infections and may facilitate the emergence of malignant cells.

Autoimmune disease

This is the response of the immune system against self and may be organ specific or systemic.

Organ specific

The immune response is set up to protect us, but for reasons that are often unexplained, an immune response targets a single organ or gland leading to an inflammatory response. The cellular structure of the organ is replaced by connective tissue and the organ function declines.

Autoimmune diseases include:

- Addison's disease affecting the adrenal gland
- Haemolytic anaemia where the red blood cell membrane is affected
- Graves disease where the production of thyroid stimulating hormone (TSH) antibody results in the over production of thyroid hormone
- Hashimoto thyroiditis where thyroid protein antibodies result in an autoimmune thyroiditis and a goitre with reduced production of thyroid hormones
- Type I diabetes mellitus where antibodies to the beta cells in the pancreas are produced, leading to the non production of insulin
- Myasthenia gravis in which ACh receptor sites are affected
- Pernicious anaemia affecting gastric parietal cells
- Juvenile arthritis, rheumatoid arthritis which affect the joints
- Transverse myelitis in the spinal cord.

Systemic autoimmune diseases

The response is directed towards a large number of target antigens and involves a number of organs and tissues. There is a defect in immune regulation, which results in hyperactive T and B cells. Tissue damage is widespread both from cell-mediated immune responses and from direct cellular damage caused by auto-antibodies.

Includes:

- Ankylosing spondylitis which affects the vertebrae.
- Multiple sclerosis where the target is the white matter in CNS.
- Systemic lupus erythematosus (SLE) where the impact can be on DNA, nuclear protein, red blood cells and platelet membranes. The immune response is directed towards a large number of target antigens and involves a number of organs and tissues.

Disease-modifying antirheumatic drugs

Drugs affecting the immune response can suppress the disease process in rheumatoid arthritis.

The first line of therapy for rheumatoid arthritis is ***methotrexates***; unlike NSAIDs (which only reduce the symptoms), disease-modifying antirheumatic drugs (DMARDs) halt or reverse the underlying disease. Their clinical effects can be slow (months in some instances). They are often combined with NSAIDs or glucocorticoid therapy, but if successful, these can be reduced.

Methotrexate is a folic acid antagonist, which has both cytotoxic and immunosuppressive qualities.

Adverse/side effects

- Bone marrow depression resulting in a drop in white blood cell and platelet counts, which can be so severe as to become life threatening.
- Liver cirrhosis.
- Folic acid administration to prevent blood disorders.

Leflunomide, sulfasalazine, penicillamine and ***ciclosporin*** are other drugs used to treat rheumatoid disease.

Cytokine modulators

These drugs are used only under specialist care and include ***adalimumab, certolizumab, etanercept, golimumab*** and ***infliximab***. They are used when the response to methotrexate or other DMARDs has been inadequate.

Canakinumab is a recombinant monoclonal antibody that selectively inhibits IL-1 β receptor binding. It is used in gouty arthritis and Still disease.

Organ transplantation

Organ transplantation is the treatment of choice for end-stage organ failure. Transplant recipients who may benefit from organ transplantation fall into the following categories:

- Heart — cardiomyopathy, ischaemic heart disease.
- Lungs for emphysema.
- Heart and lungs — cystic fibrosis.
- Liver — primary biliary cirrhosis, chronic active hepatitis.
- Kidney — polycystic kidney disease, glomerulonephritis.
- Kidney and pancreas — diabetic nephropathy.

To suppress rejection of transplanted organs

Ciclosporin, tacrolimus sirolimus and **ciclosporin** is especially useful in suppressing graft-versus-host disease following bone marrow transplantation.

Ciclosporin is a naturally occurring compound found in a fungus, which has potent immunosuppressive activity with no effect on inflammatory reaction.

Action

- Decreases proliferation of T-cells, primarily by inhibiting IL-2 (IL-2) synthesis.
- Reduces the proliferation of cytotoxic T-cells from CD8 + precursor T-cells.
- Reduces function of the effector T-cells responsible for cell-mediated immune responses.
- There is also some reduction of T-cell dependent B-cell immunity responses.

Adverse/side effects

- Nephrotoxicity.
- Hepatotoxicity and hypertension.
- Anorexia, lethargy, hirsutism, tremor, paraesthesia, gum hypertrophy.
- GIT disturbances.

Tacrolimus has a similar effect to **ciclosporin** but with a higher potency.

Azathioprine is cytotoxic and is widely used for immunosuppression; particularly for control of autoimmune diseases, such as rheumatoid arthritis, and to prevent tissue rejection in transplant surgery.

Anti-lymphocytic monoclonal antibodies are also immunosuppressants that are used to prevent rejection, alongside ciclosporin and steroid regimens. They are only used by specialists. Included is **basiliximab**.

Belimumab is sometimes used in SLE for which there are NICE guidelines (https://www.nice.org.uk/guidance/ta397).

Mycophenolate mofetil is an immunosuppressant that is a purine synthesis inhibitor. It is used to prevent organ rejection in certain cases.

Other immunosuppressants work by being T-cell activator inhibitors. An example is *belatacept*, which is used sometimes to prevent graft rejection in renal transplantation.

Anti-inflammatory drugs

NSAIDs and corticosteroids have been dealt with elsewhere in this book.

There is another group of drugs that evoke anti-inflammatory reactions, which are used for gout. This is a metabolic disease in which:

- Hyperuricaemia (raised plasma urate and uric acid concentration) causes uric crystals to be deposited in distal joints (such as the big toe), causing an inflammatory arthritis.
- Uric acid is a by-product of purine nucleotide catabolism from the breakdown of DNA molecules.
- It is an inborn metabolic error that alters uric acid homeostasis and may be due to an increased production or decreased elimination of uric acid.
- Attacks may be precipitated by excess alcohol consumption or a diet high in purine rich foods.
- The deposit of crystals stimulates an inflammatory response, which mobilizes cells and chemicals of innate immunity in an attempt to engulf and neutralize the crystals.

Allopurinol (the main prophylactic drug) or *febuxostat* are both xanthine oxidase inhibitors and work by decreasing uric acid synthesis. This reduces the concentration of insoluble urates and uric acid in tissues, urine and plasma and increases the more soluble precursors such as xanthines and hypoxanthines, reversing the build-up of uric acid crystals in joints.

Adverse/side effects

- GI disturbances.
- Allergic reactions (mainly rashes).
- Some blood problems can occur.

Uricosuric agents increase uric acid excretion by direct action on the renal tubes, and include *probenecid,* and *sulfinpyrazone*, often used if patients are allergic to allopurinol. *Benzbromarone* is available for patients with renal impairment. Aspirin and salicylates should not be used with uricosuric drugs. *Rasburicase* oxidizes uric acid in the blood converting it a more soluble substance (allantoin), which is more easily excreted.

Colchicine is extracted from the crocus plant and inhibits leukocyte and neutrophil migration into joints and tissues.

Adverse/side effects

- GI problems, haemorrhage.
- Nausea, vomiting and abdominal pain.
- Severe diarrhoea.
- Kidney damage.
- Bone marrow depression.
- Peripheral neuropathy.

Due to their anti-inflammatory and analgesic effect NSAIDs *(ibuprofen, naproxen)* and occasionally as an alternative to NSAIDs a glucocorticoid *(hydrocortisone)* are useful as combined therapy.

Antihistamine drugs

These drugs refer to the H_1-receptor antagonist that are used to treat a variety of inflammatory and allergic conditions. You will find them under the relevant sections in the book, as well as listed here.

Nasal sprays or eye drops

Antazoline, azelastine, epinastine, olopatadine and *emedastine* used in the treatment of hay fever and other allergic symptoms.

Ketotifen has other anti-inflammatory properties other than H_1-receptor antagonist actions and stabilizes mast cells.

Allergic reactions

Fexofenadine and *cetirizine* are non-sedating antihistamines and are used for allergic rhinitis or hay fever and urticaria. Topical preparations are available for insect bites, and injectable formulas can be used in conjunction with *adrenaline* in severe hypersensitive reactions to drugs and in the emergency treatment of anaphylaxis.

Antiemetics

Cyclizine, cinnarizine are antihistamines for the prevention of motion sickness and other causes of nausea, such as labyrinthine disorders.

Promethazine is occasionally used for sedation.

Adverse/side effects

- Dry mouth.
- Blurred vision.
- Constipation.
- Retention of urine.
- GI disturbances are common.
- Allergic dermatitis following topical application.

Section 9

Other areas of pharmacology

Section Outline

9.1 HERBAL MEDICINES

Herbal remedies have increased in popularity partly because the public feel that they are 'natural' and therefore healthier and safer options. This is not always the case and, as with any other medicine, they should be used with care. At last these products are being taken seriously in the UK, with results from rigorous clinical trials becoming available. In this Section some of the commoner herbal medicines will be described in alphabetical order.

Regulation

A long overdue registration scheme for herbal medicines was introduced in late 2005. Registered products have to meet standards of safety, quality and consumer information but many unlicensed products are available. The Medicines and Healthcare products Regulatory Agency (MHRA) provides advice on using herbal medicines on its website: www.mhra.gov.uk. There is a list here of all herbal medicines holding a traditional herbal registration (THA) granted by the MHRA and a list of all banned and restricted herbal ingredients.

There are two regulatory schemes for homeopathic medicines; a simplified registration scheme and the national rules scheme. Data have to be submitted to the MHRA to demonstrate the quality, safety and use within homeopathic tradition. Details of labelling and the product literature have also to be submitted.

Homeopathy is defined by the MHRA as 'a system of medicine which involves treating the individual with highly diluted substances, given mainly in tablet form. Based on their individual symptoms, a homeopath will match the most appropriate medicine to each patient' (MHRA, 2014).

A Nurse's Survival Guide to Drugs in Practice. https://doi.org/10.1016/B978-0-7020-7658-9.00009-3

Research by Lazarou and Heinrich (2019) showed that in a survey of 408 participants in the UK, herbal remedies were most popular in the 35—55-year-old age group and were used mostly for self-limiting conditions, such as for sleep and to increase well being. They were also taken as an aid to the digestive system and to boost the immune system. Some were taken for anxiety, and other popular areas were for skin conditions such as eczema.

Herbal remedies were more popular among women than men. Reasons for use mostly included that the products were natural and have fewer side effects; about one-third of those questioned grew their own plants for healthcare. Possible reasons for the increased use of herbal remedies include a greater anxiety about health but also a desire to take care of one's own health.

Drug interactions

These are becoming much more important as the number of patients taking herbal medicines increases.

Warfarin is the most common cardiovascular drug involved in interactions. It was found by Izzo et al. (2005) to interact with boldo, curbicin, fenugreek, garlic, danshen, devil's claw, don quai, ginkgo, papaya, lyceum and mango to cause possible over-anticoagulation. It may react with ginseng, green tea, soy and St John's wort to give a decreased anticoagulation effect.

Individual herbal medicines and their action

Chamomile

Daisy-like plant whose flower heads and oils are used. The oil is an ingredient of some shampoos, promoted as an agent to lighten and condition the hair.

- Chamomile is commonly used as a relaxing tea prepared by soaking the dried flowers, usually in teabags, in boiling water. It may also induce a deep sleep.
- When given in large amounts it often causes gastrointestinal colic and sometimes severe allergic reactions.
- *Apigenin*, an active component found in some chamomile extracts, has been shown to bind to the benzodiazepine receptor in the gamma-aminobutyric acid (GABA) receptor complex of the brain. This action could explain the sedative effect of chamomile.
- In Germany, chamomile is prescribed by general practitioners as a vaginal pessary to combat trichomoniasis and fungal conditions.
- In view of its coumarin content it should not be taken with *warfarin*.
- Chamomile should be avoided by those with a known hypersensitivity to members of the daisy family.

Cranberry juice

The cranberry or guelder rose, *Viburnum opulus*, bears red berries that are compounded into a juice known to have properties that help in urinary tract infections (UTIs).

- Cranberry prevents the adherence of the bacterium *Escherichia coli* (the commonest cause of UTIs) to the bladder and urethral wall.
- UTIs can cause serious kidney infections and cranberry juice is not usually recommended as a sole treatment.
- There is a possibility that cranberry may interfere with the metabolism of some drugs including warfarin. Cranberry juice contains various antioxidants, including flavonoids, which are known to inhibit cytochrome P450 enzyme activity and thus may interfere with drug metabolism.

Echinacea

- This is one of the few commonly used herbs that still carries its Greek name. The common name is coneflower.
- Used in infections such as colds, influenza and fungal infections of the skin.
- Evidence suggests that it is of little use in the prevention of the common cold, but it may be of help in treating and shortening the length of the infection. Barnes (2009) concluded that there are conflicting results in trials assessing echinacea for the prevention and treatment of upper respiratory infections (URIs).
- There is some evidence that incorporated in a gel for topical use it may suppress the itch and erythema associated with insect bites.
- Animal studies have shown that it may act as an immunostimulant on various parts of the immune system. In vitro studies have demonstrated some antibacterial (bacteriostatic) and antiviral properties.
- Should be avoided in chronic disease, such as tuberculosis, multiple sclerosis or HIV. It should also be avoided by individuals who have a known hypersensitivity to the daisy family, and by pregnant women.
- Should only be used for short periods, as tolerance develops when used continually.

Evening primrose oil

Seeds of the evening primrose, *Oenothera biennis*, contain an oil which is high in both linoleic and γ-linolenic acid. These are essential fatty acids needed for prostaglandin synthesis.

- Used in many diverse diseases such as psoriasis, premenstrual breast pain, rheumatic and arthritic conditions and Parkinson's disease.

- Some evidence of its efficacy in breast pain and dermatitis.
- Montserrat-de la Paz et al. (2013) found that dietary evening primrose oil reduced some pro-inflammatory mediators in mice and may be of benefit in chronic conditions such as fibromyalgia.
- Should be avoided in people with epilepsy or a past history of epileptic seizures, and it should be avoided in people with schizophrenia.
- Generally well tolerated but may cause mild gastrointestinal effects, such as nausea, indigestion and softening of stools.
- May cause headaches due to effect on cerebral blood vessels.

Feverfew

This is *Tanacetum parthenium*, commonly known as the tansy, and belongs to the daisy family. It is also known as 'featherfew' because of its feathery leaves and its yellow flowers bloom from June to October (Pareek et al. 2011). It is available as capsules to treat migraine.

The feverfew group of plants includes the pyrethrum, which contains pyrethrins, commonly used in insecticide sprays. These are reportedly nontoxic to humans, but are a strong irritant to the eyes and mucous membranes. It has a strong and bitter odour. Hypersensitivity reactions can occur.

- The name suggests that feverfew leaf extract would be used to counteract fevers, and this was one of the original uses. Early Greek physicians used it for 'all hot inflammations'. It is anti-inflammatory (inhibits prostaglandin synthesis) and may also be anticancer. It is very complex chemically and the reader is referred to the article by Pareek et al. (2011) for further details of its complex actions.
- Used as a migraine prophylactic and as an antiarthritic drug.
- Has also been used for allergies, asthma, tinnitus, dizziness, nausea and vomiting.
- Appears to have antiplatelet activity and should not be used in individuals on anticoagulant therapy.
- Long-term use and sudden discontinuation causes rebound headaches.
- Laboratory studies have shown some anti-inflammatory properties on the immune system, which would be useful in autoimmune conditions.
- Feverfew has some inhibitory action on the enzyme phospholipase A_2, involved in synthesis of chemicals involved in inflammation.
- Contraindicated in pregnancy because of the possibility of miscarriage.

Garlic

Garlic (*Allium sativum*) is a member of the onion family. The pharmacologically active compounds derived from the clove contain sulphur and are responsible for the strong odours associated with garlic. The sulphides are excreted on the breath and in sweat and other body secretions, enabling us to recognize that someone has eaten food containing garlic! The term *alliaceous* describes anything with this type of smell.

- A diet high in members of the onion family has long been reputed to have cardioprotective properties and the principal use of garlic is in the treatment of cardiovascular disease, where it is reported to decrease atheroma formation.
- Garlic has antiplatelet activity that is dose-dependent and may also be fibrinolytic.
- A recent meta-analysis of 14 research articles (Sun et al. 2018) came to the conclusion that garlic appears to lower plasma low-density lipoprotein (LDL) cholesterol levels and total cholesterol rather than triglycerides and high-density lipoprotein (HDL).
- Some studies have shown a blood pressure–lowering effect.
- Shown in some studies to have a hypoglycaemic effect.
- Garlic is antioxidant and is said to protect against viral infections such as the common cold as well as some cancers, but there is no conclusive evidence for this although some antibiotic-resistant bacteria are susceptible to garlic extracts in vitro.
- Patients taking *warfarin* should not take garlic as it may increase the activity of warfarin and is antiplatelet.
- In therapeutic doses, garlic should be avoided in clients on hypoglycaemic therapies and anti-inflammatory agents, such as *aspirin*.
- Garlic should be avoided by pregnant women at doses exceeding those used in foods, as it may cause miscarriage.

Ginger

Ginger is a spice derived from the rhizomes and stems of *Zingiber officinale*, a common garden plant found in the tropics and subtropics. It is used as a flavouring agent but is also used as an antiemetic.

- There is evidence that ginger helps in the nausea of travel or motion sickness, whether caused by car, plane or ship. It may also reduce nausea in pregnancy and has no known teratogenic effects.
- It does not appear to be of any value in postoperative nausea or that caused by chemotherapy.
- Research suggests that ginger extract helps to reduce pain and inflammation in osteoarthritis by 40% compared to a placebo (*Arthritis Today*, 2018).
- Occasionally causes gastric upset due to hyperacidity.
- Ginger may lower thromboxane levels in platelets, so safety with *warfarin* is in doubt.

- Other uses for ginger, such as in cancer and in infections, are unsubstantiated.
- A common sign of ginger toxicity is diarrhoea and therapy should cease if diarrhoea occurs.

Ginkgo

Ginkgo comes from the leaves of the tree of the same name, *Ginkgo biloba*, commonly called the maidenhair tree and found in China. Chinese medicine has used ginkgo for centuries as a treatment for brain disorders.

- Extracts of ginkgo have quite powerful antioxidant properties (contain bioflavonoids) and are able to scavenge free radicals in the body; this is the probable mechanism for its action.
- Many studies have shown that ginkgo can prevent tissue damage and increase the blood flow to various organs, especially the brain.
- There is evidence that ginkgo improves memory function in older people. In Germany it is used as a standardized extract to treat various dementias, including Alzheimer's disease, seemingly with considerable success.
- Ginkgo is a good alternative to caffeine for promoting alertness without the side effect of sympathetic stimulation.
- Another use is in plastic surgery, where it is used to help in skin grafting and to promote the healing of skin flaps.
- Ginkgo is potentially of value in many circulation problems, and ongoing research is seeking to support its medicinal properties.
- Side effects are mild gastrointestinal upsets and headaches, both of which are uncommon. Diarrhoea, nausea, vomiting, irritability and restlessness may occur with high doses.
- Seeds of the tree, extracts of which are sometimes used to treat urinary incontinence, are considered to be quite toxic. The use of seed preparations is inadvisable.

Ginseng

Ginseng is available in a variety of preparations, from chewing gums to liquid elixirs. The origin of ginseng is in the Far East, mainly China and Korea. The active Korean form is prepared from the root of *Panax ginseng*. Ginseng is said to have many beneficial properties. It has antioxidant properties and proposed active ingredients of ginseng are a group of steroid substances that may have slight androgenic activity.

The principal use of ginseng is as a substance that can increase stamina and well being. It is also said to have aphrodisiac properties.

- The case for ginseng as a physical and mental stimulant remains unproven, but evidence to date provides some support for these effects.

- The preparations should not be taken at night, and the heavy use of caffeine-containing drinks should be avoided in case of insomnia.
- As with most of the herbs mentioned so far, the concurrent use of *warfarin* may be contraindicated.
- Ginseng should be avoided with stimulants, antipsychotic drugs or monoamine oxidase inhibitors and in those with any acute illness or hypertension.
- A course for a few days is said to give therapeutic benefit and a prolonged course of therapy is not recommended.

Red clover

Clover is a very common weed that has a symbiotic relationship with nitrogen-fixing bacteria and is an important part of the diet for many herbivorous animals. There are several hundred different species, but the main one of interest to herbalists is the red or purple flowering variety, *Trifolium pratense*.

- Extracts are used for a variety of conditions, including skin diseases, certain cancers and coughs.
- Clover is a rich source of isoflavones, potent antioxidants and free-radical scavengers. These are the properties that are being closely examined at present.
- All isoflavones have weak oestrogenic activity which may contribute to their therapeutic action.
- Recent publications show an increase in bone density in postmenopausal women taking red clover isoflavones and they may have protective effect on the development of postmenopausal cardiovascular disease.
- Red clover should be used cautiously in individuals susceptible to bleeding problems or who are receiving anticoagulants.

Saw palmetto

This has been used for various urogenital conditions, from infections to impotence, but its main use relates to its effect on the enlarged prostate gland.

- The condition of benign prostatic hypertrophy (BPH) is very common in elderly men and can cause urinary retention.
- Saw palmetto supposedly causes a decrease in the size of the prostate gland, and many studies have shown that it is equivalent to *finasteride* (see Section 7.4) in action but without the side effects.
- A study looking at the impact of saw palmetto on lower urinary tract symptoms during treatment of prostatic cancer by radiotherapy (Sikorski et al. 2016) found no dose-limiting toxicity for saw palmetto up to 960 mg daily, but found its efficacy needed further investigation.

- Contains many fatty acids and sterols. One of these, sitosterol, inhibits the conversion of testosterone into its active form, dihydrotestosterone.
- May also block the dihydrotestosterone receptor sites.
- Could be beneficial in baldness, acne and female hirsutism.
- Side effects, if they occur, are mild and may include headaches or gastrointestinal upsets.
- Drug interactions are so far unknown, but it would be sensible not to use it with oestrogens such as the oral contraceptive pill or hormone replacement therapy.

St John's wort (Hypericum perforatum)

This herb is used as an antidepressant and preparations are standardized according to their hypericin (the active component) content. It is popular in Germany where it is prescribed for depression but is not licensed to be sold OTC in the United States.

- Some studies have shown the herb to be as good as tricyclic or selective serotonin reuptake inhibitor (SSRI) antidepressants without so many unwanted effects.
- Probably acts by modifying the dopaminergic, noradrenergic or serotonergic receptor activity in the brain and benefit may not be seen for 3–4 weeks following commencement of therapy.
- Should not be used in combination with other antidepressants, sedatives or alcohol. It is dangerous to take with other antidepressants which may actually work on serotonin transmission and so produce an additive effect.
- Photosensitivity may occur and precautions should be taken in the sun.
- Should be avoided in pregnancy as it has abortifacient and teratogenic properties in high doses.
- A metanalysis (Ng et al. 2017) looked at evidence from 27 clinical trials and concluded that St John's wort had similar efficacy to an SSRI for mild-moderate depression but had a lower dropout rate in the studies. As the length of the studies was from 4 to 12 weeks, evidence for long-term efficacy and safety is not available in this analysis.

9.2 PAEDIATRIC PHARMACOLOGY

This is a specialist area and there is a British National Formulary (BNF) for children available online at www.bnfc.org. The reader is referred to this text for details of drug dosages in children. This is a complex area where age may range from premature babies at 24 weeks' gestation to adolescents. Many drugs in the adult BNF are not licensed for use in children. Occasionally paediatric specialists may use unlicensed drugs if there is no alternative.

Medicines are not given to children unless absolutely necessary and following the discussion of treatment options with the parents or child's carers.

Licensing of medicines

Many manufacturers write disclaimers that their products should not be used in children.

Some medicines do have proven problems, but it is usually due to a lack of clinical trials in paediatrics (they can be ethically difficult, and additional cost to manufacturer may not be recouped).

Some medicines are used unlicensed (off-label) and it is not unusual for babies in neonatal units to receive at least one unlicensed medicine during their hospital stay. Over 50% of drugs used in children may not have been studied in this age group and the BNF does include advice on the use of off-label medicines.

The MHRA also has a section on medicines for children available at www.mhra.gov.uk, where they emphasize the need for more trials so that safe dosages and the correct formulation may be supplied for medicines in children. EU regulation on paediatric medicines was adopted at the end of 2006 and the European Commission published a 10-year report in 2017 on the implementation of the paediatric regulations. This did show an overall increase in authorized medicines in children but with some areas weaker than others. Infectious diseases and rheumatology were doing well but oncology and neonatology need to develop further. There is a European database of clinical trials.

Paediatric dosage considerations

- Dose administered to a child is never equivalent to that administered to an adult and the relationship between adult and paediatric doses is not linear.
- Doses based on age bands are used for drugs with a wide therapeutic index.
- Age and body weight may be used to calculate dosage (Table 9.1). Body surface area is a more reliable indicator as it reflects cardiac output, renal function and fluid requirements better than weight. In practice, surface area

TABLE 9.1 Age ranges and definitions.

Preterm newborn infants	Born at <37 weeks' gestation
Term newborn infants	0–27 days
Infants and toddlers	28 days to 23 months
Children	2–11 years
Adolescents	12 to 16–18 years

is only occasionally used for drugs with a low therapeutic index, such as cytotoxic agents.

- The recommended dose has usually been calculated by the manufacturer and is in the BNF for children, taking into account all the above factors.

Pharmacokinetic factors in children

There are age-related differences in the body's handling of drugs, and this may lead to different dose requirements.

Absorption and drug action

- In the first 6 months of life there is slower peristalsis and gastric emptying allowing greater drug absorption and sometimes higher plasma levels.
- Activity and concentration of gastric secretions is less in the newborn. Gastric pH at birth is between 6 and 8. It remains relatively high until falling to adult levels by about age 2–3. This means there is reduced absorption of acidic medicines, such as phenytoin.
- Low levels of bile in the newborn may impair absorption of some fat-soluble drugs.
- Parenteral absorption via an intramuscular injection is unpredictable in both the very young and very old due to poor tissue perfusion and reduced muscle mass. This method is also painful and should be avoided.
- Topical administration in the very young may lead to high drug absorption, as their skin has fewer waterproof and protective layers.

Distribution and drug action

- Lower concentration of plasma proteins and therefore a higher concentration of unbound drug available.
- Capacity of plasma proteins to bind drug is well below adult levels for about 2 years.
- Bilirubin can be displaced from albumin by drugs that strongly bind. This is especially important in the neonatal period because the blood–brain barrier is not yet fully developed and bilirubin may enter the brain.
- Levels of body fluid decrease with age and the levels of fat increase.
- Total body water in the premature neonate is 92% and 75% in the term newborn baby.
- Fat content in preterm babies in very low at about 3%. In full-term babies it is 12%, in 1-year-olds it is 30% and in adults it is about 18%.
- Level of extracellular fluid will affect the level of the drug actually reaching the receptor. This will be a lower concentration in the neonate and a diminished response will result.
- Fat-soluble drugs will accumulate less in fat reservoirs in the young and will tend to have a faster but briefer action because of this.

Metabolism and drug action

- The activity of drug-metabolizing enzymes does not reach adult level until about 3 years of age.
- Before this, the capacity of neonates and young children to metabolize drugs is poor. Hepatic clearance is reduced and half-lives increase.
- May mean some drugs are administered only once daily in newborns, instead of twice daily.
- Some metabolic pathways may be different, for example, paracetamol metabolism.

Excretion and drug action

- Rates of glomerular filtration and renal blood flow are lower in the neonate than the adult.
- Clearance of drugs dependent on the renal route is lower and extended dose intervals may be required.
- Renal function usually reaches adult level after about a year.

Administration of medicines

The child should be involved in decisions about medication where age and circumstances allow this. Obtaining co-operation is essential and more likely if a parent or friend is giving the medicine.

There may be difficulty taking the medication as the correct formulation may not be available. Liquid forms of many medicines do not exist.

An oral syringe is supplied when the dose is less than 5 mL and is used to calculate doses accurately and to administer the drug in a controlled manner.

Care must be taken when trying to disguise the taste of a medicine as some drugs may interact with various foods. It is better to give a drink after the medicine has been taken if possible.

Sugar-free medicines should be provided when possible to prevent dental caries. If the medicine is not sugar free, parents should be advised on dental hygiene in long-term use.

The intravenous route is usually preferred if a drug cannot be given orally.

Intramuscular injections should be avoided when possible, but certain drugs such as vaccines are only administered intramuscularly.

9.3 DRUGS AND THE ELDERLY

The elderly form an increasingly large percentage of those requiring health-care. Chronic conditions often warrant long-term pharmacological therapy but you may not be aware of the extent of prescribing to the elderly. Although those over 65 years of age made up about 20% of the UK population in 2018, they received nearly half of all prescribed medication, with about one-third taking three or more different medications. The risk of falls increases by about 14% for every extra medication taken over the first four, so care with prescribing is essential.

Polypharmacy is the norm, not the exception. Possible reasons include:

- multiple pathologies
- increasing range of drugs available
- inappropriate prescribing
- lack of medication review
- increased emphasis on preventative treatments.

The increased availability of OTC drugs must also be remembered and the elderly could well be taking herbal remedies and vitamin preparations that may interact with their prescribed drugs. An example is cranberry juice. This is very popular for its antiseptic properties within the urinary system and its antioxidant properties but there is a possibility that it may interfere with the metabolism of warfarin, making the latter less effective (see Section 5.7).

There is a correlation between increasing age and adverse drug reaction (ADR) rate and the elderly are more susceptible to ADRs because of:

- exposure to more medication
- age-related physiological changes in pharmacokinetics
- age-related changes in pharmacodynamics
- increased pathological changes due to disease processes
- impaired homeostasis
- poor compliance that may be due to poor memory, failing sight, bad hearing, declining dexterity and decreased mobility.

It is a challenge for those in healthcare to provide appropriate treatment for multiple conditions while minimizing side effects and the risk of iatrogenic disease.

New signs and symptoms in the elderly should always be regarded as possible adverse reactions to medication already taken (e.g. thiazide-induced gout, phenothiazine-induced parkinsonian tremor, increased incidence of falls due to hypnotics or antihypertensives) (Box 9.1).

BOX 9.1 Drugs in the elderly

- Doses need to be tailored to the client – often a lower dose is needed
- Repeat prescriptions should be reviewed regularly and unnecessary drugs withdrawn
- Drugs that are needed should not be withheld: for instance, aspirin as secondary prevention for a myocardial infarction, warfarin for atrial fibrillation
- Start low, go slow, is good advice but sometimes drugs are underprescribed and so do not control the condition (e.g. angiotensin converting enzyme inhibitors in heart failure, tricyclics for depression)

Changes in pharmacokinetics

All pharmacokinetic parameters — absorption, distribution, metabolism and elimination — may be significantly altered. These changes should be taken into account and are even more important if a drug has a narrow therapeutic window.

Absorption

We may expect this to be impaired due to:

- reduced gastric acidity
- reduced surface area for absorption
- reduced blood flow to the gastrointestinal tract
- reduced gastrointestinal motility
- delayed gastric emptying.

Although the overall absorption may be slightly lower, these effects are rarely important.

Distribution

May be influenced by the following changes:

- Significant decrease in the lean body mass: standard dose of drug therefore provides a greater amount of drug per kg of body weight.
- Total body water may decrease by as much as 15%: distribution of water-soluble drugs therefore decreased (e.g. digoxin, theophylline, antibiotics), leading to higher plasma concentrations.
- Body fat is increased so lipid-soluble drugs may have a larger volume of distribution and this may prolong their half-lives (e.g. benzodiazepines, psychotropics).
- In general, standard doses of drugs may need reduction.
- Plasma albumin is normally well maintained, but may be reduced by up to 25% in chronic disease, resulting in higher levels of drugs normally protein bound (e.g. warfarin, phenytoin, diazepam, furosemide).

Metabolism

Hepatic metabolism is reduced in the elderly due to:

- loss of liver mass
- reduced blood flow to the liver.

Other disease states will further reduce liver blood flow, such as heart failure.

First-pass metabolism of drugs with a high extraction ratio (e.g. propranolol) is impaired. A dose reduction of between 30% and 40% may be needed for such drugs.

Liver enzyme activity may also be impaired and so it is necessary to monitor drugs with a narrow therapeutic index especially carefully (e.g. digoxin, warfarin, theophylline).

Renal elimination

This is the most important age-related change in pharmacokinetics.

- Renal function deteriorates with age. Glomerular filtration rate decreases by approximately 1% per year over the age of 40 years.
- Reduced clearance of renally excreted drugs may lead to accumulation and toxicity.
- Renal impairment may not be obvious, as decreasing muscle mass means that plasma creatinine levels may be normal.
- Drugs with a low therapeutic index are most dangerous (e.g. digoxin, lithium).
- Other diseases (e.g. diabetes, heart failure) may adversely affect renal function.
- Acute illnesses may lead to a rapid decline in renal function.
- Some drugs are best avoided completely in the elderly, such as long-acting hypoglycaemics (e.g. glibenclamide) and long-acting benzodiazepines (e.g. diazepam). Age-related accumulation may occur due to their long half-lives.

Changes in pharmacodynamics

Changes may occur due to the change in responsiveness of the target organs and altered receptor sensitivity.

- There is increased sensitivity to some drugs. The elderly are especially sensitive to drugs acting on the central nervous system (CNS), such as benzodiazepines, opioids and antiparkinsonian drugs.
- Cholinergic transmission in the brain declines with age and the elderly may be more prone to drug-induced confusion.
- Side effects of slowed gastrointestinal motility and retention of urine tend to be greater with anticholinergic drugs such as tricyclic antidepressants (e.g. amitriptyline).
- More sensitive to warfarin, due to greater inhibition of vitamin K-dependent clotting factors.
- More sensitive to diuretics due to impaired ability to maintain homeostasis.
- More prone to drug-induced hypotension.
- Thermoregulatory mechanisms may be impaired and this means that hypothermia may occur with certain drugs (e.g. phenothiazines and opioids).

- Response to some drugs may be reduced due to downregulation of receptors or reduced drug–receptor binding (e.g. beta-blocker function declines with age).

Adverse drug reactions in the elderly

Due to the factors listed above, the elderly are especially predisposed to ADRs. The majority of ADRs are dose-dependent and therefore predictable but still many admissions to acute elderly care units are due to ADRs. Adverse reactions also tend to be more severe when they do occur in the elderly.

The main drug groups involved in ADRs are:

- cardiovascular drugs
- nonsteroidal anti-inflammatory drugs (NSAIDs)
- psychotropics.

Patients in residential care often receive more medication than those living independently and may see several different doctors, thus lacking continuity of care. Box 9.2 lists drugs most commonly prescribed in the elderly.

Drugs acting on the central nervous system

The half-life of diazepam alters from 20 hours in a 20-year-old to 90 hours in an 80-year-old. The drugs take longer to be metabolized and may remain in the body for long periods of time. The elderly may remain partially sedated the following day after taking a hypnotic and this has a cumulative effect, leading to increased drowsiness and confusion.

Administration of benzodiazepines is a well-identified risk factor for increased falls resulting in a fractured neck of femur.

Other drugs associated with falls include antipsychotics such as *chlorpromazine*. These drugs tend to make the patient drowsy and used to be called 'major tranquillizers'. They are used to treat psychoses such as schizophrenia.

BOX 9.2 Drugs most commonly prescribed in the elderly

Diuretics
Antihypertensives
Hypoglycaemics
Nitrates
Beta blockers
Digitalis
Antianxiety agents
Antidepressants

Depression in the elderly

Depression is the most common mental health problem of older people. It is underdiagnosed and is the most common factor precipitating suicide in the elderly. Deaths from suicide are higher than in any other age group, ranking in the top 10 causes of death, yet depression is eminently treatable.

Certain illnesses in the elderly are associated with high rates of depression (e.g. Parkinson's disease).

Although antidepressants are the key for some, their use may also be associated with an increased risk of falls. It must be noted, though, that the negative effects of drug use on falling are frequently studied but the beneficial results of drug therapy often tend to be ignored.

Analgesics

An increased incidence of falls may be associated with opioid analgesia especially and drugs such as morphine may cause drowsiness. Some research has shown an increase in falls associated with the use of NSAIDs.

Antihypertensive drugs

One-third of the population in Britain over the age of 50 is hypertensive. This means a high proportion of the elderly should be on treatment for raised blood pressure.

The autonomic nervous system does not always function as efficiently in the elderly, and drugs are a major cause of postural hypotension. Included would be any drugs prescribed for their antihypertensive action.

Other drugs associated with a drop in blood pressure include:

- nitrates used for angina
- antiparkinsonian drugs (e.g. levodopa)
- antidepressants and antipsychotics.

Although the problem of polypharmacy is enormous, it is frequently overlooked as the causative factor when an elderly client falls.

Nonspecific complaints in the elderly such as confusion, lethargy, weakness, dizziness, incontinence, depression and falling should all prompt a close look at the patient's drug list.

The key to successful medication regimens in the elderly, as in all client groups, is communication. Planning care with the person and careful explanation in understandable terms of how the drugs work and why they are needed are essential. Discussing how the person feels on their new medication is essential. We want to know whether it actually improves their lifestyle or perhaps they may even feel worse since they commenced the drug.

Guidelines given in the BNF (2019) for prescribing in the elderly include careful consideration whether a drug is actually indicated at all. Recommendations are:

- To limit the range of drugs prescribed so that familiarity of their use and effects of the drugs in the elderly are understood.
- To reduce the dose in the elderly compared with that in young people. Sometimes 50% of the adult dose may be prescribed.
- Regular tablet reviews in case it is possible to discontinue some medications. Blood tests to assess renal function can sometimes indicate that a lower dose is required due to poor elimination.
- Try and simplify drug regimens to avoid a confusing array of dosages.
- Explain very clearly what the drugs are for and how they should be taken. Ensure instructions are given in full on each prescription and packaging.
- Make sure the patient understands how to obtain repeat prescriptions and involve a relative or friend if necessary.

New drugs should not be prescribed without thoughtful decision-making based on the individual and it should be remembered that the aim of prescribing in the elderly is to improve general well being and restore functional dependence. An improved quality of life is the treatment goal, not just prolongation of life.

9.4 TOPICAL DRUGS

Topical drugs are applied to surfaces of the body, usually as creams or lotions, for their local action. They usually have two components, a base and an active ingredient. Examples include eye drops and ointments, ear drops, nose drops and all the lotions and creams that are applied to the skin.

The skin

The skin is susceptible to many diseases including inflammatory conditions that may be allergic or infective in nature. Although the skin has properties that ensure it is virtually waterproof, some chemicals can be absorbed and pass through the skin with relative ease once they have penetrated the keratinized epidermis. This is partly dependent upon the base that is used to carry the drug, commonly as a lotion, cream or ointment, which may also be important in hydrating the skin. These are briefly described in Section 1.4.

Ointments, creams and lotions

Ointments are oily with a high fat content whereas creams are thinner and aqueous, having a water base. Creams disappear rapidly due to evaporation of the water content when applied to the surface of the skin. Any oil in them is absorbed, softening the keratin layer of the skin and making it feel softer. This property has led to their use as cosmetics.

- Creams are aqueous when oil is dispersed in water and oily if water is dispersed in oil. Barrier creams are used to protect the skin against water or sunlight.
- Ointments are greasy and adhere to the skin. They are more occlusive than creams and not so readily absorbed. Ointments are useful in dry, scaly conditions and may also be used as protection, an example being lip balm. There are water-soluble ointments that do not stain clothing, emulsifying ointments such as lanolin, used to retain the chemical in contact with the skin, and nonemulsifying ointments that do not mix with water. The latter often have paraffin as a base and are used when the skin is dry and scaly in such conditions as psoriasis, eczema and chapped hands.

Lanolin is wool fat and some people become sensitized to lanolin with prolonged use.

- Lotions are liquids applied to the skin and evaporate quickly. They may be used for cooling or antiseptic actions and often contain alcohol to increase speed of evaporation. They are often preferred for hairy areas of the body. Shake lotions contain a powder that is left on the skin after the lotion has evaporated (e.g. *calamine lotion*).
- Pastes contain a large amount of powder and can be applied to small areas of the skin such as the lesions in psoriasis. They are less occlusive than ointments.
- **Emollients** are used to hydrate, smooth and soothe the skin in such conditions as eczema. They need frequent application even when the condition has improved. Examples are *aqueous cream* which is readily absorbed and more greasy preparations such as *white soft paraffin.*

Some emollient bath products contain tar (useful in psoriasis and eczema), others contain oatmeal (useful in eczema and dry skin) whilst some contain paraffin. Urea is sometimes added as a keratin softener and hydrating agent, which may be useful in the elderly.

MHRA warning (2018) that there can be a fire risk with paraffin-based skin emollients covered by a dressing or clothing and patients should not use a naked flame or smoke near these.

- Barrier preparations often contain water repellent substances and are protective. They are used on the skin around stomas, on unbroken pressure areas in the elderly and to prevent nappy rash. They may contain a water repellent such as **dimeticone**. Examples include **Sudocrem**, **Drapolene** and **zinc cream**.

Active ingredients

Corticosteroids

- Frequently prescribed as they suppress the local immune or inflammatory response.
- They may be given alone in contact dermatitis, atopic eczema and insect stings or may be combined with a bactericidal or antifungal agent for infections of the skin.

If there is an infection present, corticosteroids should never be used alone as they will suppress the inflammatory response but allow spread of the infective agent.

- Corticosteroids are not curative and when the cream is stopped the condition may reappear.
  Examples are:
  - **hydrocortisone 1%** − a mild corticosteroid
  - **betnovate RD** − moderately potent
  - **betamethasone valerate 0.1%** − potent
  - **clobetasol propionate 0.05%** − very potent.

The least potent corticosteroid at the lowest strength necessary should always be used and they should normally be applied sparingly, no more than twice a day, only to the affected area.

Nappy rash

- The first line of treatment is always to ensure nappies are changed regularly and tight-fitting waterproof protection is avoided.
- The rash may clear with the use of exposure followed by a barrier cream.
- A mild corticosteroid (0.5%) may be used (not in neonates) if the inflammation and rash is causing discomfort and the barrier cream is applied after the steroid cream.
- The steroid should be used for no longer than a week.

- An antifungal may be required if there is a candidal infection (thrush); cotrimazole cream is an example.

Coal tar

This is anti-inflammatory and antimitotic. It was widely used years ago but now has been largely replaced by corticosteroids. Coal tar remains valuable in eczema and psoriasis and preparations are available that can be added to the bath. Coal tar pastes may be used in eczema, and in psoriasis ***dithranol*** is used.

Antimicrobial agents

Antibacterial, antiviral and antifungal agents are all available as creams to apply to the skin.

Antibacterial preparations

In a bacterial infection, the infective organism should be identified before treatment.

Prolonged treatment can lead to sensitization and penicillin and sulphonamides should never be used on the skin due to high risk of sensitization. Infections of the skin are often treated with systemic antibiotics.

- Cellulitis is a rapidly spreading inflammation of the skin and subcutaneous tissue that requires systemic treatment and often involves a staphylococcal infection.
- Erysipelas is usually due to a streptococcal infection and is superficial with clearly defined edges to the lesions. It also requires systemic antibiotics.
- Impetigo is due to staphylococcal infection and if there is only a small lesion it may be treated with ***fusidic acid*** applied topically. If extensive, a systemic antibiotic (e.g. flucloxacillin), is needed.
- Not all skin conditions that are oozing or have pustules are infected and antibacterials should be avoided in leg ulcers unless used as a short course for a defined infection.

Fungal infections

Localized fungal infections are treated with topical antifungals. Treatment should always be continued for 2 weeks after the lesion has disappeared to prevent relapse. The agent is often combined with a mild corticosteroid.

- Ringworm can infect the scalp, the body, the hand, the foot (athlete's foot) or the nail. In nail and scalp infections, a systemic antifungal is usually needed.

- Agents used include the imidazole antifungals such as *clotrimazole, econazole* and *ketoconazole. Terbinafine* cream is effective but more expensive.
- Candidiasis (thrush) may be treated with imidazole antifungals or *nystatin.*
- Sometimes refractory candidiasis needs systemic treatment with a triazole such as *fluconazole.*

Antiviral preparations

Cold sores are due to herpes simplex infection and once the virus is present the cold sores will recur under certain conditions such as exposure to strong sunlight.

Aciclovir (Zovirax) cream is used to treat cold sores. The person usually knows when the cold sore is developing and early application is needed for successful treatment. If infection is frequent, systemic treatment may be required.

Parasiticidal preparations for the skin

Scabies (itch mite). This is an infection by the *Sarcoptes scabiei* mite that reproduces on the skin and burrows into the skin to lay its eggs. Scabies can be transmitted without body contact via shared clothing, towels or bedding.

Permethrin is used and *malathion* if permethrin is unsuitable. All members of the infected household should be treated simultaneously and treatment should be applied to the whole body.

The itch remains often for weeks after the parasite has been eliminated and *crotamiton* can be used for this. A topical corticosteroid may help but take care that the mite has actually been eliminated.

Head lice (Pediculus humanus capitis)
These are wingless insects that spend their entire lives on the human scalp and feed exclusively on human blood. They are about the size of a sesame seed. Head lice eggs are called nits and can be seen attached to individual hairs. They are either brown or white (empty shells). They cause itching and there may be a feeling of something moving in the hair. They are very common and spread easily. They are not associated with poor hygiene. Special fine-tooth combs are used to identify the lice.

Treatment is with *dimeticone* which coats the lice and prevents their excretion of water. Treatment has to be repeated after 7 days as it is less effective against eggs. *Malathion* is an organophosphorus insecticide that is an alternative, but resistance has been reported. Infected members of the family should be treated at the same time.

The MHRA issued a warning (2018) that these products may be flammable and there is a risk of serious burns if hair is exposed to flames or ignition.

Eczema (dermatitis)

The commonest form is atopic and is associated with hay fever and asthma. This often occurs in childhood and has a familial component. The skin affected is red, scaly and dry. There may be weeping areas where vesicles have formed and crusting over of the skin surface.

Dry skin needs an emollient to be applied regularly and liberally. Examples include aqueous cream and E45. This should continue if the condition improves and also alongside other agents being used to treat the eczema.

Topical corticosteroids are used. Only mild forms should be used on the face and neck. Elsewhere the potency prescribed depends on the severity of the condition.

Lichenification due to repeated scratching is treated with potent corticosteroids. Bandages containing *ichthammol paste*, to reduce pruritis, may be applied over the steroid. Sometimes coal tar and ichthammol are used in chronic eczema.

Severe refractory eczema is managed by a specialist and may involve treatment with drugs that reduce the immune response such as *ciclosporin*, *pimecrolimus* or *tacrolimus*. Long-term safety of the topical agents is still being evaluated so they are not first-line options.

Alitretinoin is used in severe refractory hand eczema that does not respond to corticosteroids. Contraception must be used to prevent pregnancy in women of child-bearing age.

Psoriasis

Skin lesions occur due to rapid proliferation of cells in the epidermis producing thickening and scaling. Epidermal cells usually divide about every 28 days, but in psoriasis this may be reduced to every 3–4 days so that the cells do not mature. It is an immune reaction, but the antigen is unknown. Psoriatic plaques tend to occur on the elbows, knees, lower back, buttocks, scalp and nails. It is difficult to produce a long-term remission.

Psoriasis may occasionally be provoked by certain drugs including lithium, chloroquine, NSAIDs, beta blockers and ACE inhibitors.

- Emollients such as *E45* are used to reduce scaling and itching. They are also useful alongside other treatments.
- Topical corticosteroids may be used for localized acute lesions.
- Vitamin D preparations are used in chronic plaque psoriasis. They affect cell division and should only be applied to the lesions. They may be irritant and hands must be washed after application. Examples are *calcipotriol* and *tacalcitol.*
- Coal tar derivatives may be valuable, such as *coal tar paste* and calamine and coal tar ointment. Shampoos and impregnated dressings are also available.
- *Dithranol* decreases cell division and heals plaques but can burn healthy skin so has to be applied as a thick paste. It is also available combined with yellow soft paraffin and can be applied at home and washed off after 30 minutes. It leaves brown staining on healed areas for a few days due to oxidization products and will stain clothing or bedclothes purple.
- *Tazarotene* is a retinoid with similar efficacy to vitamin D but it causes more irritation usually. It does not stain and is odourless. It should be applied sparingly over the plaques to try and avoid irritation.
- Phototherapy using ultraviolet B radiation is available in specialist centres under the care of a dermatologist. It is useful in chronic psoriasis but may irritate inflammatory psoriasis.
- Systemic drugs are available in severe resistant psoriasis under specialist care. *Acitretin* is a vitamin A derivative and needs to be combined with other forms of treatment. It is teratogenic and this remains a risk for up to 3 years after use so women of childbearing age must be counselled and contraception used. Liver function must also be monitored.

Drugs affecting the immune system are used in both eczema and psoriasis. Systemic drugs are only used under specialist care. Ciclosporin given orally can be used in severe psoriasis or sever eczema.

Methotrexate (alongside folate) may be used for severe psoriasis. The dose has to be adjusted according to the severity of the condition and the blood measurements.

Drugs that inhibit the activity of tumour necrosis factor (TNF) such as *etanercept, adalimumab* and *infliximab,* can be used by specialist in severe plaque psoriasis.

Acne

Needs to be treated early to avoid scarring.

Patients should be told that improvement may take at least 2 months.

Topical preparations are used in mild to moderate acne. If these are ineffective or if the acne is severe, oral antibacterials are used.

- Topical preparations include **benzoyl peroxide**. This produces local skin irritation at first but this often subsides as treatment continues. It is also available combined with an antibacterial.
- **Azelaic acid** is an alternative that may be less irritant. It has antimicrobial properties.
- Antibacterial resistance of *Propionibacterium acnes* is increasing. Topical antibacterials are often not effective and should be used in those who do not wish to take systemic antibiotics or cannot tolerate them. They include **erythromycin (Zineryt)** and **clindamycin**. There is often cross-resistance between these two drugs.
- Advice is to use non-antibiotic antimicrobials such as **benzoyl peroxide** when possible and to avoid treatment with different topical and systemic antibiotics at the same time. Treatment should not be continued longer than is necessary but is needed with topical antibiotics for at least 6 months.
- Hormone treatment with an antiandrogen decreases sebum secretion and also reduces hirsutism as hair growth is also androgen dependent. **Co-cyprindiol (Dianette)** is used and will also provide contraception.
- Oral antibiotics used include **tetracycline** and **doxycycline**. If there is no improvement after 3 months an alternative should be used. Treatment may need to be continued for 2 years or longer in some cases.
- Topical **retinoids** such as **adapalene** and **tretinoin** are useful. They may cause some redness at first with skin peeling and treatment should be continued until no new lesions develop. Exposure to sunlight should be avoided. They are contraindicated in pregnancy and women of child-bearing age should use contraception.
- If severe and unresponding, the patient should be referred to a dermatologist who may prescribe **isotretinoin** orally. This reduces sebum secretion and the associated risks, especially teratogenicity, have already been described. This is a toxic drug that should only be prescribed by an expert dermatologist. It is given for 16 weeks usually.
- **Adalimumab** (an inhibitor of TNF activity) is licensed for the treatment of acne inversa.

Drugs acting on the ear

These are often applied in the form of drops for the softening of ear wax or for otitis externa (inflammation of the external ear).

Instillation of ear drops

- The drops should be at about blood heat.
- The head should be turned with the affected ear uppermost.
- Drops are instilled and the head is kept in this position for several minutes.

Otitis externa

An inflammatory condition of the skin in the meatus. Infection may also be present. Cleansing and medication of the meatus need to be regular and the meatus must be cleared of discharge for the treatment to be effective.

Sometimes a ribbon gauze wick is inserted to keep the lotion in contact with the meatus.

- Drugs used include *corticosteroid* ear drops with an astringent such as *aluminium acetate* solution.
- If infection is present a topical antibiotic such as *neomycin* or *clioquinol* may be used, but only for about a week as there is danger of a fungal infection occurring.
- A solution of *acetic acid 2%* is used as an antibacterial and antifungal in the ear canal. It is sold OTC as *EarCalm* spray.
- For pain, a systemic analgesic such as *paracetamol* or *ibuprofen* should be used.
- Sometimes a systemic antibiotic may be needed.

Otitis media

Inflammation in the middle ear, usually in young children, with rapid onset of signs and symptoms of an ear infection.

- It may be caused by viruses or bacteria or both.
- There is usually pain in the ear, rubbing of the ear and fever with crying and loss of appetite.
- Symptoms usually subside within 3–7 days without any antibacterials.
- Common complications such as perforated eardrum and short-term hearing loss are not prevented by the use of antibiotics.
- Paracetamol and ibuprofen may be used for the fever and pain.
- If the child is systemically very unwell or if there is a discharge following perforation of the ear drum, then antibiotics are used.

Removal of ear wax

Wax (cerumen) is produced by modified sweat glands in the ear and is anti-septic. It only needs removal when it causes hearing difficulty or prevents sight of the ear drum.

- Ear irrigation with warm (body heat) water must be done by a trained person and not attempted in a child or if there is a history of otitis media in past six weeks, perforation of the ear drum or chronic otitis externa. A person with hearing only in one ear should not have that ear irrigated as the small risk of damage is too high.

- Wax may be softened by the use of almond oil ear drops, olive oil ear drops or sodium bicarbonate twice daily for a few days before irrigating.

Drugs acting on the nose

These are used in allergic rhinitis, perennial rhinitis, as nasal decongestants or for infection.

Nasal sprays and drops are used in hay fever and other allergic reactions.

Many sprays contain sympathomimetic such as ephedrine and these may damage the nasal cilia.

Topical corticosteroids

Beclometasone dipropionate, budesonide, flunisolide, fluticasone, mometasone

- Used to prevent and treat allergic rhinitis.
- They need to be used regularly to be effective.
- They should not be used in untreated infection of the nose or after nasal surgery.
- More than the prescribed dose should not be used as the drugs can be absorbed and side effects of systemic corticosteroids may occur (see Section 6.1 and 7.2).
- When used in children, height must be monitored.
- Systemic effects of a spray may be less than drops.
- Local side effects include epistaxis, dryness and irritation of the nose and throat and taste disturbances.

The antihistamine *azelastine* (*Rhinolast*) may be used as a nasal spray for breakthrough symptoms in allergic rhinitis.

MHRA warned in 2017 that chorioretinopathy which is a serious disease of the retina has been reported after nasal administration of corticosteroids. Patients should be advised to report any blurred vision or visual disturbances when on any form of steroid therapy.

Nasal decongestants

Sodium chloride 0.9% as drops may help to relieve nasal congestion by liquefying mucous secretions.

- In rhinitis caused by the common cold a decongestant can be used but not for longer than 7 days.

- Decongestants all contain sympathomimetics such as *ephedrine* that vasoconstrict the blood vessels in the mucosa, reducing oedema. They are often not useful as they can cause rebound congestion due to vasodilation when they are stopped. This leads to further use of the decongestant and a vicious circle develops.
- They must not be used with a monoamine oxidase inhibitor (see Section 4.5) or a hypertensive crisis may occur.
- Side effects include headaches, tolerance and occasionally cardiovascular effects.

Nasal staphylococci

Nasal staphylococci and other organisms can be eliminated by the use of *chlorhexidine* with *neomycin*.

Recolonization by the bacteria frequently occurs.

In resistant cases there is a nasal ointment containing *mupirocin (Bactroban Nasal)* usually reserved for methicillin-resistant *Staphylococcus aureus* (MRSA). Treatment should be only for 5−7 days to avoid resistance. The course can be repeated once if the sample is positive.

Topical applications to the eye

Local treatment of eye disease is usually by the application of drops or ointments to the surface of the eye.

Preparations for the eye are sterile and once eye drops have been opened they should not be used more than a month after the opening date because of the risk of infection. In hospital they are usually discarded a week after opening.

If drops are applied to both eyes they should have their own labelled container to avoid cross contamination. Single-application containers are available for use in clinics.

- Hands must always be washed before the application of eye drops.
- The head is bent backwards and the lower lid gently pulled down.
- The patient is told to look upwards.
- The dropper is held above the eye and one drop squeezed inside the lower eyelid without touching the eye or skin with the applicator.
- The patient is told to close the eye for a short while and excess liquid is wiped away.

Drops may be absorbed into the circulation from the blood vessels in the conjunctiva or from the nose when drops pass down the lacrimal ducts. Ointments are less likely to be absorbed.

Eye lotions such as saline 0.9% are used to irrigate the conjunctiva and flush out foreign bodies or irritants. In an emergency, clean water may be used.

Anti-inflammatory preparations

Corticosteroid eye drops and ointments are used in some inflammatory conditions and following eye surgery.

- They should not usually be used in a red eye where the diagnosis has not been made as they can mask infection and worsen the condition, which may be due to Herpes simplex virus and could lead to corneal ulceration. Herpes simplex infection requires *acyclovir* (see below).
- Steroids may be combined with anti-infective agents in drops for use after eye surgery to reduce inflammation and the risk of infection.
- Prolonged use of steroid eye drops may lead to cataract formation and, in some patients, glaucoma.
- Preparations include *betamethasone*, *dexamethasone* and *prednisolone*.

Antihistamine eye drops are used in allergic conjunctivitis and sometimes in hay fever, for example, *antazoline (Otrivine)*.

Lodoxamide, nedocromil and *sodium cromoglicate* are mast cell stabilizers that are sometimes used in inflammatory conjunctivitis.

Immunosuppressants such as *cyclosporine* drops inhibit the release of lymphokines and thus suppress the cell-mediated immune response. They are sometimes used in severe keratitis (inflammation of the cornea) in dry eye disease, but only by a specialist.

Dry eyes

Lack of tears leads to soreness of the eyes.

- *Hypromellose* drops are used for tear deficiency and may need to be instilled every hour in order to give relief. Hypromellose may be combined with a mucolytic such as *acetylcysteine* or a *carbomer* (e.g. *carmellose*) which clings to the surface of the eye and may mean less frequent administration (perhaps four times daily).
- Other preparations are available such as *povidone*, and eye ointments such as *paraffin* may be applied at night to prevent corneal erosion.

Anti-infective eye preparations

Conjunctivitis is common and may be caused by staphylococci or streptococci. It is usually treated with *chloramphenicol* eye drops with ointment applied at night. *Fusidic acid* is used for staphylococcal infection.

- Corneal ulcers may be treated with intensive application of *ciprofloxacin* throughout the day and night, especially for the first 2 days.
- Other antibiotic eye drops are available such as *gentamicin*, *neomycin* and *polymyxin*.
- Herpes simplex infections can cause corneal ulcers. The virus is treated with *aciclovir* eye ointment five times daily for at least 3 days.

Drugs affecting pupil size

Mydriatics dilate the pupil.

- They may be antimuscarinic, such as cyclopentolate, homatropine or atropine.
- Rarely precipitate acute-angle glaucoma, usually in long-sighted individuals over 60 years old.
- Sympathomimetics such as phenylephrine may be used, especially where dilation is difficult.

Miotics constrict the pupil and include *pilocarpine* that is used to treat glaucoma.

Treatment of glaucoma

Glaucoma may be asymptomatic and can lead to blindness if untreated. It is usually associated with a raised intraocular pressure and the optician now measures this during an eye test.

- Glaucoma is treated by drugs that lower intraocular pressure and these include beta blockers such as *timolol*, *betaxolol* or *levobunolol*. They may be absorbed systemically and so should not be used in patients with asthma, bradycardia or heart block.
- Prostaglandin analogues such as *latanoprost* and *travoprost* may be used. They may increase the brown pigment in the iris leading to a change in eye colour.
- Sympathomimetics such as *adrenaline* (epinephrine) or the prodrug *dipivefrine* reduce the rate of production of aqueous humour and increase its outflow but are contraindicated in some types of glaucoma because they dilate the pupil.
- Oral carbonic anhydrase inhibitors such as *acetazolamide* and *brinzolamide and dorzolamide* (to the eye) reduce aqueous humour production. They are used alongside other treatments and cause a slight diuresis when given orally.
- Miotics such as *pilocarpine* are also used to constrict the pupil.
- Prostaglandin analogues may also be used locally, for example, *bimatoprost, latanoprost and tafluprost*.

Local anaesthetics

These include *lidocaine, oxybuprocaine, proxymetacaine* and *tetracaine*. They are used for minor surgical procedures such as removal of corneal sutures. For surgery, retrobulbar injections may be used.

Macular degeneration

This is a degenerative condition that affects the central area (macula) of the retina. It usually occurs over the age of 55 years and is a common cause of loss of vision in older people. It is a progressive loss of central vision that makes the recognition of faces difficult and impacts on driving, reading and writing.

There are two types of degeneration, dry and wet. Dry macular degeneration is slow to progress but with wet macular degeneration new blood vessels develop below and within the retina. This can lead to rapid sight loss.

The aim of treatment is to try and slow down the progression of vision loss. This will be under the care of a specialist.

Drug treatment is only recommended in certain cases of wet progressive macular degeneration and involves specialist intravitreal injections of antivascular endothelial growth factor (VEGF), for example, *afliberecept.*

There are NICE guidelines (2018f) for age-related macular degeneration that are available on their website (www.nice.org.uk/guidance/ng82).

9.5 EMERGENCY TREATMENT OF POISONING

Toxicology is the study of harmful interactions between chemicals and biological systems: that is, the study of poisons. A poison is any substance which has a harmful effect on a living system.

The study of poisons must have begun by 1500 BCE when the earliest collection of medical records, the *Ebers Papyrus*, was written; it contains many recipes and references to poisons. The ancient Egyptians distilled prussic acid from peach kernels; in ancient Greece experiments were carried out into various poisons using condemned criminals as subjects. Poisons were studied and used for murder, political assassination and suicide. In 399 BCE Socrates was ordered to commit suicide by taking hemlock.

Toxicology is now much more than the study of poisons and their antidotes. There are over 65,000 man-made chemicals in the environment, each potentially toxic. The difference between the therapeutic and the toxic properties of substances may be indistinguishable except for the dose.

There were 4359 deaths in England and Wales related to drug poisoning in 2018. This is the highest annual increase (16%) since 1993 when these figures were first collected (Office for National Statistics, 2019).

- Two-thirds of these deaths were related to drug misuse. More than half of drug poisoning deaths involve more than one drug and sometimes alcohol.
- Over half these deaths (51% in 2018) involve an opiate. Other drugs include cocaine (rising for the past 7 years with 637 deaths in 2018), amfetamines, benzodiazepines, antidepressants and paracetamol.
- In 2018 there were also 125 deaths involving new psychoactive substances (NPS), known as legal highs. This was an increase from 61 deaths in 2017.

- Two-thirds of drug poisonings in 2018 were male (2984 male deaths compared with 1375 female deaths).
- Intentional self-poisoning was responsible for 30% of female deaths and 16% of male deaths (All figures from the Office for National Statistics, 2019).

Accidental poisoning

This may be encountered at any age, but the causes differ. In children it is commonest between the ages of 1 and 5 when they like to explore the environment with their mouth as well as their eyes and fingers. The main cause of hospital admission is medicines (70%) and household products (20%). Accidental poisoning from medicines peaks at age two (Public Health England, 2018).

In older children and adults it is usually a mishap at school or at work such as inhalation of gases or fumes from organic solvents. For accidents involving household or industrial products, the National Poisons Information Service (NPIS) should be consulted.

The elderly, especially if confused, may forget they have taken a dose of their drug or make mistakes with doses.

Most cases of accidental poisoning occur following drug misuse, which is highest in those aged between 30 and 49 years (Office for National Statistics, 2019).

Deliberate self-poisoning

Those who have features of poisoning should usually be admitted to hospital, especially if the drug taken has delayed action (e.g. paracetamol, tricyclic antidepressants). Some of these patients may appear well but should be admitted even if free of symptoms.

Usually poisoned adults are able to tell us what they have taken but signs and symptoms of a drug overdose may also be present.

Further advice

TOXBASE is the database of the NPIS and is available to registered users at www.toxbase.org. It provides information on the treatment of those exposed to drugs, household products and also agricultural or industrial chemicals. The UK National Poisons Information Service gives 24-hour specialist advice on treatment of poisoning. Their telephone number is 0344 892 0111. Help with identifying tablets or capsules is also given.

Some common features seen in drug overdose

The actual medication taken and the dose are often not known and most care is symptom management. There are very few specific antidotes to be administered but these are available for paracetamol, opioids and iron.

A full history should be taken but information given by both the patient and relatives may not be totally reliable. Sometimes symptoms may be those of other illnesses and so careful assessment is required.

Coma

This is one of the common signs of poisoning and is usually due to CNS depression by:

- opioid analgesics
- hypnotics
- antidepressants
- anticonvulsants
- tranquillizers
- alcohol.

It does not occur with paracetamol poisoning unless another drug has been taken as well.

Convulsions

Caused by CNS stimulation by anticholinergics, sympathomimetics, tricyclic antidepressants and monoamine oxidase inhibitors.

Single, short-lasting convulsions do not need treatment but if they are lengthy or are repeated *lorazepam* or *diazepam*, as an emulsion, may be given by slow intravenous injection into a large vein. If the IV route is not available, intramuscular injections should not be used and *midazolam* oromucosal solution can be given buccally or *diazepam* rectally.

Respiratory features

In an unconscious patient the airway may be obstructed and may require immediate attention. Most drugs that impair consciousness are also respiratory depressants and sometimes assisted ventilation may be necessary.

- Cough, wheeze and breathlessness often occur after inhalation of irritant gases such as ammonia, chlorine and smoke from fires.
- Cyanosis may be due to a combination of factors in the unconscious patient. Can also be due to methaemoglobinaemia caused by poisons such as chlorates, nitrates, nitrites, phenol and urea herbicides. Methaemoglobinaemia should be treated with *methylthionium chloride* if the methaemoglobin concentration is 30% or above, or if hypoxia is present even with oxygen therapy (BNF, 2019). This reduces the ferric iron and methaemoglobin back to the ferrous iron of haemoglobin.

- Hypoventilation is common with any CNS depressant. Usually respiration gets shallower rather than slower. A marked reduction in rate is likely to be due to opioids.
- Hyperventilation may be due to salicylate poisoning and occasionally to CNS stimulant drugs and cyanide.
- Pulmonary oedema may follow inhaled poisons or some herbicides such as *paraquat* (herbicide banned in the EU that is lethal if taken in small quantities and has been linked to Parkinson's disease in those working with it).

Cardiovascular features

- Tachycardia may be due to anticholinergics, sympathomimetics and salicylates.
- Bradycardia may be caused by digoxin and beta blockers.
- Cardiac conduction defects and arrhythmias may be caused by a variety of drugs, especially tricyclic antidepressants, some antihistamines and some antipsychotics. Many antiarrhythmic drugs actually cause arrhythmias if taken in excess. Correction of underlying conditions such as hypoxia, acidosis or other biochemical abnormalities may be sufficient but ventricular arrhythmias need specialist treatment.
- Hypotension may occur in any severe poisoning. A systolic blood pressure of less than 70 mmHg may lead to irreversible brain damage or acute tubular necrosis and so must be corrected. The foot of the bed should be raised and an intravenous infusion of sodium chloride or a colloid is likely to be commenced.
- CNS depressants may lower the systolic blood pressure.
- Diuretics lower the blood pressure by depleting the blood volume.
- Hypertension is uncommon in overdosage but may occur following sympathomimetics such as amfetamines, phencyclidine and cocaine.

Pupil changes

- Very small and pinpoint pupils, especially if the respiratory rate is slowed, suggest opioid analgesics.
- Dilated pupils suggest tricyclic antidepressants, other anticholinergics or antihistamines.

Body temperature

- Hypothermia may develop if patients have been unconscious for some hours but is more likely following phenothiazines or barbiturates and is commoner in the elderly.

- Hyperthermia can develop if CNS stimulants such as amfetamines have been taken. Children and the elderly may also get hyperthermia following anti-muscarinics.
- A fan should be used after the removal of unnecessary clothing and tepid sponging may be required. The NPIS may need to be consulted, especially if serotonin syndrome is the cause.

Antidotes

Most important here is **naloxone** which is the antidote to all narcotic drugs. It may completely reverse a coma within 1–2 minutes and will increase the respiratory rate.

Flumazenil is the antidote for benzodiazepines.

Acetylcysteine is given in paracetamol overdose.

Screening for poisons

The purpose is to identify and quantify poisons if treatment is available. There is no point in doing an emergency screening if the result has no bearing on the treatment that will be given. *Paracetamol* is the drug that is most likely to be screened for.

Minimizing the absorption of ingested poisons

There are three methods:

- emptying the stomach – rarely used
- administering activated charcoal
- whole bowel irrigation has been used in overdoses of certain enteric-coated formulations and in lithium and iron overdose but is only used on the advice of the NPIS.

Gastric lavage

Rarely used and should never be attempted if the patient is very drowsy or comatose or when a corrosive material has been ingested.

- Gastric lavage is of doubtful value if it is conducted more than an hour after ingestion and there is danger of inhalation of stomach contents. The airway must always be protected.
- It should only be used if a **life-threatening amount** has been taken within the last hour of a substance that cannot be effectively removed by other methods. Examples are iron and lithium that are not adsorbed by charcoal.

- Induction of vomiting with emetics such as ipecacuanha is not recommended as this may lead to aspiration and there is no evidence that it affects absorption.

Activated charcoal

- Taken by mouth, the charcoal is not absorbed and combines with some drugs in the gastrointestinal tract to reduce their absorption.
- The sooner it is given, the more effective it will be.
- It is best given within the first hour of ingestion but may be effective up to 2 hours after ingestion and longer if modified-release preparations are taken.
- It is a tasteless, black, gritty slurry and patients do not like to take it.
- It does not adsorb all toxins but is good for paracetamol, benzodiazepines and digoxin. It is useful for poisons that are toxic in small amounts such as tricyclic antidepressants.
- It can enhance the elimination of some drugs when they have been absorbed and repeated doses are given for overdoses of carbamazepine, dapsone, phenobarbital, theophylline and quinine overdoses. If vomiting occurs an antiemetic should be given.
- Activated charcoal should not be used with petroleum distillates, corrosive substances, alcohols, malathion, cyanides or metal salts including iron and lithium salts.

Other techniques to increase elimination of poisons include:

- haemodialysis for salicylates, phenobarbital, sodium valproate, methanol, ethylene glycol and lithium
- alkalization of the urine in salicylate poisoning.

Effects of some common drugs taken as an overdose

Paracetamol

Paracetamol (acetaminophen in the United States) was marketed in 1956, and in 1966 toxicity causing jaundice and fatal hepatic necrosis was reported. It became apparent that liver damage was a dose-related effect.

Paracetamol is contained in over 100 OTC preparations worldwide and is one of the most common pharmaceutical products taken in overdosage in the UK. Acute hepatic failure due to paracetamol overdose is the most common cause of acute liver failure requiring transplantation in the UK (about 40% of cases). England and Ireland remain the two countries in Europe with the highest rates of liver failure from paracetamol overdose.

Toxicity can occur at low doses. The recommended maximum dose for an adult is 4 g in 24 hours; that is 2 tablets 6-hourly. Double this dose can cause toxicity.

Deaths from paracetamol overdosage have decreased since the packet size available for purchase OTC was decreased in 1998. In 2017 there were only 39 deaths due to paracetamol overdose in England, compared with 85 deaths in 2000 (Office for National Statistics, 2019).

Paracetamol metabolism

In therapeutic doses paracetamol is metabolized by the liver largely to harmless conjugates, but about 5% is metabolized by cytochrome P450 enzymes in the liver to a highly toxic intermediate, *N*-acetyl-*p*-benzoquino-neimine (NAPQI). This is rapidly bound to glutathione in the liver and inactivated as shown in Fig. 9.1.

- In high doses of paracetamol the normal metabolic route becomes saturated and larger amounts of this poisonous metabolite are formed.
- The liver stores of glutathione needed to bind NAPQI are rapidly depleted.
- When glutathione levels fall to less than 30%, NAPQI is free to combine with liver hepatocytes and causes cell death and necrosis.
- It also causes renal failure from acute tubular necrosis in a small percentage of cases.
- Antidotes consist of sulphydryl donors such as methionine and *N*-acetylcysteine which act as precursors of glutathione.

In children the risk of hepatotoxicity is reduced as the formulations taken tend to be paediatric ones and children may metabolize paracetamol in a different way to adults.

Identifying those at risk of liver damage

The amount of paracetamol ingested Severe damage is likely if more than 250 mg paracetamol/kg body weight has been ingested. Hepatotoxicity may occur if 150 mg/kg has been taken within 1 hour. Rarely it may develop after a single dose of 75 mg/kg in less than 1 hour. The fatal dose for an adult may be as little as 12 g (24 tablets). It is important that body weight is taken into account to avoid underestimating the impact of the overdose. In obese patients over 110 kg, a body weight of 110 kg should be used.

The time since ingestion is critical

The severity of paracetamol overdosage is best determined by the plasma paracetamol concentration related to the time from ingestion (Fig. 9.2). Plasma concentrations taken within 4 hours of ingestion are not reliable as the drug is still being absorbed. If the plasma paracetamol concentration is above the normal treatment line the patient is given acetylcysteine. The graph is not

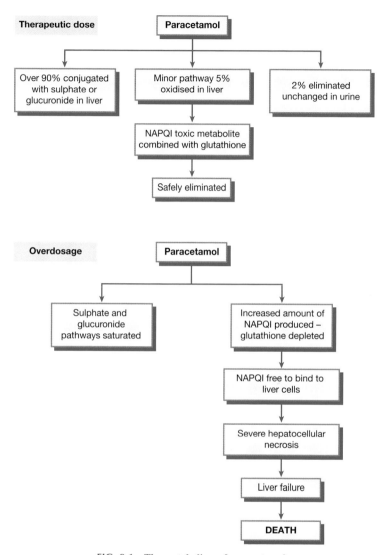

FIG. 9.1 **The metabolism of paracetamol.**

reliable if a staggered overdose over more than 1 hour has been taken. If there is any doubt, acetylcysteine should be commenced.

It used to be thought that those who are on drugs that induce liver enzymes are at increased risk. Such drugs include anticonvulsants, rifampicin and St John's wort. Alcohol also induces liver enzymes and toxicity is likely to occur with lower doses in chronic heavy drinkers. Although there is evidence that this may have an impact, the CSM has advised that this should no longer be taken into account when assessing paracetamol toxicity.

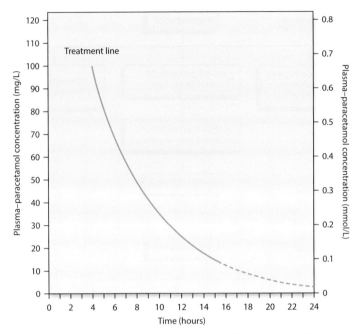

FIG. 9.2   **Treatment graph for paracetamol overdosage.** Patients whose plasma paracetamol concentrations are above the normal treatment line should be treated with acetylcysteine by intravenous infusion. The prognostic accuracy after 15 hours is uncertain but a plasma paracetamol concentration above the treatment line should be regarded as carrying a serious risk of liver damage.

Clinical features

There is usually a 24-hour delay before there are any symptoms of hepatotoxicity.

● The only early features are anorexia, nausea and vomiting. These may occur within a few hours of the overdose but usually settle within 24 hours. Liver enzymes are already rising.

● Loss of consciousness is not a feature.

● 24–72 hours after ingestion, there may be right upper abdominal pain and tenderness over the liver. Liver enzymes are peaking with bilirubin levels and prothrombin time (measured as international normalized ratio [INR]) also raised.

● 72–96 hours after ingestion, liver damage is maximal and jaundice occurs. In severe cases hepatic encephalopathy and acute renal failure may be present and death may follow.

● Features of hepatic failure may include vomiting and abdominal pain, confusion, hyperventilation, hypoglycaemia, cerebral oedema and bleeding.

- If the patient survives, recovery occurs between 96 hours and 14 days. The liver regenerates and heals.

Patients who have taken an overdose of paracetamol should be taken to hospital urgently even if they have no symptoms. Severe liver damage may be caused by 20–30 tablets.

Treatment

Activated charcoal may be administered if more than 12 g of paracetamol or 150 mg/kg have been ingested in the past hour.

Acetylcysteine This drug provides virtually complete protection against liver damage if it is taken in the first 8 hours after ingestion. Its efficacy declines after this period, but it offers protection up to 24 hours after ingestion and possibly beyond this.

Late treatment is not contraindicated and does appear to reduce morbidity and mortality. Advice from the NPIS should be sought if more than 24 hours have elapsed.

The drug is given in a total dose that is divided into 3 consecutive intravenous infusions over a total of 21 hours. Dosage tables can be seen in the BNF (2019).

Adverse/side effects

- Hypersensitivity reactions that are anaphylactoid in nature and most common in the first hour of treatment may occur. The infusion rate is decreased or administration stopped until the reaction settles.
- Nausea and flushing.
- Rashes may be treated with antihistamines.
- Wheezing may be treated by salbutamol by nebulizer. Caution required in asthma but treatment should not be withheld.
- Angioedema and respiratory distress are relatively rare.

Aspirin

This used to be commonly taken in overdose before paracetamol became the most popular analgesic.

Aspirin (salicylic acid) can produce serious toxicity and death at high doses. Half a 325 mg tablet per kg produces mild toxicity whereas more than 1 tablet per kg can produce serious toxicity, for example, 70 tablets or more in a 70-kg man. Chronic toxicity can occur with 100 mg/kg per day for 2 days.

Effects of overdosage

Symptoms can begin 1—2 hours after ingestion but may be delayed for 4—6 hours or longer if tablets are sustained release or enteric coated.

- Common symptoms include tinnitus, nausea and vomiting, deafness, sweating, vasodilation, hyperventilation, lethargy and dehydration.
- Salicylate centrally stimulates the respiratory system producing hyperventilation.
- Respiratory alkalosis follows with a compensatory metabolic acidosis and dehydration. Hypokalaemia may occur.
- Lactic acidosis also occurs and the acidic nature of salicylate adds to the acidosis.
- At normal doses, aspirin is an antipyretic, but an overdose of salicylate increases heat production, oxygen use and glucose use. Fever results with tachycardia and hypoglycaemia.
- Alters platelet function and may result in bleeding, especially from the gastrointestinal tract.
- Rare features include pulmonary oedema and renal failure.
- Coma uncommon but does indicate very severe poisoning.

Treatment

- Must be in hospital where salicylate levels, pH and electrolytes can be monitored.
- Fluid needs to be replaced.
- Sodium bicarbonate (1.26%) is given to alkalinize the urine if salicylate level is above 500 mg/L in an adult. This hastens elimination.
- In severe poisoning haemodialysis may be used.

NSAIDs

Ibuprofen is the commonest

- It causes nausea, vomiting and abdominal pain.
- Serious toxicity is rare.
- Activated charcoal if more than 400 mg/kg taken within the past hour.
- Symptomatic measures otherwise.

Opioids

These are discussed in Section 3.2. An overdose causes coma and respiratory depression. The pupils will be pinpoint.

Naloxone is the specific antidote, but its half-life is shorter than many opioids and it may need to be given by infusion.

Tricyclic antidepressants, for example, amitriptyline, dosulepin

These are the most dangerous antidepressants in overdose and less than 10 times the normal dose results in serious toxicity. There are still approximately 200 deaths a year in the UK from overdose, although the safer SSRIs are being prescribed more as alternatives. There are approximately 43 deaths per million prescriptions issued for tricyclics.

The patient requires rapid transfer to hospital as deterioration from a talking patient to an unconscious, convulsing one may occur within an hour.

Clinical features

- Early signs of overdose are anticholinergic symptoms such as a dry mouth, dilated pupils and sometimes urinary retention.
- The skin will be dry and warm.
- Tachycardia and hyperthermia may be present.
- Jerky limb movements.
- Hypotension. Tricyclics are sympathomimetic but block the alpha-adrenergic receptor on blood vessels, resulting in vasodilation.
- Drowsiness, ataxia and nystagmus may be present.
- Increased muscle tone and reflexes.
- Respiratory depression.
- Loss of consciousness.
- Convulsions may occur. Associated hypoxia may lead to acidosis, more prolonged seizures and increased cardiac toxicity.
- Cardiac arrhythmias. The drugs have a sodium channel-blocking effect like some antiarrhythmic agents, for example, *quinidine*. The effect on the electrocardiogram is a widened QRS complex and the width is linked to the severity of the overdose. Wide-complex tachycardia may be followed by more fatal arrhythmias such as ventricular tachycardia, torsades de pointes and atrioventricular dissociation.

Management

- No antidote.
- Activated charcoal within an hour. Careful management of the airway and breathing is required.
- The patient will always be attached to a cardiac monitor.
- Intravenous *diazepam* may be given to control convulsions.
- Sodium bicarbonate by infusion is given if necessary to alkalinize the plasma. This increases protein binding of the tricyclic so that less free drug is available to bind with the myocardium. It also corrects acidosis making serious arrhythmias less likely when there is a wide-complex tachycardia.
- Antiarrhythmic drugs are not used as these can increase the incidence of fatal arrhythmias.

- Counteracting the cholinergic effects such as hallucinations with a cholinesterase inhibitor such as *physostigmine* is contraindicated as this may precipitate convulsions or asystole.
- *Flumazenil* must not be given even if the patient has also taken an overdose of benzodiazepines. Seizures will occur.

Venlafaxine, a selective noradrenaline (norepinephrine) reuptake inhibitor, is also dangerous.

Selective serotonin reuptake inhibitors fluoxetine (Prozac) and others

These are much safer antidepressants with only 4.3 deaths per million prescriptions. They still resulted in 310 deaths in the 10 years between 1993 and 2003 but many more times the therapeutic dose needs to be taken. Ingestion of up to 50 times the normal dose produces toxicity and deaths have followed ingestion of 150 times the normal dose.

Clinical features

- Nausea and vomiting.
- Agitation, tremor and nystagmus.
- Drowsiness.
- Sinus tachycardia.
- Convulsions may occur.
- Occasionally **serotonin syndrome** with neuropsychiatric effects, neuromuscular hyperreactivity and autonomic instability. Hyperthermia, rhabdomyolysis, renal failures and clotting disorders may develop.

Management

- Supportive − no antidote.
- Activated charcoal within an hour.
- Diazepam if needed to prevent convulsions, and also in serotonin syndrome when the NPIS should be contacted for advice.

Benzodiazepines diazepam, temazepam, lorazepam and related drugs

Death from benzodiazepines alone is extremely rare. They have a high therapeutic index but do potentiate the effects of other CNS depressants such as alcohol.

- They produce CNS depression ranging from mild drowsiness to a short period of unconsciousness.
- Respiratory depression can occur with large doses but is not common.

- There is likely to be ataxia, dysarthria and nystagmus.
- Potentiate the effects of other drugs acting on the CNS.
- Antidote is ***flumazenil*** but this is rarely used as the patient may be benzodiazepine-dependent or may have taken more than one type of drug. If tricyclics have been taken the ***flumazenil*** may precipitate seizures.

Beta blockers

Therapeutic overdose may result in bradycardia and hypotension with resultant dizziness and sometimes syncope. Heart failure may be precipitated or increased in severity.

Clinical features

Effects of overdosage vary with different drugs.

- Bradycardia and hypotension.
- Cardiac effects include atrioventricular block, conduction delay, ventricular arrhythmias and cardiac arrest.
- Pulmonary oedema, bronchoconstriction and hypoglycaemia may occur.
- Convulsions and coma if lipid-soluble drugs; most common with ***propranolol***.
- ***Sotalol*** may cause torsade de pointes and ventricular arrhythmias.

Management

Large overdoses require expert advice.

- Activated charcoal binds well.
- Intravenous ***atropine*** is administered to treat bradycardia.
- Cardiogenic shock is treated with ***glucagon*** in glucose given intravenously. Raises cyclic AMP and is not dependent on the adrenergic receptor to do this. The raised cyclic AMP increases intracellular calcium levels and so increases the strength of cardiac contractions.
- Occasionally ***isoprenaline*** is used and is available from specialist importing companies.
- A cardiac pacemaker may be required.

Calcium channel blockers

Rate-limiting drugs are the most dangerous, with ***verapamil*** at the top of the list. Profound cardiovascular collapse may occur that does not respond well to treatment.

As little as 1 tablet may produce symptoms in children.

Clinical features

- *Verapamil* is a negative inotrope and so decreases cardiac contractility, sometimes leading to complete heart block and asystole. Hypotension occurs and some vasodilation. *Diltiazem* produces similar effects.
- Dihydropyridine drugs such as *amlodipine* cause severe hypotension due to vasodilation.
- Symptoms after standard preparations usually occur within 1—4 hours. With sustained preparations it may be as long as 24 hours before symptoms are produced.
- Nausea and vomiting.
- Dizziness, agitation and confusion.
- Metabolic acidosis.
- Hyperglycaemia due to blocking calcium channels on beta cells causing decreased insulin release.
- Cardiogenic shock.
- Coma in severe poisoning.

Management

- Activated charcoal within an hour. Repeated doses if a slow-release preparation has been taken.
- *Calcium chloride* or *gluconate* by injection in severe cases.
- *Atropine* for symptomatic bradycardia.
- In severe cases an insulin and glucose infusion may be required to manage hypotension and heart failure.
- Inotropes may be used but hypotension is treated differently depending on whether it is due to vasodilation or myocardial depression. The BNF suggests the NPIS should be contacted for advice.

Digoxin
Chronic toxicity

- May occur with therapeutic doses as a result of the drug slowly building up, especially in the elderly and if there is poor kidney function.
- Hypokalaemia and hypomagnesaemia seen with diuretic use increase toxicity.
- Toxicity may occur when serum levels of digoxin are only slightly raised or even within normal limits.
- Acute toxicity is rarely seen but can be fatal.

Clinical features

- Anorexia, nausea and vomiting.
- Dizziness, fatigue, confusion, lethargy and delirium can occur.

- Changes in colour vision so that there is increased perception especially of yellow and green colours.
- Other visual disturbances including blurring or halos.
- Electrocardiogram changes.

Acute toxicity

May not have symptoms for the first 6 hours. Serious arrhythmias occur within 24 hours or 5 days if sustained action.

- Heart block and bradycardia.
- Hyperkalaemia due to blockade of Na^+/K^+ ATPase pump.

Management

- Activated charcoal is given.
- Serum potassium is monitored. Hyperkalaemia is treated.
- Atropine may be given for bradycardia.
- Antidote is the Fab antibody. This binds free digoxin within minutes to an hour. The full effect takes several hours. It is used in severe cases.
- Calcium must not be given as treatment for hyperkalaemia as it can increase arrhythmias.

Stimulant drug poisoning

Amfetamines, cocaine, ecstasy and theophylline

Amfetamines

Stimulants that cause wakefulness, paranoia, hallucinations, excessive activity and hypertension. This may be followed by exhaustion, convulsions, hyperthermia and coma.

Early stages can be treated and controlled by diazepam or lorazepam but advice from the NPIS is recommended for the treatment of hypertension.

Tepid sponging maybe required for the hyperthermia and anticonvulsants may be required. Sometimes artificial respiration is needed.

Cocaine This is a CNS stimulant and so causes agitation, dilated pupils, tachycardia, hyperthermia, hypertension, hypertonia, hallucinations and hyperreflexia.

Intravenous diazepam is used to control agitation and cooling methods should be used for the hyperthermia but expert advice is needed for the cardiac effects of an overdose.

Ecstasy (MDMA) This can be a problem even when the dose taken has been tolerated in the past. It can cause severe reactions which include delirium, coma, convulsions, ventricular arrhythmias, hypothermia, rhabdomyolysis, acute renal failure and acute hepatitis. Other effects may be disseminated intravascular coagulation (DIC), adult respiratory distress syndrome (ARDS), hypotension and intracerebral haemorrhage.

Treatment is supportive as there is no antidote. Diazepam can be used to control severe convulsion and agitation. The patient should be closely monitored, including by ECG.

Self-induced water intoxication may also be a problem and should be watched for. Ecstasy may increase the levels of antidiuretic hormone (ADH) and so may cause fluid retention and hyponatraemia.

Iron salts These are usually accidental and in children. They cause nausea, vomiting, abdominal pain, haematemesis, diarrhoea and rectal bleeding. An overdose can be fatal and hypotension, coma, shock and metabolic acidosis may occur. Mortality is reduced by the antidote, *desferrioxamine mesylate,* which chelates iron. The serum iron can be taken as an emergency but in a very severe overdose, the antidote should be given immediately.

In the limited space available here, only common drugs taken in overdosage have been described. The reader is referred to texts in the further reading list for more details.

Appendix

Drug measurement and calculations

The International System of Units (SI) is used for drug doses and concentrations and patient data (including weight and body surface area), drug levels in the body, and other measurements.

WEIGHT

Grams (g) and milligrams (mg) are the units most often encountered in drug dosages. Doses of less than 1 g should be expressed in milligrams, e.g., 250 mg rather than 0.25 g. Similarly, doses less than 1 mg should be expressed in micrograms, e.g., 200 micrograms rather than 0.2 mg. Whenever drugs are prescribed in microgram dosages, the unit should be written in full, e.g., digoxin 250 micrograms, as the use of the contracted term, μg or mcg, may in practice be mistaken for mg and, as this dose is 1000 times greater, disastrous consequences may follow.

Drug dosages are often described in terms of unit dose per kilogram of body weight, i.e., mg/kg, μg/kg, etc. This method of dosage is frequently used for children and allows dosages to be tailored to the individual patient's size.

VOLUME

Liters (l or L) and milliliters (ml or mL) account for almost all measurements expressed in unit volume for the prescription and administration of drugs.

CONCENTRATION

When expressing the concentration of dosages of a medicine in liquid form, several methods are available.

- Unit weight per unit volume describes the unit of weight of a drug contained in unit volume, e.g., 1 mg in 1 mL, 40 mg in 2 mL. Examples of drugs in common use expressed in these terms are pethidine injection, 100 mg in 2 mL; chloral hydrate mixture, 1 g in 10 mL; phenoxymethylpenicillin oral solution, 250 mg in 5 mL.

- Percentage (weight in volume) describes the weight of a drug, expressed in grams, that is contained in 100 mL of solution, e.g., calcium gluconate injection 10%, which contains 10 g in each 100 mL of solution, or 1 g in each 10 mL, or 100 mg (0.1 g) in each 1 mL.
- Percentage (weight in weight) describes the weight of a drug, expressed in grams, that is contained in 100 g of a solid or semisolid medicament, such as ointments and creams, e.g., fusidic acid ointment 2%, which contains 2 g of fusidic acid in each 100 g of ointment.
- Volume containing "1 part": a few liquids, and to a lesser extent gases, particularly those containing drugs in very low concentrations, are often described as containing 1 part per "x" units of volume. For liquids, "parts" are equivalent to grams and "volume" refers to milliliters, e.g., an adrenaline injection 1 in 1000 contains 1 g in 1000 mL or, expressed as a percentage (w/v), 0.1%.
- Molar concentration: only very occasionally are drugs in liquid form expressed in molar concentration. The mole is the molecular weight of a drug expressed in grams, and a 1 molar (1 M) solution contains this weight dissolved in each liter. More often the millimole (mmol) is used to describe a medicinal product, e.g., potassium chloride solution 20 mmol in 10 mL indicates a solution containing the molecular weight of potassium chloride in milligrams × 20 dissolved in 10 mL of solution.

BODY HEIGHT AND SURFACE AREA

Drug doses may be expressed in terms of micrograms, milligrams, or grams per unit of body surface area. This is frequently the case where precise dosages tailored to individual patients' needs are required. Typical examples may be seen in cytotoxic chemotherapy or in drugs given to children. Body surface area is expressed as square meters or m^2 and drug dosages as units per square meter or units/m^2, e.g., cytarabine injection 100 mg/m^2.

FORMULAE FOR CALCULATION OF DRUG DOSES AND DRIP RATES

Oral drugs (solids, liquids)

$$\text{Amount required} = \frac{\text{strength required} \times \text{volume of stock strength}}{\text{stock strength}}$$

Parenteral drugs

(a) Solutions (intramuscular, intravenous injections)

$$\text{Volume required} = \frac{\text{strength required} \times \text{volume of stock strength}}{\text{stock strength}}$$

(b) Powders

It is essential to follow the manufacturer's directions for dilution, then use the appropriate formula.

(c) Intravenous infusions

$$\text{Rate (drops / min)} = \frac{\text{volume of solution} \times \text{number of drops per ml}}{\text{time (min)}}$$

1. Using standard giving sets (20 drops/mL): clear fluids

$$\text{Rate (drops / min)} = \frac{\text{volume of solution (ml)} \times 20}{\text{time (min)}}$$

2. Using filtered giving sets (15 drops/mL): blood

$$\text{Rate (drops / min)} = \frac{\text{volume of solution (ml)} \times 15}{\text{time (min)}}$$

(d) Infusion pumps

$$\text{Rate (ml / h)} = \text{volume (ml)} \div \text{time (h)}$$

(e) Intravenous infusions with drugs

$$\text{Rate (ml / h)} = \frac{\text{amount of drug required (mg/h)} \times \text{volume of solution (ml)}}{\text{total amount of drug (mg)}}$$

N.B. After selecting the appropriate formula, ensure that all strengths are in the same units, otherwise convert.

1% solution contains 1 g of solute dissolved in 100 mL of solution.

The term 1:1000 means 1 g in 1000 mL of solution; therefore, 1 g in 1000 mL is equivalent to 1 mg in 1 mL.

ACKNOWLEDGMENTS

The measurement section was adapted from Henney et al., 1995, *Drugs in Nursing Practice*, fifth edition, Churchill Livingstone, Edinburgh, with permission, and the formulae from Havard, 1997, *A Nursing Guide to Drugs*, fourth edition, Churchill Livingstone, Edinburgh, with permission.

References

Agency for Healthcare Research and Quality (AHRQ). Hospital survey on patient safety culture: 2014 user comparative database report: Chart 5-2, Item-level average per cent positive response-database hospitals. https://www.ahrq.gov/professionals/quality-patient-safety/patient-safetyculture/hospital/2014/hosp14chart5-2html/index.html; 2014.

Aissaoui N, Puymirat E, Tabone X, et al. Improved outcome of cardiogenic shock at the acute stage of myocardial infarction: a report from the USIK 1995, USIC 2000, and FAST-MI French Nationwide Registries. *Eur Heart J*. 2012;33:2535−2543.

Arthritis Foundation. Health Benefits of Ginger for Arthritis, Living with arthritis blog. Online at: http://blog.arthritis.org/living-with-arthritis/health-benefits-of-ginger/; 2018.

Banja J. The normalization of deviance in healthcare delivery. *Bus Horiz*. 2010;53(2):139.

Barnes J. Charms & Harms: Echinacea. *J Prim Health Care*. 2009;1:146−147.

Bates DW. Preventing medication errors: a summary. *Am J Health Syst Pharm*. 2000;64(14):S3−S9.

Beckett NS, Peters R, Fletcher AE, et al. Treatment of hypertension in patients 80 years of age or older. *Nat Eng J Med*. 2008;358:1887−1898.

Bonsall L. 8 rights of medication administration. Clinical Nursing Resources. NursingCenter. https://www.nursingcenter.com/ncblog/may-2011/8-rights-of-medication-administration; 2011.

British Heart Foundation. High blood pressure: How can we do better? https://www.bhf.org.uk/for-professionals/healthcare-professionals/data-and-statistics/bp-how-can-we-do-better; 2016.

British Heart Foundation. Heart and circulatory disease statistics. http://www.bhf.org.uk/what-we-do/our-research/heart-statistics/heart-statistics-publications/cardiovascular-disease-statistics-2019; 2019.

British Heart Foundation. Cardiovascular Disease Statistics − BHF UK Factsheet. https://www.bhf.org.uk/what-we-do/our-research/heart-statistics; Found at: bhf-cvd-statistics-uk-factsheet%20(7).pdf; 2020.

British National Formulary (BNF) 78. Joint Formulary Committee. London: BMJ Publishing and the Royal Pharmaceutical Society; 2019.

British Thoracic Society. British guideline on the management of asthma: a national clinical guideline. First published 2003. Revised edition published July 2019. https://www.brit-thoracic.org.uk/quality-improvement/guidelines/asthma/.

British Thoracic Society. Guideline for oxygen use in healthcare and emergency settings. https://www.brit-thoracic.org.uk/quality-improvement/guidelines/emergency-oxygen/; 2018.

Cabilan CJ, Hughes JA, Shannon C. The use of contextual, modal and psychological classification of medication errors in the emergency department: a retrospective descriptive study. *J Clin Nurs*. 2017;26:4335−4343.

The CAPRICORN Investigators. Effect of carvedilol on outcome after myocardial infarction in patients with left ventricular dysfunction: the CAPRICORN randomised trial. *The Lancet*. May 05, 2001;357(Issue 9266). P1385-1390. https://www.thelancet.com/journals/lancet/article/PIIS0140673600045608/fulltext

Chomchai S. Insecticides: organophosphates and carbamates. In: Ling L, Clark R, Erickson T, Trestall J, eds. *Toxicology Secrets*. Philadelphia: Hanley and Belfus; 2001:186.

Cox J. Quality medication administration. *Contemp Nurse*. 2000;9(3−4):3−8.

Crane J, Crane FG. Preventing medication errors in hospitals through a systems approach and technological innovation: a prescription for 2010. *Hosp Top*. 2006;84(4):3−8.

Diabetes UK. Diabetes Prevalence 2019. https://www.diabetes.org.uk/about_us/news/diabetes-prevalence-2019; 2019.

Diabetes UK. Flash glucose monitoring. Guide to diabetes https://www.diabetes.org.uk/guide-to-diabetes/managing-your-diabetes/testing/flash-glucose-monitoring; 2020.

Durham B. The nurses' role in medication safety. *Nursing*. 2015;45(4):1−4.

Dwornik M. Circulatory support in cardiogenic shock: a focused update for a general cardiologist. 21 January, 2016. *BCS Editorial*. https://www.bcs.com/pages/news_full.asp?NewsID=19792461.

Edwards S, Axe S. The ten 'Rs' of safe multidisciplinary drug administration. *Nurse Prescrib*. 2015;13(8):352−360.

Edwards S, Axe S. Medication management: reducing drug errors, striving for safer practice. *Nurse Prescrib*. 2018;16(8):404−412.

Elliott M, Liu Y. The nine rights of medication administration: an overview. *Br J Nurs*. 2010;19(5):300−305.

Freeman DJ, Norrie J, Sattar N, et al. Pravastatin and the development of diabetes mellitus − evidence for a protective treatment effect in the West of Scotland Prevention Study. *Circulation*. 2001;23;103(3):357−362.

Fowler SB, Sohler P, Zarillo DF. Bar-code technology for medication administration: medication errors and nurse satisfaction. *Medsurg Nurs*. 2009;18(20):103−109.

Gao WQ, Quan-Zhou F, Yu-Feng L, et al. Systematic study of the effects of lowering low-density lipoprotein-cholesterol on regression of coronary atherosclerotic plaques using intravascular ultrasound. *BMC Cardiovacs Disord*. 2014;14:60. http://www.biomedcentral.com/1471-2261/14/60.

Goddard K, Roudsari A, Wyatt JC. Automation bias: a systematic review of frequency, effect mediators, and mitigators. *J Am Med Inform Assoc*. 2012;19:121−127.

Guardian. Hunt to crack down on NHS drug errors linked to up to 22,000 deaths. 2018. https://www.theguardian.com/society/2018/feb/23/jeremy-hunt-pledges-crackdown-on-drug-errors-in-nhs.

Hansson L, Zanchetti A, Carruthers SG, Dahlof B for the HOT Study Group 1998. Effects of intensive blood pressure lowering and low dose aspirin in patients with hypertension: principal results of the Hypertension Optimal Treatment (HOT) Trial. HOT Study Group. *Lancet*. 1998;351(9118):1755−1762.

Izzo AA, Di Carlo G, Borrelli F, Ernst E. Cardiovascular pharmacotherapy and herbal medicines: the risk of drug interaction. *Int J Cardiol*. 2005;98:1−14.

Johnson M, Sanchez P, Langdon R, et al. The impact of interruptions on medication errors in hospitals: an observational study of nurses. *Nurs Manag*. 2017;25(7):498−507.

Jones SW. Reducing medication administration errors in nursing practice. *Nurs Stand*. 2009;23(50):40−46.

Kapur N, Parand A, Soukup T, et al. Aviation and healthcare: a comparative review with implications for patient safety. *JRSM Open*. 2016;7(1).

Lampert L. 8 Rights of medication administration: avoid medication errors. Pennsylvania: Ausmed Education; 2016. https://www.ausmed.com/articles/8-rights-of-medication-administration/.

Law M. Plant sterol and stanol margarines and health. *Est J Medicine*. 2000;173:43−47.

Lazarou R, Heinrich M. Herbal medicine: who cares? The changing views on medicinal plants and their roles in British lifestyle. *Phytother Res*. 2019;33:2409−2420.

Lenzer J. FDA is incapable of protecting US 'against another Vioxx'. *BMJ*. 2004;329:1253.

Macdonald M. Patient safety: examining the adequacy of the 5 rights of medication administration. *Clin Nurs Special*. 2010;24(4):196−201.

McDougall C, Brady AJ, Petrie JR. ASCOT: a tale of two treatment regimens. *BMJ*. 2005;331(7521):859−860.

McNaughton R, Huet G, Shakir S. An investigation into drug products withdrawn from the EU market between 2002 and 2011 for safety reasons and the evidence used to support the decision-making. *BMJ Open*. 2014;4(1).

MHRA. Banned and restricted herbal ingredients. https://www.gov.uk/government/publications/list-of-banned-or-restricted-herbal-ingredients-for-medicinal-use/banned-and-restricted-herbal-ingredients; 2014.

MHRA. *Rules and guidance for pharmaceutical manufacturers and distributors 2017*. London: GovUK: 2017.

MHRA. Emollients: new information about risk of severe and fatal burns with paraffin-containing and paraffin-free emollients. https://www.gov.uk/drug-safety-update/emollients-new-information-about-risk-of-severe-and-fatal-burns-with-paraffin-containing-and-paraffin-free-emollients; 2018.

MHRA. Herbal medicines granted a traditional herbal registration. https://www.gov.uk/government/publications/herbal-medicines-granted-a-traditional-herbal-registration-thr; 2019.

Ming L, Wu L, Terrar DA, et al. Circulation. SYSTEMATIC REVIEW Modernized Classification of Cardiac Antiarrhythmic Drugs ©2018 The Authors. Circulation is published on behalf of the American Heart Association, Inc., by Wolters Kluwer Health, Inc. This is an open access article under the terms of the Creative Commons Attribution License, which permits use, distribution, and reproduction in any medium, provided that the original work is properly cited, 2018.

Montserrat-de la Paz S, García-Giménez MD, Ángel-Martín M, Marín-Aguilar F, Fernández-Arche A. Dietary supplementation evening primrose oil improve symptoms of fibromyalgia syndrome. *J Funct Foods*. 2013;5:1279−1287.

MRC Working Party. Medical research council trial of treatment of hypertension in older adults: principal results. *BMJ*. 1992;304:405−412.

Nathan DM. Some answers, more controversy, from UKPDS. United Kingdom prospective diabetes study. *Lancet*. 1998;352(9131):832−833.

National Patients Safety Agency (NPSA). Release of organization patient safety incident reports. http://www.nrls.npsa.nhs.uk; 2012.

Ng QX, Nandini V, Ho CYX. Clinical Use of Hypericum Perforatum (St John's Wort) in Depression: A Meta-Analysis. *J Affective Disorders*. 2017;210:211-221.

NHS England. Patient safety alert stage three: directive: improving medication incident reporting and learning. https://www.england.nhs.uk/wp-content/uploads/2014/03/psa-med-error.pdf; 2014.

NHS Patient Safety Strategy. NHS England and NHS improvements. https://improvement.nhs.uk/documents/5472/190708_Patient_Safety_Strategy_for_website_v4.pdf; 2019.

NHS. Wolff-Parkinson-White Syndrome. Online at: https://www.nhs.uk/conditions/wolff-parkinson-white-syndrome/; 2020.

NICE. Acute kidney injury: prevention, detection and management. Clinical Guideline cg169. https://www.nice.org.uk/guidance/cg169; 2013

NICE. Obesity: identification, assessment and management. Clinical Guideline cg189. www.nice.org.uk/guidance/cg189; 2014.

NICE. Insulin therapy in type 2 diabetes. https://cks.nice.org.uk/insulin-therapy-in-type-2-diabetes#!scenario; 2016.

NICE. Adverse drug reactions. https://cks.nice.org.uk/adverse-drug-reactions; 2017.

NICE. Antiplatelet treatment. https://cks.nice.org.uk/antiplatelet-treatment; 2018a.

NICE. Chronic heart failure in adults: diagnosis and management. https://www.nice.org.uk/guidance/ng106; 2018b.

NICE. Chronic obstructive pulmonary disease in over 16s: diagnosis and management. www.nice.org.uk/guidance/ng115; 2018c.

NICE. Dementia: assessment, management and support for people living with dementia and their carers. NICE guidelines [NG97]. http://www.nice.org.uk/guidance/ng97; 2018d.

NICE. NICE recommends wider use of statins for prevention of CVD. https://www.nice.org.uk/news/article/nice-recommends-wider-use-of-statins-for-prevention-of-cvd; 2018e.

NICE. Age-related macular degeneration, NICE guideline (NG82). www.nice.org.uk/guidance/ng82; 2018f.

NICE. Anticoagulation—oral. https://cks.nice.org.uk/anticoagulation-oral; 2019a.

NICE. Hypertension in adults: diagnosis and management. http://www.nice.org.uk/guidance/ng136; 2019b.

NICE. Motor neurone disease: assessment and management. NICE guidelines [NG42]. http://www.nice.org.uk/guidance/ng42; 2019c.

NICE. Obesity management in adults. https://pathways.nice.org.uk/pathways/obesity/obesity-management-in-adults; 2019d.

NICE. Surveillance of gastro-oesophageal reflux disease and dyspepsia in adults: investigation and management (NICE guideline CG184). https://www.nice.org.uk/guidance/cg184; 2019e.

NICE Oxygen. https://bnf.nice.org.uk/treatment-summary/oxygen.html; 2019f.

NICE. Surveillance of diabetes (NICE guidelines NG17, NG18, NG19 and NG28). https://www.nice.uk/guidance/ng28/resources/2019-surveillance-of-diabetes-nice-guidelines-ng17-ng18-ng19-ng28-pdf-8862045321157; 2019g.

Nursing and Midwifery Council (NMC). *The Code: Professional Standards of Practice and Behaviour for Nurses and Midwives.* London: NMC; 2015.

O'Connor A, Schug SA, Cardwell H. A comparison of the efficacy and safety of morphine and pethidine as analgesia for suspected renal colic in the emergency setting. J Accid Emerg Med. 2000;17:261−264.

Office for National Statistics. Deaths related to drug poisoning in England and Wales Statistical Bulletins: 2018 registrations. https://www.ons.gov.uk/peoplepopulationandcommunity/birthsdeathsandmarriages/deaths/bulletins/deathsrelatedtodrugpoisoninginenglandandwales/2018registrations; 2019.

Office for National Statistics. The number of suicides by the method of drug poisoning, where paracetamol was mentioned on the death certicifate, by sex and age-group, England, registered between 2000 and 2017. Available at: https://www.ons.gov.uk/peoplepopulationandcommunity/birthsdeathsandmarriages/deaths/adhocs/009814thenumberofsuicidesbythemethodofdrugpoisoningwhereparacetamolwasmentionedonthedeathcertificatebysexandagegroupenglandregisteredbetween2000and2017; 2019.

Pahan K, Chandra SJ, Jana M. Aspirin induces Lysosomal biogenesis and attenuates Amyloid plaque pathology in a mouse model of Alzheimer's disease via PPARα. *J Neurosci.* 2018;38(30):6682−6699.

Pandor A, Ara RM, Tumur I, et al. Predicting the effect of Fenofibrate on cardiovascular risk for individual patients with type 2 diabetes mellitus. *J Intern Med.* 2009;265(5):568−580.

Pareek A, Suthar M, Rathore G, et al. Feverfew (*Tanacetum parthenium* L.): a systematic review. *Pharmacogn Rev.* 2011;5(9):103−110.

Public Health England (PHE). Reducing unintentional injuries in and around the home among children under five years. https://assets.publishing.service.gov.uk/government/uploads/system/uploads/attachment_data/file/696646/Unintentional_injuries_under_fives_in_home.pdf; 2018.

Public Health England (PHE). Ambitions set to address major causes of cardiovascular disease. https://www.gov.uk/government/news/ambitions-set-to-address-major-causes-of-cardiovascular-disease; 2019.

Redman DD. Reducing medication errors in the OR. *AORN J.* 2017;105(1):106−109.

Resuscitation Council. Resuscitation guidelines. https://www.resus.org.uk/resuscitation-guidelines/; 2015.

Riaz MK, Riaz M, Latif A. Review—medication errors and strategies for their prevention. *Pak J Pharm Sci.* 2017;30(3):921−928.

Ritter JM, Flower R, Henderson G, et al. *Rang and Dale's Pharmacology.* 9th ed. Edinburgh: Elsevier; 2019.

Roughead EE, Semple SJ, Rosenfield E. The extent of medication errors and adverse drug reactions throughout the patient journey in acute care in Australia. *Int J Evid Based Healthc.* 2016;14:113−122.

Scally B, Emberson JR, Spata E, et al. Effects of gastroprotectant drugs for the prevention and treatment of peptic ulcer disease and its complications: a meta-analysis of randomised trials. *Lancet.* 2018;3(4):231−241.

Shuvy M, Atar D, Steg PG, et al. Oxygen therapy in acute coronary syndrome: are the benefits worth the risk? *Eur Heart J.* 2013;34:1630−1635.

Sikorskii A, Safikhani A, McVary KT, et al. Saw Palmetto for symptom management during radiotherapy for prostate cancer. *J Pain Symp Manag.* 2016;51(6):1046−1054.

Snowden A, Barron D. Medicines management in mental health. *Nurs Stand.* 2011;26(3):35−40.

Stockley IH. Drug Interactions, 7th edn. The Pharmaceutical Press, London. 2005.

Stroke Association. Atrial Fibrillation and Stroke. Information leaflet https://www.stroke.org.uk/resources/atrial-fibrillation-af-and-stroke; 2019.

Struthers AD. Pathophysiology of heart failure following myocardial infarction. *Heart.* 2005;91:14−16.

Sun YE, Wang W, Qin J. Anti-hyperlipidemia of garlic by reducing the level of total cholesterol and low-density lipoprotein A meta-analysis. *Medicine.* 2018;97(18): e0255.

Taylor CJ, Ordonez-Mena JM, Roalfe AK, et al. Trends in survival after a diagnosis of heart failure in the United Kingdom 2000−2017: population based cohort study. *BMJ.* 2019;364:l223.

Teo KK, Yusuf S, Furberg CD. Effects of prophylactic antiarrhythmic drug therapy in acute myocardial infarction: an overview of results from randomised controlled trials. *JAMA.* 1993;270:1589−1595.

Thomas SJ, Booth N, Chen D, et al. Cumulative incidence of hypertension by 55 years of age in blacks and whites: the CARDIA Study. *J Am Heart Assoc.* 2018;7(14): e007988. https://doi.org/10.1161/JAHA.117.007988.

UK Prospective Diabetes Study (UKPDS) Group. Effect of intensive blood glucose control with metformin in overweight patients with type 2 diabetes (UKPDS 34). *Lancet.* 1998;352:854−865.

Vinogradova Y, Coupland C, Hill T, et al. Risks and benefits of direct oral anticoagulants versus warfarin in a real world setting. *BMJ.* 2018;362:k2505.

Vrbnjak D, Denieffe S, O'gorman C, et al. Barriers to reporting medication errors and near misses among nurses: a systematic review. *Int J Nurs Stud.* 2016;63:162−178.

Waller D, Sampson A. *Medical pharmacology and therapeutics.* 5th ed. Edinburgh: Elsevier; 2017.

Wann LS, Curtis AB, Ellenbogen KA, et al. 2011 ACCF/AHA/HRS focused update on the management of patients with atrial fibrillation (update on dabigatran): a report of the American College of Cardiology Foundation/American Heart Association Task Force on Practice Guidelines. *Circulation.* 2011;123(10):1144−1150.

Westbrook JI, Woods A, Rob MI. Association of interruptions with an increased risk and severity of medication administration errors. *Arch Int Med.* 2010;170(8):683−690.

Williams N. The MRC breathlessness scale. *Occup Med.* 2017;67(6):496−497.

Williams V. A classification of antiarrhythmic actions reassessed after a decade of new drugs. *J Clin Pharmacol.* 1984;24:129−147.

World Health Organization (WHO). *Medication Errors; Technical series on Safer Primary Care.* Geneva, Switzerland: WHO; 2016.

World Health Organization (WHO). Diabetes Key facts. https://www.who.int/news-room/fact-sheets/detail/diabetes; 2018. WHO. Geneva, Switzerland.

World Health Organization (WHO). *World Health Organization Model List of Essential Medicines: 21st List.* Geneva, Switzerland: WHO; 2019.

Wright K. Do calculation errors by nurses cause medication errors in clinical practice? A literature review. *Nurse Educ Today.* 2010;30(1):85−97.

Yamauchi K, Ogasawara M. The role of histamine in pathophysiology of asthma and the clinical efficacy of antihistamines in asthma therapy. *Int J Mol Sci.* 2019;20(7):1733.

Further Reading

Asher J, Houston M. Ezetimibe monotherapy for cholesterol lowering in 2,722 people: systematic review and meta-analysis of randomized controlled trials. *J Clin Hypertens (Greenwich).* 2007;9(8):622−628.

Digger T, Viira DJ. Anaesthesia and surgical pain relief—the ideal general anaesthetic agent. *Pharm J.* 1 August, 2008. https://www.pharmaceutical-journal.com/learning/learning-article/anaesthesia-and-surgical-pain-relief-the-ideal-general-anaesthetic-agent/10030510.article?firstPass=false.

Gao WQ, Law MR, Wald MJ, et al. Quantifying effect of statins on LDL cholesterol, ischaemic heart disease and stroke: systematic review and meta-analysis. *BMJ.* 2003;326:1423.

Koopal C, Visseren FLJ, Westerink J, et al. Predicting the effect of fenofibrate on cardiovascular risk for individual patients with type 2 diabetes. *Diabetes Care.* 2018;41(6):1244−1250.

Lewis SR, Pritchard MW, Evans DJW, et al. Colloids versus crystalloids for fluid resuscitation in critically ill people. *Cochrane Database Syst Rev.* 2018;8:CD000567. https://doi.org/10.1002/14651858.CD000567.

Mallet C, Eschalier A, Daulhac l. Paracetamol: Update on its analgesic mechanism of action. https://www.intechopen.com/books/pain-relief-from-analgesics-to-alternative-therapies/paracetamol-update-on-its-analgesic-mechanism-of-action.

National Cancer Registration & Analysis Service and Cancer Research UK. *Chemotherapy, Radiotherapy and Tumour Resections in England: 2013−2014 workbook.* London: NCRAS; 2017.

Ognibene S, Vazzana N, Giumelli C, et al. Hospitalisation and morbidity due to adverse drug reactions in elderly patients: a single-centre study. *Intern Med J.* 2018;48(10):1192−1197.

Olsen MH, Angell SY, Asma S, et al. A call to action and life course strategy to address the global burden of raised blood pressure on current and future generations: the Lancet, Commission on hypertension. *Lancet.* 2016;388:2665−2712.

Public Health England. Health matters: combating high blood pressure. https://www.gov.uk/government/publications/health-matters-combating-high-blood-pressure; 2017.

Public Health England. Hypertension prevalence estimates for local populations. https://www.gov.uk/government/publications/hypertension-prevalence-estimates-for-local-populations; 2016.

Sikorskii A, Safikhani A, McVary KT, et al. Saw Palmetto for symptom management during radiation therapy for prostate cancer. *J Pain Symp Manag.* 2016;51(6):1046−1054.

Taylor CJ, Ordonez-Mena JM, Roalfe AK, et al. Trends in survival after a diagnosis of heart failure in the United Kingdom 2000—2017: population based cohort study. *BMJ*. 2019;364:l223.

WHO. Hypertension: key facts. www.who.int/news-room/fact-sheets/detail/hypertension; 2019.

Xiang Q, Venkatanarayanan N, XianHo Y. Clinial use of Hypericum perforatum (St John's wort) in depression: a meta-analysis. *J Affect Disord*. 2016;210:211—221.

Useful Websites

www.nice.org.uk.

www.gov.uk/mhra.

www.medicines.org.uk/emc.

www.nice.org.uk/guidance/cg61.

www.qrisk.org.

www.jbs3risk.com/pages/risk_calculator.htm.

www.nhs.uk/conditions/high-cholesterol/.

https://www.stroke.org.uk/professionals/atrial-fibrillation-information-and-resources.

https://www.nhs.uk/conditions/wolff-parkinson-white-syndrome/.

https://www.resus.org.uk/resuscitation-guidelines/peri-arrest-arrhythmias/.

https://www.diabetes.org.uk/about_us/news/new-stats-people-living-with-diabetes.

https://www.who.int/news-room/fact-sheets/detail/diabetes.

https://www.diabetes.org.uk/guide-to-diabetes/managing-your-diabetes/testing/flash-glucose-monitoring.

https://www.ons.gov.uk/peoplepopulationandcommunity/birthsdeathsandmarriages/deaths/bulletins/deathsrelatedtodrugpoisoninginenglandandwales/2018registrations.

https://assets.publishing.service.gov.uk/government/uploads/system/uploads/attachment_data/file/696646/Unintentional_injuries_under_fives_in_home.pdf.

Index